Mind-Body Wellness

Susan M. Henney • Justin D. Hackett

Mind-Body Wellness

A Science-Based Approach

Springer

Susan M. Henney
The University of Houston - Downtown
Houston, TX, USA

Justin D. Hackett
Pennsylvania Western University
California, PA, USA

ISBN 978-3-031-91610-6 ISBN 978-3-031-91611-3 (eBook)
https://doi.org/10.1007/978-3-031-91611-3

This Springer imprint is published by the registered company Springer Nature Switzerland AG
The registered company address is: Gewerbestrasse 11, 6330 Cham, Switzerland

For Ryan and Walker, always, and for my mother, the wellspring of well-being.
Susan Henney

For my amazing wife Mandy, our boys Aidan, Collin, and Nathan, and my parents Gary and Donna for being the unwavering bright spots in my life.
Justin Hackett

Preface

Wellness in general, and mind–body wellness in particular, is no longer at the fringes of academia. Many degrees and certificates with a wellness emphasis are being developed at universities and colleges all over the world. Now, more than ever, students yearn to know more about how to increase their own sense of mental and physical wellness, as well as that of family, friends, and clients. Academic courses in mind–body wellness typically explore the dynamic interaction between our minds and physical bodies, with a focus on behaviors, techniques, and approaches that impact the development and maintenance of health and well-being. Such classes also address the ways in which our assumptions and beliefs about the interconnection of mind and body relate to how we view health and illness. This evidence-based text is designed to support learning, self-reflection, and behavior change in such courses by exploring how human well-being is related to dimensions of mind–body wellness.

The healthcare sector is growing, with more than 2.5 million more jobs expected through 2030. However, the face of healthcare is changing, with conventional medicine commonly being supplemented by mind–body wellness approaches. These approaches broadly include healthy eating, fitness promotion, mindfulness practices, stress management, workplace wellness, mental health promotion, and more. This growing industry sector generates trillions in revenues, and students in relevant programs require appropriate science-based training to promote wellness in a variety of settings.

As popular as the field of wellness is in contemporary discourse, it is particularly subject to misinformation, disinformation, and pseudoscience. Emotional appeals, presentation of information that "looks and sounds scientific," suspicion about the motives of the medical and pharmaceutical establishments, social media marketing disguised as wellness, and cognitive biases toward "natural" and "alternative" solutions to ill health are all reasons why people can be deceived by the pseudoscientific aspects of wellness culture. Becoming a more critical consumer of information can help us wade through the complexities of how wellness culture is marketed to us.

The textbook begins with an overview of the mind–body connection, approaches to defining wellness, and what wellness means to people. Subsequent chapters cover the foundational topics relevant to training in this field, such as science vs pseudoscience, daily hassles, environmental wellness, wellness in relationships, spirituality, and wellness programming. The book ends with consideration of how mind–body wellness can not only impact our personal well-being but also societal well-being.

The promise of mind–body wellness is not guaranteed, even when we focus extensively on improving it. As you will discover through this text, focusing on our health and wellness is more involved than you may think, and yet focusing on improving wellness can bring positive changes to our lives. Our minds and our bodies are intricately connected and supporting one often positively impacts the other. Living in wellness is a journey—we will have successes, and we'll have moments where we fall short of our goals—yet the process of thriving and flourishing in all parts of life is so worth it.

Houston, TX, USA Susan M. Henney
California, PA, USA Justin D. Hackett

Acknowledgements

Thank you to Dr. Rueben Brock and Dr. Michael Baranski for reviewing early drafts of this work and to our student assistants who contributed their time and talents to the project, particularly Lauren Garris.

The time to research and write this manuscript would not have been possible without the support of the College of Health Sciences and Human Services at Pennsylvania Western University and the Department of Social Sciences at the University of Houston-Downtown.

Contents

Chapter 1
The Mind-Body Connection

The promise of a long life filled with health and wellness attracts people to wellness-related behaviors, practices, procedures, and products they believe will help fulfill this promise. Globally, the health and wellness market is a $4.5 trillion industry, with the beauty and personal care sector alone accounting for a fourth of this number (Statista, 2024). This sector is expected to grow to more than $6 trillion annually by 2025. However, the pursuit of wellness also poses a dilemma. How do we know what works and what does not? How can we distinguish a safe product from a harmful one? If we work in the healthcare field or the wellness space, what healthful, safe, and effective wellness products and practices can we recommend to our clients? The purpose of this book is to provide a science-based perspective on these issues, one which can enhance our own wellness, and also give us the tools to make effective purchases, engage in productive planning for our health needs, and furnish others with appropriate resources and best practices to enhance their wellness journey.

There are different views on the connection between mind and body. The contrasting views create the "mind-body problem." The central conflict within the mind-body debate is whether the mental is the physical or if the mental is something beyond the physical (Van Gelder, 1998). Are the mind and body two separate entities, or are they one? The two most notable theories in this debate are monism and dualism. The theory of monism is that the mental is the physical and that it is a single unit. Monism is featured more often in non-Western schools of thought. This idea of monism revolves around inclusiveness and holism (Scheper-Hughes & Lock, 1987). One of the core beliefs of monism "is not that the whole has no parts, but rather that the whole is prior to its parts" (Schaffer, 2010). It rejects any splitting between mind and body. According to a monistic view, the mental and physical worlds live together, have a synergistic nature, and are not either mental or physiological. Rather, our mental experiences are *also* physiological ones. Monism is divided into two groups of thought—idealists and materialists. Idealists believe that

S. M. Henney, J. D. Hackett, *Mind-Body Wellness*,
https://doi.org/10.1007/978-3-031-91611-3_1

only our minds and mental processes exist, and materialists believe that only matter exists.

On the other hand, dualism is a more Western philosophy. Dualism revolves around the idea of dichotomies, such as mind vs. body, spirit vs. matter, and unreal vs. real (Scheper-Hughes & Lock, 1987). However, if the mind and body are separate, then how are they related? Do they interact? Do they influence one another? Dualism suggests the mind and body are two distinct entities. We have a physical aspect, the brain and the body, and we have our minds, the nonphysical aspect of who we are. This perspective creates a dichotomy between "the mental" and "the physical." This separate nature of mind and body is why we can have unique, individual experiences. Dualism does leave the question open of whether the mind controls the body, or if the body controls the mind. Descartes believed that the mind thinks, and the body is an extension of that. An example of this is that the soul is to the body as a captain is to a ship; the soul is in charge of directing the motion of our bodies (Gorham, 1994).

While these viewpoints provide contrasting perspectives on the connections between our minds and bodies, evidence does support the Monism view of a close relationship connecting them. For instance, many of us have experienced the pain of a broken heart—something we can literally feel all over our body. There is research showing that this emotional pain can be diminished by acetaminophen—the active ingredient in Tylenol (Dewall et al., 2010). An over-the-counter-medicine used to treat headaches and fevers helps to dull emotional pain as well! Feelings of love activate the same neurological reward centers in our brain as cocaine. In fact, several euphoria-inducing chemicals are released when we experience love. It is no wonder then that the pain we experience from a broken heart impacts our entire body—it's like we are experiencing withdrawal symptoms. Clearly, the connection between our mind and body is a complex, multifaceted one. Many books exist discussing the mind-body problem, and no doubt these conversations still happen late into the evenings in dorm rooms across the world. While we will not settle this debate in this book, we certainly hope to add some more information to inform the conversation.

What Is the Mind-Body Connection?

The Mind

The functions of our mind include what we know (or think we know), feel, think, believe in, value, like, and dislike, as well as our attitudes and outlook on life. These are powerful forces for both health and growth or illness and decline, because how we feel in the mind affects how we feel in the body. The brain is a physical and biological entity, but the mind is an awareness that arises from the physical operation of the brain. Consciousness itself is an active interchange between the body, the brain, and the environment, with our emotions both shaping and being shaped by the artifacts of consciousness (e.g., Damasio, 1999). The brain is part of the body…it is not separate from it, but a functional whole with the rest of the body. This means that the conscious expression of the brain—the mind—is intertwined with the functioning of the body, just as the physical brain is.

Neuropsychologists have been studying the influence of the brain on the rest of the body for many years. For example, scientists have determined that there are neural networks that connect the brain's cortical areas that control motor functions, thought, and emotion to the adrenal glands above your kidneys. Among other functions, the adrenal glands produce hormones that influence blood pressure and the stress response (Dum et al., 2016). Why is this important? It is evidence that there is some cognitive control over our stress responses, even the "fight or flight" response, indicating that our "instinctual" responses to stress may be more under our control than most people believe. Even in high-stress, high-anxiety situations, with the appropriate preparation and mind-body skills, we can moderate our body's response.

Our social or work worlds are important contexts for us, and these contexts can affect how our body functions, via our interpretation and evaluation of events and happenings within these contexts. For example, metabolic syndrome is a group or cluster of symptoms and conditions that are related to or may even be precursors to heart disease, stroke, and diabetes. Some of the indicators of metabolic syndrome that are important if tracking together include high blood pressure, accumulated body fat around the waist area, high blood sugar, and abnormal cholesterol readings. Metabolic syndrome is increasingly common; in the United States up to a third of people have indicators of metabolic syndrome. Large epidemiological studies in the United Kingdom called the Whitehall studies found that people who worked in low-level jobs characterized by high stress and low autonomy had almost twice the risk of developing metabolic syndrome as those in higher-level jobs (Chandola et al., 2006). Research of this nature implies that psychosocial stressors in our daily lives can influence our heart health and the collective functioning of multiple key areas of our bodies. How we interpret and process our external world brings the stressors of the world inside, which is then related to our physiological health and wellness.

The Body

What we put in our bodies, how and how often we move our bodies, our chronic and acute illnesses, the functioning or malfunctioning of our organ systems, accidents and injuries, and even our dental health and vision affect our physical selves. Our perception of our own health and wellness depends on the bodily sensations we receive. Does my body feel invigorated, full of energy, and pain free? Does my body feel sluggish, tired, and painful? Or do I just feel "unwell?"

The extent to which people monitor and are reactive to their own bodily sensations varies quite a bit. Some people do not seem to physically feel pain in the same way or to the same intensity as others. Researchers who use real-time MRI scans while people are experiencing painful sensations have found that sensitivity to pain can be associated with the amount of grey matter (the type of brain material that is full of neuron cells) in specific areas of the brain (Emerson et al., 2014). In other words, it appears that there are measurable structural differences in the brain that relate to how we perceive pain. The brain of your friend who can go to work and function adequately with tooth pain might be different structurally from another person who is immediately reactive to dental pain and unable to perform the duties of their job or complete routine daily tasks. This then results in differential behaviors—one makes an immediate appointment with the dentist, while the other puts it off and waits to see how bad it gets.

Another line of research connecting what is happening in our bodies to the physical structure of the brain comes from research examining the long-term impact of chronic pain. Long-term experiences of chronic pain can change your brain structure over time. When studied with advanced imaging techniques, chronic back pain patients show significant decreases in gray matter. This decrease is seen most acutely in the prefrontal cortex of our brain and is similar to the loss we typically see over 10–20 years (Apkarian et al., 2004). The good news is that these appear to be neuroplastic changes, which may be reversible if better pain management is achieved. Intervening and assisting people experiencing chronic pain is essential to help mitigate these consequences.

Dynamic Interconnectivity

However, your mind and body do not operate separately from one another. The mind and body affect each other in an ongoing, multifaceted, and complicated feedback loop. Our concentration might be on one or the other; there might be a problem with one that is extreme in the sense that it overrides the other, or they both might be in crisis. Alternatively, our mind and body may both be extremely well functioning. Even if they appear at first glance to be operating independently, we are finding more and more connections between the activity of the body and the functioning and structure of the brain. Indeed, the various systems of the body "speak" the same biochemical language, and they are in continuous communication within and across systems. This communication can result in minute changes in hormone or neurotransmitter levels that can be undetectable to us, or it can result in larger, more pronounced changes, such as thirst and a bad headache when dehydrated. It can result in changes that make us feel great, or changes that make us want to stay in bed. At the extreme, the communication can be an emergency "all hands on deck" call across your body systems, such as when exposure to an allergic agent results in severe anaphylactic shock or a severe infection causes a cytokine storm leading to multiorgan failure.

It is interesting that some people focus on the negative side of the mind-body connection, specifically that negative thoughts or feelings can cause physical symptoms or that a physical symptom can cause negative feelings or thoughts. However, the system works both ways in that positive outlooks, beliefs, feelings, and experiences can affect our bodies positively, allowing us to feel more bodily energy, to interpret pain differently, and to perceive a lessening of stress. In other words, when our bodies feel good, we feel better mentally. When our bodies are relaxed, we perceive ourselves as less stressed. When we physically smile or belly laugh, we can feel "happier," more positive, and the world, quite literally, seems like a better place.

One example of this is the relationship between physical activity and mood. You probably have heard that one way to cope with feeling down or blue is to get your body moving and get some exercise. It turns out that even a relatively small physical effort can have a big effect on your mood. Specifically, it matters less how hard you work out or for how long, instead what really matters is that you exercise regularly. A light walk for 30 min can lift your mood, but the most notable and sustainable results happen if you do it every day (Craft & Perna, 2004). For many people, just getting into the habit is the hard part. Once you have a physical exercise routine built into your daily schedule, the benefits are likely to keep you motivated!

We can even use physical exercise to help us control our cravings for sweet foods. Research highlights that short, brisk walks can reduce the cravings for sweets in both average weight and overweight persons. That is, physical activity influences a person's perception of their own desire for sweets. In overweight individuals, exercise can even attenuate these cravings when we desire food as a way to cope with stressors. Exercising can help us burn more calories while simultaneously encouraging healthier decision-making with food by attenuating cravings (Ledochowski et al., 2015; Oh & Taylor, 2012).

There also appears to be a dynamic relationship between sleep and mood. Both amount and quality of sleep are related to depression and anxiety, with all aspects of sleep disturbance—difficulty falling asleep, difficulty staying asleep (early waking), and reduced sleep quality being associated with mood problems. Addressing sleep problems through a combination of behavioral interventions, education on sleep hygiene, sleep monitoring, and even medical interventions is often a positive step toward better mood. Thus, physical activity is a realistic target for intervention in the treatment of depressed mood and sleep should be addressed in the treatment of mood disorders. Can the body treat the mind? Yes. Using the body to *treat and heal* the mind is gaining traction in mainstream medical and psychological communities.

Sleep also has a bi-directional relationship with obesity. Sleep deprivation, when we do not sleep as much as our bodies need us to, typically occurs when we sleep less than 7 hours. When we are not sleeping enough, our bodies experience metabolic changes that lead to weight gain (Cooper et al., 2018). Feeling drained and exhausted from lack of sleep likely negatively impacts our ability to engage in physical exercise. Moreover, obesity increases the risk for sleep disorders that make it hard to get a good night's sleep. This creates the bi-directional nature between sleep and weight gain. Not sleeping well causes weight gain, and weight gain makes it difficult to sleep well.

A Look at the Gut Biome

The "gut" is how we informally describe the digestive system that runs from the mouth to the anus. Did you know that your gut is its own unique and vitally useful environment? The gut biome refers to all of the microorganisms that live in your intestines; these might include bacteria, viruses, and fungi—by some estimates there are up to 1000 different bacteria that can live in the human digestive tract. All of this constitutes a complex and dynamic ecosystem that lives with us symbiotically and has an essential role in our digestive functioning. The gut microorganisms also impact our immune systems, both by providing a physical barrier to invasive bacteria and by influencing inflammatory processes in the bowels. Bacteria in your gut help to synthesize certain vitamins and minerals and make others more bioavailable. Furthermore, the gut microbiome looks different in different people; there is some evidence that people who are obese may have a different microbiome than lean people (Turnbaugh et al., 2009).

However, did you know that there is preliminary evidence that your gut microbiome "communicates" with your brain and vice versa? Researchers now study the microbiota–gut–brain (MGB) axis and its relationship to our mental health and life functioning. Research teams around the world are studying the idea that the MGB axis continuously transmits, interprets, and responds to information via neural, immune, and endocrine pathways. Depressed patients, for example, have been noted to show fewer bacteria overall and fewer types of bacteria (Liu et al., 2023). Over several different studies, patients with bipolar disorder were also found to have significantly less specific types of bacteria (e.g., Sublette et al., 2021). Both the oral and fecal biome of children with autism spectrum disorders can be different from neurotypical children, with some bacteria being overrepresented and some underrepresented (Vuong & Hsiao, 2017). More research needs to be done in these areas, especially regarding causal pathways and the exact composition of the dysbiosis (the imbalance in the natural gut flora).

Increasing both the number of beneficial bacteria AND the diversity of beneficial bacteria may be a target of intervention to improve mood, reduce anxiety, and increase wellness in both clinical samples and healthy people. This can be done through changes in diet, the use of pro or prebiotics, and even fecal transplantation. Think about it this way: if the composition of the microbiome changes, the type and nature of the communication along the MGB pathway changes, as does the response or reaction to the changed information. This is a fantastically interesting area of research that opens up many new possibilities for intervention and treatment of both mental and physical illness.

Mind-Body Pathways

There is a variety of research that points to a dynamic relationship between the functioning of the mind and the body. However, it is also true that we know more about the functional relationship than we know about how these relationships between mind and body work. In other words, we know the connections are there, but how they operate tends to be less clear.

Allostatic load (McEwen & Stellar, 1993): Allostatic load is the accumulated wear and tear on the body and brain when they are repeatedly or chronically exposed to stressors with the resultant hormonal and catecholamine response. This is related to research findings that chronic stress alters the structure and functioning of the brain, gut, nerves, cardiovascular system, and endocrine system. This shows that there is a brain-body basis for stress-related illness.

Stress response system: When people are exposed to stressors, a cascade of responses occur. One of the well-known pathways for stress responses is a hormonal feedback loop, which is a systematic process initiated in the brain and eventually triggering most of the major body systems. When we identify a hazard or stressor impacting us, the brain immediately jumps into action, with the amygdala (which interprets visual and auditory cues) alerting the hypothalamus, which signals the adrenal glands to release adrenaline. Subsequently, heart rate goes up, breathing gets faster, extra oxygen floods the brain to sharpen focus, and sugar floods the bloodstream to provide energy. At the same time, a complementary system called the HPA axis (hypothalamus–pituitary–adrenal) activates, wherein the hypothalamus signals the pituitary to release a hormone that tells the adrenal glands to release cortisol. This keeps the body and mind activated and on high alert over longer periods of time.

Inflammation: More research evidence is accumulating to indicate that ongoing stress may be related to chronic inflammation, and that even mild chronic inflammation plays a very important role in breaking down bodily systems, reducing functioning, and preventing repair and recovery. For example, there is evidence that stress may induce or worsen neurodegenerative diseases and even cancer via a pathway related to peripheral inflammation or neuroinflammation. Patients with major depression who are otherwise medically healthy have been repeatedly observed to have activated inflammatory pathways (Liu et al., 2017).

In the end, all of this should lead you to reflect on the realities of the mind-body connection and what science has to say about it. While not every sensationalistic thing you hear or see on social media or in marketing campaigns about the mind-body connection is scientifically valid, there is plenty of good, solid research out there so that you can find sound and persuasive evidence about the interrelationship between your mind and your body.

Wellness and the Medical Model

You may have heard of biopsychology or neuropsychology or maybe even biological psychology…what these fields have in common is a focus on research and practice related to the biological basis of behavior and mental and emotional functioning. The medical field also has many doctors who are focused in this area, both in research and treatment. This work is improving the quality of life for people around the world. But how does this medical model differ from a wellness perspective? Table 1.1 contrasts these two approaches.

The medical model of health is pervasive and largely accepted without major challenge within the American healthcare system. The medical model is based on the premise that all illness, disease, and disorders have a biological cause and disease process which, if we subject it to scientific scrutiny, will result in evidence-based diagnosis and treatment. While the strongly evidence-based foundation of the medical model is imperative when dealing with health, this model also generally ignores or downplays psychological and contextual factors. This focus on biological factors has been criticized as prioritizing treatment of the disease, rather than treatment of the whole person, and has directly resulted in preference for chemical, surgical, and other physical treatments rather than evaluating the psychological and social determinants of health (e.g., Barbour, 1995). The psychological and social determinants of health are aspects of life that we know impact people's health throughout the lifespan, such as autonomy, resilience, availability of high-quality education, accessible and affordable healthcare, safe and attainable housing, clean air and water, ability to procure nutritious food and to be physically active, as well as the ability to avoid racism, inequality, violence, trauma, and environmental toxins

Table 1.1 A wellness approach is qualitatively different than the medical model

Medical model	Wellness approach
The physical body is prone to dysfunction and disease	The physical body trends toward health, if purposeful health-seeking and health-affirming behaviors are the norm
Practitioners focus on biological explanation for and treatment of disease and disorders	Practitioners look at multiple factors for explanations for bodily dysfunction, including body, mind, relationships, stress, and social or contextual factors
Chronic disorders and disability lower quality of life	Meaningful quality of life is a result of positive emotional world, good coping skills, functional physical activity, and informed self-care
The medical professional is the expert and "sage" regarding the person's health; individual agency is minimized	Individuals are powerful agents in their own health and wellness, and practitioners are facilitators and scaffolders of healthy behaviors
Management of symptoms is common intervention	Symptoms speak to where healthy behaviors can have an impact; when appropriate, balance medical treatment with complimentary care
Health is a status to be measured and achieved	Health is a process that lasts a lifetime

(U.S. Department of Health and Human Services, Office of Disease Prevention and Health Promotion, 2024).

Let's consider the example of mental health treatment. For many years, the dominant approach to understanding, assessing, and treating mental illness has been the biomedical model. However, there has been a notable lack of progress on improving mental health outcomes for people who seek psychiatric services, even though mental health treatment is used now more than ever (e.g., Stupak & Dobroczynski, 2021). In 2021, 50% of Americans reported recent symptoms of anxiety or depressive disorder, and these issues were not unique to the United States (Xiong et al., 2020). Residents in China, Spain, Italy, Iran, Turkey, Nepal, and Denmark all reported significant symptoms of anxiety, depression, post-traumatic stress disorder, psychological distress, and stress. Universities around the world are seeing an increase in mental health-related issues amongst college students. Thus, even though psychiatric medication and psychological intervention are widely available, people remain notably distressed. When we respond to poor living conditions, jobs that devalue and overwork us, unending reports of violence, unacknowledged systemic discrimination, poverty, food insecurity, and a complex and crushingly expensive medical system with anxiety, depression, and mental distress, should we be medicating these symptoms or looking at the systems that bring them forth? The answer is probably both. People need good, sound mental health care, which can include the judicious use of medication, but they also need healthy food, safe housing, and good jobs in order to thrive. This is the balance sought by the wellness approach.

Health and Wellness Practitioner Perspectives

There are so many names for and ways to describe health and wellness practitioners and their areas of practice that it can become very confusing. Conventional medicine, alternative medicine, complementary medicine, and integrative medicine are all ways to describe different approaches to health and wellness assessment, diagnosis, treatment, and education.

Conventional medicine (also called allopathic medicine): It uses scientific research to identify safe and effective practices that are used in the diagnosis and treatment of diseases and to alleviate human pain and suffering. Conventional medicine is aligned closely with the medical model, and treatments and interventions tend to be biological and/or biochemical in nature. This is the type of medical approach most commonly used across healthcare settings.

Traditional medicine: It is based on the collective knowledge, beliefs, and practices of different cultures and is typically handed down either by oral or written tradition. The practices involved in traditional medicine frequently use the natural world (plants, herbs, animals, minerals, etc.) and/or spiritual practices to prevent, diagnose, and treat symptoms and disorders in the mind and body.

Complementary and alternative medicine (CAM): CAM is the modern term for when complementary and alternative medicines are classified together under an umbrella discipline. Complementary medicine encompasses an array of treatments that are used alongside conventional medical approaches. Alternative medicine treatments are used in place of conventional medicine. Together under the CAM umbrella, complementary and alternative approaches have received some mainstream acceptance, particularly in larger medical centers and among insurance providers.

Integrative medicine: Refers to the purposeful combining of CAM with conventional medicine in an integrated patient care plan that has evidence-based practice at its core. Integrative medicine approaches are in great demand across the country, and academic medical programs, medical centers, and insurers are struggling to keep up with demand (Ross et al., 2017).

Mind-body medicine: Grounded in the belief that treating the whole person—mind, body, and behavior together—is the best way to enhance wellness and to humanely treat the causes of human suffering. You may be wondering where mind-body medicine would fit into today's medical infrastructure? In modern practice, it is often difficult to discern a difference between CAM and integrative medicine, and one could recognize mind-body medicine as a subfield of either approach.

In modern practice, it is no longer possible to discern between what "is or is not" an intervention specific to either CAM, integrative medicine, or mind-body medicine. These approaches may be called different names in different places, but virtually all programs, centers, and departments offer a similar array of services, which can include any or all of the approaches in Table 1.2. We will discuss some of these interventions in depth in later chapters. However, we will focus on those that have established science or strong preliminary science behind them. Many wellness interventions lack a base of rigorous research, which is necessary for making reasonable evaluations of the benefits and risks of wellness interventions and sensible decisions about them. We will not further address pseudoscientific interventions, such as homeopathy. Homeopathy is not medicine, and it is not a treatment, cure, or remedy for any known symptom or disorder. Homeopathy, and fads like it, rely primarily on the placebo effect—people believe it will alleviate their symptoms and so it does, for a time.

It should be noted that any or all of these treatments and interventions, both those classically characterized as healthcare and those under a wellness approach, should also be understood relative to their purpose. Curative care has the purpose of curing a disorder or disease with a return to full wellness or delaying disease progression to such an extent as to have positive quality of life. Examples of the former would be antibiotic or antiviral treatment, surgery for an ACL tear, or a cast for a broken bone, whereas examples of the latter could be dialysis or medication for multiple sclerosis. Preventive care is that which promotes healthy lifestyle choices and

Table 1.2 Typical wellness interventions

Name	Description
Acupuncture and acupressure	Thin needles are inserted into the body (acupuncture) or physical pressure is applied (acupressure) in order to balance energy flow within the body for the purpose of pain and/or symptom relief
Aromatherapy	Inhaling or absorbing essential oils to promote well-being
Autogenic training	Inducing deep relaxation via the combination of visualization and body awareness
Ayurveda	Based in the belief that all bodily systems and the person's consciousness must be in balance for wellness to be achieved. Diet, herbal medicine, yoga/yogic breathing, and other interventions are used to bring alignment to our natural energy sources (the three doshas)
Biofeedback	Involuntary bodily functions are brought under voluntary control through training via the use of electronic or instrument monitoring
Chiropractic	Concerned with the mechanics of the musculoskeletal system, chiropractic utilizes adjustments, manipulation, massage, and other techniques to bring symptom and pain relief and to return clients to desired levels of functioning
Herbal medicine	The use of preparations and products that utilize plants, plant materials, and plant derivatives to treat or prevent illness and/or to enhance wellness
Massage	There are many ways to practice massage, but the common denominator is the purposeful manipulation of the body, typically the muscles, for the purpose of reducing pain, inducing relaxation, and/or reducing stress
Meditation	Can involve training attention, regulating awareness, and/or clearing the mind for the purpose of relaxation, stress reduction, or to manage psychological or physical symptoms, like anxiety
Movement-based practices, like Yoga, Tai chi, and Qigong	Use of body movements as a spiritual, mental, and physical discipline to harmonize mind and body, increase peace and serenity, and enhance self-understanding
Progressive muscle relaxation	Intentional tensing and relaxation of muscles in the body, typically from toes to head or head to toes
Spirituality	Connecting with something greater than ourselves and using the purpose, meaning, and value of the human spirit (sometimes called the soul) to promote healing and well-being
Visualization/guided imagery	Either individually or with the help of a practitioner, these techniques use mental images that evoke all five senses to facilitate relaxation, stress relief, symptom relief, or to create scenes of healing and comfort

health-promoting behaviors, detects potential health problems, and intervenes in minor health issues before they become major ones. Examples include vaccination, mammograms, colonoscopy, established dietary practices (like controlling portion sizes and eating fruits, vegetables, and whole grains), and regular exercise. Palliative care is concerned with people who have serious or life-limiting diseases. Palliative care centers around reducing human suffering through pain and symptom management, stress reduction, and maintaining quality of life. Examples include palliative chemotherapy (to shrink tumors in order to relieve pain), a medication pump for pain relief, caregiver support, and chaplain visits.

Finally, it's useful to discuss licensure and certification for those in the wellness space. In any situation where you find yourself ill or experiencing symptoms, it is best to seek out licensed healthcare professionals for best practice-based assessment and treatment. Table 1.3 provides a list of different licensed and/or certified practitioners and whether they have medication prescribing authority. Wellness or Holistic "doctors," holistic health practitioners, and holistic healers are sometimes trained physicians or osteopaths, but they can also be trained in other disciplines or have received minimal or informal training. It is important to ask the qualifications of your health and wellness providers and to balance risk versus benefit of any treatment offered; if anything is described to you as being a no-risk and no-side-effect intervention, you should ask many questions about it.

Table 1.3 Health and wellness providers

Provider	Licensed or certified?	Prescribing authority?
Advanced practice registered nurses (APRN), including nurse practitioner (NP), nurse anesthetist (CRNA), clinical nurse specialist (CNS), and certified nurse midwives (CNM)	Yes	Prescribing authority varies by jurisdiction
Allied health, including physical therapists, occupational therapists, dieticians/nutritionists, speech and language pathologists	Yes, for those listed	No
Chiropractor	Yes	No
Dentist (DDS)	Yes	Yes
Naturopath (ND)	23 states and some territories regulate the work of NDs, requiring either licensure or registration for practice	Limited, depending on jurisdiction
Osteopath (DO)	Yes	Yes
Physician (MD), including psychiatrists	Yes	Yes
Physician assistant (PA)	Yes	Yes (except controlled drugs in KY)
Podiatrist (DPM)	Yes	Yes
Psychologist (PhD)	Yes	Limited, in some jurisdictions can prescribe only specific psychoactive medications

Employment in the Wellness Field

In the United States, we have a government agency charged with supporting research and disseminating information about the mind-body connection (among other topics), called the National Center for Complementary and Integrative Health (NCCIH), under the auspices of the National Institute of Health. This agency provides millions of dollars in research funding at hundreds of academic and clinical sites around the country and disseminates the findings from these studies.

COVID-19, and the ensuing global pandemic, brought many health-related issues to the forefront and changed the wellness field. While many of the issues emerging from the crisis are certainly not new, the pandemic amplified the attention these issues receive. Underlying health issues increased the likelihood that one may die from the virus, and this concern made healthy behavior salient for many of us. Sales of home gym equipment rose significantly. Governments mandated masks to help attenuate the spread of the virus. Additionally, the lockdowns and subsequent isolation of people around the world increased the focus placed on mental health. Due to the impact of COVID-19 as well as demographic and societal changes, we see a growing recognition amongst many of the importance of our physical and mental well-being.

According to the U.S. Bureau of Labor Statistics employment in health-related areas is expected to grow 17% between 2020 and 2030. This growth, with an emphasis on health behaviors, is heavily influenced by the COVID-19 pandemic. Large numbers of employers anticipate investing more in health and well-being programs for employees. These programs will surely help address health care costs but also highlight the growing recognition of the importance of health—including not only physical health but also mental health and resources that can help people confront a variety of stressors. The good news is that all of this means that solid and stable careers are available in the health and wellness field for people with bachelor's degrees, such as:

- Corporate Wellness Coordinator/Manager
- Consumer Health Services Manager
- Patient Support Manager
- Patient Access Manager
- Community Health Worker
- Health and Wellness Educator
- Health Center/Facility Manager
- Fitness Center Manager/Director
- Behavioral Health Case Manager
- Wellness Coach
- Life Coach
- Fitness Coach
- Content Creator

With additional training and certification, the field opens up even more:

- Physical Therapist or Occupational Therapist Assistant
- Physical Education Teacher
- Compliance Manager
- Benefits Manager
- Athletic Trainer
- Personal Trainer
- And many more…

Mind-body wellness is no longer on the fringes of academia and this book explores some of the growing areas of research and thought in the wellness field. We'll review work on mind, body, and the connection between them. We also review everyday wellness and the role of our environment and relationships on sense of well-being.

Wellness Tip: Mind Your Mindset

You can understand mindset by thinking of it as your outlook on life or your "way of being" within your life context. Mindset is the sum total of our beliefs, assumptions, and attitudes that make up how we approach the world. When we are children, our mindset is very changeable, depending on who we are with and where we are (adults tend to forcefully define and reinforce a certain mindset in children). As we get older, our mindset tends to solidify or become more rigid, because the message of the people around us and society is that we must "be THIS way" to be successful or happy or worthy.

Think about whether this is the only approach. Do we have to be so set in our way of thinking—inflexible and rigid about our attitudes and assumptions about ourselves and our abilities? Do we have to put ourselves or others in a "box" of abilities and characteristics? Ask yourself if your mindset is helping you or holding you back? Is it moving you toward your goals or keeping you where you are? What would happen if you worked on changing your mindset to a growth mindset? Would that be easy, scary, impossible, liberating?

Luckily, we do not have to live with a rigidly set mindset. Carol Dweck (2006), one of the foremost researchers on mindset, defines two types of mindsets as "fixed" vs "growth." As shown in Fig. 1.1, people with a fixed mindset have strict expectations about themselves and others; they believe that intelligence, ability, and motivation are set and unchangeable, and they can be pessimistic and have low motivation to change or learn. Those with a growth mindset search for ways to improve themselves, their work, and their relationships; they can be resilient and flexible in the face of challenges.

Examining one's mindset is one of the key ingredients of therapy and even informal counseling. This is accomplished by encouraging a person to examine their thoughts, assumptions, and beliefs to see which ones are helpful (and they should keep) and which ones are causing them pain (and they should change). Dweck says

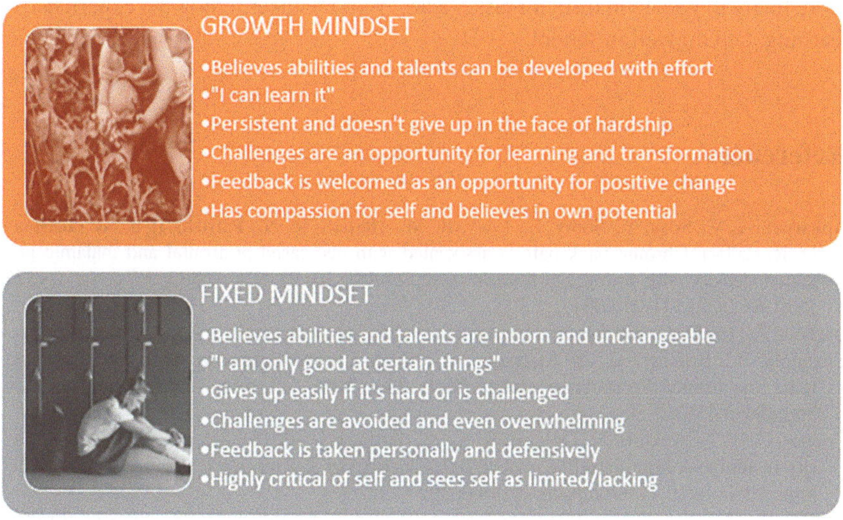

Fig. 1.1 Growth vs. fixed mindset

that we can develop or maintain a growth mindset by adopting the word "yet" into our self-evaluations ("I am not successful yet" and "I do not have my own house yet") and by replacing our negative thoughts about ourselves and the world with positive ones.

A change of mindset is a useful way to look at the therapeutic process, as it avoids all sorts of psycho-jargon and intimidating interactions! This change of mindset can go all the way back to our first interactions with our parents; in other words, parents and other teaching figures can do a lot to help children to develop a resilient, sturdy, and growth-oriented mindset. This, of course, prepares us to then provide the same assets to the children in our own lives, as Dweck (2012) states:

> Parents think they can hand children permanent confidence—like a gift—by praising their brains and talent. It doesn't work, and in fact has the opposite effect. It makes children doubt themselves as soon as anything is hard or anything goes wrong. If parents want to give their children a gift, the best thing they can do is to teach their children to love challenges, be intrigued by mistakes, enjoy effort, and keep on learning. That way, their children don't have to be slaves of praise. They will have a lifelong way to build and repair their own confidence.

Growing and developing is part of how children mature into young adults. In considering growth, we recognize physical and cognitive changes—kids grow in size and in their abilities to think deeply about issues. For kids who develop a fixed mindset, they view their abilities as set and unchangeable. When they view intelligence, including their own, as a permanent feature of who they are and as something that cannot be changed, this negatively impacts their motivation to work toward a goal. If a growth mindset is developed, intelligence is likely to be viewed as an aspect of who they are that can grow and develop, just like them. These kids are more likely to persist in difficult tasks, learn from mistakes, enjoy the experience of learning, and do well in school.

References

Apkarian, A. V., Sosa, Y., Sonty, S., Levy, R. M., Harden, R. N., Parrish, T. B., & Gitelman, D. R. (2004). Chronic back pain is associated with decreased prefrontal and thalamic gray matter density. *The Journal of Neuroscience, 24*(46), 10410–10415. https://doi.org/10.1523/JNEUROSCI.2541-04.2004

Barbour, A. (1995). *Caring for patients: A critique of the medical model.* Stanford University Press.

Chandola, T., Brunner, E., & Marmot, M. (2006). Chronic stress at work and the metabolic syndrome: Prospective study. *BMJ, 332*(7540), 521–524. https://doi.org/10.1136/bmj.38693.435301.80

Cooper, C. B., Neufeld, E. V., Dolezal, B. A., & Martin, J. L. (2018). Sleep deprivation and obesity in adults: A brief narrative review. *BMJ Open Sport & Exercise Medicine, 4*(1), e000392. https://doi.org/10.1136/bmjsem-2018-000392

Craft, L. L., & Perna, F. M. (2004). The benefits of exercise for the clinically depressed. *Primary Care Companion to the Journal of Clinical Psychiatry, 6*(3), 104–111. https://doi.org/10.4088/pcc.v06n0301

Damasio, A. R. (1999). *The feeling of what happens: Body and emotion in the making of consciousness.* Harcourt Brace.

Dewall, C. N., Macdonald, G., Webster, G. D., Masten, C. L., Baumeister, R. F., Powell, C., Combs, D., Schurtz, D. R., Stillman, T. F., Tice, D. M., & Eisenberger, N. I. (2010). Acetaminophen reduces social pain: Behavioral and neural evidence. *Psychological Science, 21*(7), 931–937. https://doi.org/10.1177/0956797610374741

Dum, R. P., Levinthal, D. J., & Strick, P. L. (2016). Motor, cognitive, and affective areas of the cerebral cortex influence the adrenal medulla. *Proceedings of the National Academy of Sciences, 113*(35), 9922–9927. https://doi.org/10.1073/pnas.1605044113

Dweck, C. S. (2006). *Mindset: The new psychology of success.* Random House.

Dweck, C. S. (2012). *Mindset: Changing the way you think to fulfill your potential.* Robinson.

Emerson, N. M., Zeidan, F., Lobanov, O. V., Hadsel, M. S., Martucci, K. T., Quevedo, A. S., Starr, C. J., Nahman-Averbuch, H., Weissman-Fogel, I., Granovsky, Y., Yarnitsky, D., & Coghill, R. C. (2014). Pain sensitivity is inversely related to regional grey matter density in the brain. *Pain, 155*(3), 566–573. https://doi.org/10.1016/j.pain.2013.12.004

Gorham, G. (1994). Mind-body dualism and the Harvey-Descartes controversy. *Journal of the History of Ideas, 55*(2), 211–234. https://doi.org/10.2307/2709897

Ledochowski, L., Ruedl, G., Taylor, A. H., & Kopp, M. (2015). Acute effects of brisk walking on sugary snack cravings in overweight people, affect and responses to a manipulated stress situation and to a sugary snack cue: A crossover study. *PLoS One, 10*(3), e0119278. https://doi.org/10.1371/journal.pone.0119278

Liu, L., Wang, H., Chen, X., Zhang, Y., Zhang, H., & Xie, P. (2023). Gut microbiota and its metabolites in depression: From pathogenesis to treatment. *eBioMedicine, 90*, 104527. https://doi.org/10.1016/j.ebiom.2023.104527

Liu, Y.-Z., Wang, Y.-X., & Jiang, C.-L. (2017). Inflammation: The common pathway of stress-related diseases. *Frontiers in Human Neuroscience, 11*, 1–11. https://doi.org/10.3389/fnhum.2017.00316

McEwen, B. S., & Stellar, E. (1993). Stress and the individual. Mechanisms leading to disease. *Archives of Internal Medicine, 153*(18), 2093–2101.

Oh, H., & Taylor, A. H. (2012). Brisk walking reduces ad libitum snacking in regular chocolate eaters during a workplace simulation. *Appetite, 58*(1), 387–392. https://doi.org/10.1016/j.appet.2011.11.006

Ross, C., Blau, M., & Sheridan, K. (2017). *Medicine with a side of mysticism: Top hospitals promote unproven therapies.* STAT. Retrieved from www.statnews.com/2017/03/07/alternative-medicine-hospitals-promote/

Schaffer, J. (2010). Monism: The priority of the whole. *The Philosophical Review, 119*(1), 31–76. https://doi.org/10.1215/00318108-2009-025

Scheper-Hughes, N., & Lock, M. M. (1987). The mindful body: A prolegomenon to future work in medical anthropology. *Medical Anthropology Quarterly, 1*(1), 6–41. https://doi.org/10.1525/maq.1987.1.1.02a00020

Statista. (2024). *Size of the wellness market worldwide from 2017 to 2022, with a forecast to 2027.* Retrieved from https://www.statista.com/statistics/491362/health-wellness-market-value/

Stupak, R., & Dobroczynski, B. (2021). From mental health industry to humane care. Suggestions for an alternative systemic approach to distress. *International Journal of Environmental Research and Public Health, 18*(12), 6625. https://doi.org/10.3390/ijerph18126625

Sublette, M. E., Cheung, S., Lieberman, E., Hu, S., Mann, J. J., Uhlemann, A. C., & Miller, J. M. (2021). Bipolar disorder and the gut microbiome: A systematic review. *Bipolar Disorders, 23*(6), 544–564. https://doi.org/10.1111/bdi.13049

Turnbaugh, P. J., Hamady, M., Yatsunenko, T., Cantarel, B. L., Duncan, A., Ley, R. E., Sogin, M. L., Jones, W. J., Roe, B. A., Affourtit, J. P., Egholm, M., Henrissat, B., Heath, A. C., Knight, R., & Gordon, J. I. (2009). A core gut microbiome in obese and lean twins. *Nature, 457*(7228), 480–484. https://doi.org/10.1038/nature07540

U.S. Department of Health and Human Services, Office of Disease Prevention and Health Promotion. (2024). *Healthy people 2030.* Retrieved from https://odphp.health.gov/healthypeople/objectives-and-data/social-determinants-health

Van Gelder, T. (1998). Monism, dualism, pluralism. *Mind & Language, 13*(1), 76–97. https://doi.org/10.1111/1468-0017.00066

Vuong, H. E., & Hsiao, E. Y. (2017). Emerging roles for the gut microbiome in autism spectrum disorder. *Biological Psychiatry, 81*(5), 411–423. https://doi.org/10.1016/j.biopsych.2016.08.024

Xiong, J., Lipsitz, O., Nasri, F., Lui, L. M. W., Gill, H., Phan, L., Chen-Li, D., Iacobucci, M., Ho, R., Majeed, A., & McIntyre, R. S. (2020). Impact of COVID-19 pandemic on mental health in the general population: A systematic review. *Journal of Affective Disorders, 277*, 55–64. https://doi.org/10.1016/j.jad.2020.08.001

Chapter 2
A Scientific Approach to Wellness

One of the most important skills that we learn from academic work is how to be good consumers of information. Information comes at us fast and from so many different sources that it can be hard to discern what is fact from what is fiction. Critical thinking and a strong ability to identify and ward against cognitive biases are part of the thinking skills that we should master as college graduates.

What Is Science and Why Is It Important?

Use of what we call the scientific method is critical because it allows us to understand the world around us and how it works, while minimizing the influence of bias. Humans filter everything we observe, experience, and learn through our beliefs, attitudes, values, and assumptions; the human factor is a primary source of bias in science. Because the scientific method is systematic, empirical, and transparent, it guards against bias, and it makes the process of science open to observation and analysis.

The steps of the scientific method are relatively straightforward, and it all starts with an observation of something interesting. The steps are:

Observation: A scientist observes something in the real world and wonders about it.

Question: The scientist develops a research question to study some aspects of what they observed.

Research: The scientist does a lot of research reviewing previously published work to see if this question or ones like it have been studied before. This allows scientists to examine preexisting evidence prior to engaging in the steps to acquire more or advanced knowledge. The scientist is always concerned with advancing science forward by asking unique, important questions and by studying topics that will help us to approach issues with more relevant information.

S. M. Henney, J. D. Hackett, *Mind-Body Wellness*,
https://doi.org/10.1007/978-3-031-91611-3_2

Hypothesis development: The scientist makes one or more specific and testable statements about what they have observed, considering the research. One way to think about a hypothesis is that it is an answer or explanation to the question that you have asked.

Experiment: The scientist designs a way to test the hypothesis. This involves identifying *independent variables* (the variables that you control and change), *dependent variables* (variables that you measure), a sample (the participants in your experiment), and a method (how you are manipulating and measuring your variables and minimizing bias).

Data analysis: Typically, the scientist will record the data and analyze it using the correct statistical method. The goal is to determine if the results could be found by chance or whether change in the independent variable is related to change in the dependent variable.

Conclusion: The scientist will report their results and their interpretations of these results to the scientific community. Through a process called peer review, the scientific community will evaluate whether the methodology of the study followed the scientific method and whether the results were reliable, valid, and interpreted in a reasonable way.

We all seek ways to make sense of what we observe in the world around us. Figure 2.1 provides a real-world example of how the scientific process unfolds, using a high school-based intervention for chronic stress in adolescents. However, not all ways of observing the world result in equally valid and reliable conclusions.

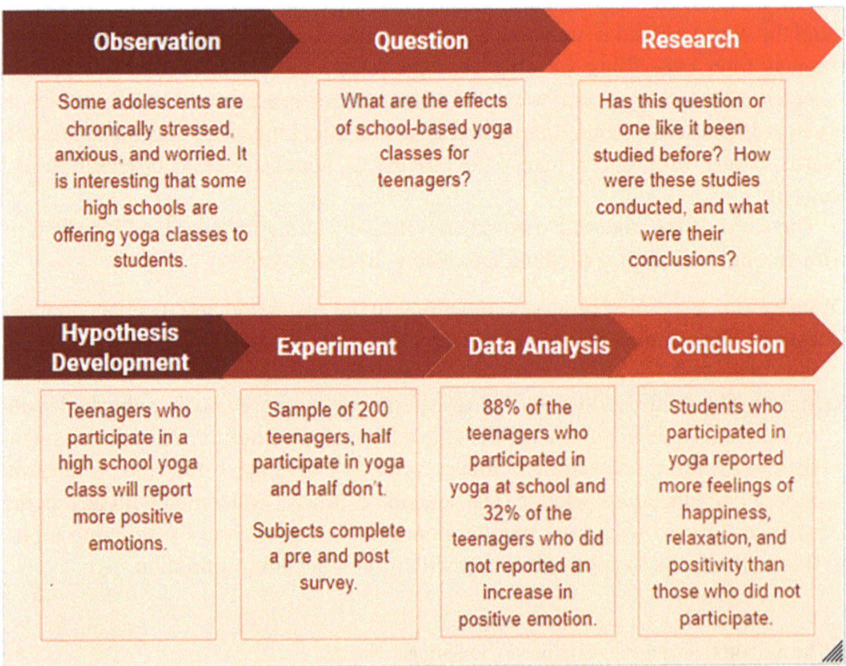

Fig. 2.1 The scientific method in action

Without the scientific method, our conclusions about the world remain biased, idiosyncratic, and unable to be replicated. Replication—when the same conclusion is reached after a question is studied by different scientists—is important because it tells us that a conclusion is sturdy and reliable, and we are therefore more confident in applying it in the real world. If a scientific result cannot be replicated, it tells us that our understanding of the issue is incomplete and that we need a different approach to studying it prior to implementing it in the real world.

Science related to the medical field helps to determine which treatments, procedures, and pharmaceuticals are safe and effective. Consumers and patients rely on their providers, insurance companies, and regulatory bodies to know which interventions will be effective for their medical issues and which ones have a positive risk-to-reward profile (this means that the benefits of receiving the intervention outweigh the side effects and risks). Evaluations of this type rely on the principles of robust and well-executed scientific investigation. On the other hand, shoddy science and pseudoscientific claims result in consumers and patients receiving interventions that have no effect at best and are actively harmful at worst or in patients refusing best-practice treatments in favor of a pipe dream.

Sometimes you might read about a "study" of a particular treatment that says it "proves" that the treatment is effective or painless or side-effect free, but it is based on casual or quasi-scientific methods. How will you know if the study is based on the scientific method? Check the Methods section of the study. Is the study described in a way that conforms to the scientific method? Is the sample that is used described in detail and appropriate to the question? Are the variables used described fully, and is the measurement of the variables reasonably related to the research question? Is the study from a known scientific source, such as a university or hospital? While none of these things guarantee a scientifically sound research study, their absence should make you question the results and seek more information from legitimate science-based sources.

How Can I Tell if Something Is Pseudoscience?

Look at the source—Personal, governmental, religious, academic, news, etc.

Look at the funding—Who has a stake in this information? In many ways, this is the most important issue. Even scientists can sometimes be funded by people who have a stake in a certain outcome.

Look at the method used to establish efficacy—Do they describe it? Will they let you look at the data? Is it published in a peer-reviewed setting? Many times, pseudoscience is not transparent at best and actively hostile to questions and criticism at worst.

Look for grandiose claims—If something sounds too good to be true, it probably is. This can also come in the form of physically impossible claims or unrealistic guarantees.

Look for "scienceploitation"—Uses big, scientific-sounding words and jargon to explain concepts that should be easy to define for the lay public.

Does it claim to be "exclusive knowledge"—There is nothing exclusive about science. It's been around forever and, if legitimate, is done via a set of clear expectations. It's never secret or something "doctors don't want you to know" or something that's been "hidden" from you.

Evidence-Based Practice

There is an important relationship between scientific investigation, science-based findings, and effective and ethical practice in medicine, allied medicine, and wellness. Rigorous scientific investigation and the subsequent findings result in what we call scientific knowledge. In other words, our reliable and replicable understanding of the world based on years of study using the scientific method represents our accumulated scientific knowledge. Our base of scientific knowledge is typically divided into laws, theories, and hypotheses. Scientific laws, which represent a description of how an aspect of the natural world actually operates, require the highest level of scientific evidence, including many years of empirical studies and replication studies accumulated over multiple researchers. An example of a scientific law is Newton's Third Law of Motion (for every action there is an equal and opposite reaction), which has been studied so extensively that it is an accepted explanation for natural forces.

Theories, while not as comprehensively studied as laws, are broader statements about how phenomena are related to each other and how they operate in the real world. A theory is tested over time, and it is the accumulation of the best evidence that can be collected on the phenomenon. Behavioral theory, for example, has been extensively studied over many years and provides one explanation for human behavior by analyzing what comes before and after a behavior in order to describe why the behavior is occurring and to predict future behavior. It is important to avoid the common usage of the word "theory" (i.e., "That is just your personal theory—it doesn't mean anything.") when looking at issues of health and wellness. The word "theory," as we will use it in this book, is a powerful statement about the weight of the accumulated evidence in favor of a certain explanation for phenomena.

A hypothesis is a clear, testable, and reasonable explanation for a specific phenomenon. Sometimes, hypotheses are described as our "best guess" or "educated guess" about the relationship between variables, but this is misleading. A hypothesis is not a guess at all, as it is derived from a comprehensive search of the existing literature in the area and also the expertise of the researchers in their field. A hypothesis is a preliminary or tentative prediction, subject to being disproved, rather than a guess. The study's hypothesis will be stated as a null—a statement of no effect. Examples of hypotheses include:

- In a clinical trial of a new weight management drug: "People taking drug X will have the same weight change over the study as people taking a placebo."
- In a study of yoga: "People practicing four to six yoga poses once per day will report daily positive and negative emotions at the same rate as people reading daily or going about their normal daily lives."
- In a clinical trial of a new pneumonia vaccine: "Those taking the new vaccine will have a similar rate of infection over time as those taking a placebo vaccine or an existing vaccine."

Once we have studied a phenomenon and tested our hypotheses, we still have to transform the results into actual practice. This is where evidence-based practice becomes essential—it is how we take scientific findings and integrate them with practical expertise in order to provide effective interventions that have known risks and benefits. When practitioners use evidence-based practices, the delivery of assessments, advice, and treatments is informed by our most rigorous evidence. This is most likely to result in the best available outcomes for patients. Evidence-based practice doesn't guarantee positive outcomes, but it makes them more likely than interventions with no evidence. It is important to note that even though evidence-based practice is based on science, it is not devoid of context. Evidence-based practice should always be provided within the priorities and value system of the patient, and it continually strives to be culturally relevant and humane.

There is a lot of concern, however, that research results are very slow to reach practical, public-facing applications. We may know a lot about treatments, interventions, or practices related to a certain disease or disorder, but we may not have translated this knowledge into practice. People are hungry, sometimes desperate, for new and better treatments for the illnesses afflicting themselves and their loved ones, but even when solid research exists it is slow to come to public use. Some researchers estimate that the lag time between scientific discovery and public use tends to be around 17 years (Morris et al., 2011).

What Is Pseudoscience?

Pseudoscience is a belief, idea, conclusion, theory, or method that is labeled as scientific but is not. Pseudoscience is the ultimate "fake news"—it is designed to fool you and, particularly, to manipulate you politically, socially, and/or economically. Pseudoscience typically reflects a belief system, and its purpose is to convert you to that belief system. In contrast, science doesn't require belief because it rests on a method—the same organized, visible, and rigorous method across all questions. Students aren't asked to "believe" in science, rather to understand the method by which valid and reliable results are obtained and be able to identify this type of result when they see it.

Pseudoscientific belief comes in several forms. Science denialism is used to question a finding, a branch of science, or even the scientific method itself. Science deniers are more than just skeptics—rational skepticism should be a part of science—rather, they are typically resistant to facts and/or are dogmatic true believers in whatever position they have assumed. Most people have relatively firm beliefs about what knowledge is, how it comes to be, and, particularly, who to trust as a source of knowledge. Yet misunderstandings about what science is and how it is conducted are common; for example, the fact that scientific findings can be updated with new evidence is a good part of science that allows knowledge to grow, but a science denialist would say that because science changes, it is too "tentative" to trust. Such misunderstandings of science have led to denial of the science behind climate change, vaccination, psychiatric medication, and cancer treatment, among many others. In terms of medical denialism, people focus their disbelief largely on behaviors they perceive as “voluntary” or on behaviors associated with “personal beliefs,” such as vaccination, diet, supplements, and even chemotherapy and HIV treatment.

Another form of pseudoscience that has a firm foothold in social media and marketing practices is pseudo-scientific theory, or promotion of a theory or explanation of how something works to the exclusion of any other science-based theory. People want, desperately and wholeheartedly, for their theories and beliefs to be true—they believe in miracle cures because they or someone they love is sick or they believe in “alternative treatments” for cancer because they are afraid of chemotherapy. This has led to a cottage industry in pseudo-scientific theory-making for homeopaths, flat earthers, vaccine deniers, and the like. It is noteworthy that science deniers and believers in pseudo-scientific theories don’t necessarily deny all scientific endeavors, as most still want airplanes to be designed safely, buildings not to collapse, and for surgeons and doctors to save their life after a heart attack or car accident.

A final progenitor of pseudoscience belief that pervades all realms of scientific inquiry is the denial of the role of experts and expertise in science. Pseudoscience almost always presents claims as “facts” without scientific or empirical evidence to back the claim. In other words, pseudoscience relies on confirmation (“this is true because I say it’s true”) rather than evidence. This means that pseudoscience is unfalsifiable, and one must believe it’s true rather than evaluating evidence.

What follows are descriptions of some hallmarks of pseudoscience, and Table 2.1 provides real-world examples of these concepts:

Table 2.1 Examples of cognitive bias

COGNITIVE BIAS	Real-World Examples
ANECDOTES	"Once I found out that my body parts are ruled by different Zodiac signs, I started following an astrology diet, and I feel great!"
TESTIMONIALS	"I tried 'The Awesome Cure,' and in just one week it reduced my anxiety, cleared up my skin, eliminated my acid reflux, and saved my marriage."
APPEALS TO EMOTION	Anti-vaccination efforts often target parents' love and concern for their children by asking "don't you care about your kids" or "don't your kids deserve the 'real truth'?"
GASLIGHTING	"You are crazy to believe in what your pediatrician says. Doctors are all in the pocket of Big Pharma. You sound like you love your kids, but listening to doctors is child abuse."
KERNEL OF TRUTH	"Abstinence is the only way to stop abusing alcohol. If you have a history of alcohol abuse, you will always abuse alcohol whenever you drink." [Abstinence is *one* way to stop abusing alcohol..]
CHERRY PICKING	"After using our breakthrough weight loss supplement for just one week, June lost 8 pounds and Juan lost 10 pounds! [This is not to mention Tonya, Maria, and Taveris, who took the supplement and lost no weight.]
EXTRAORDINARY CLAIMS	"The Awesome Cure" is your one stop for wellness. You don't need ten pills and supplements – in one pill, "The Awesome Cure" will make you thin, strong, and healthy."
WORD OF MOUTH	"A lot of people are saying that the 5G towers are dangerous. People in my neighborhood are saying they know people living by the 5G towers who have cancer."

Anecdotes: When people explain their understanding of the world through short stories or accounts of their own or others' experiences. Anecdotes are always subjective and reflect personal experience as the storyteller sees it. All information that doesn't fit the teller's worldview is left out or ignored, and there is limited or no ability to confirm the events or conclusions.

Testimonials: Similar to anecdotes, testimonials are longer and more detailed, and they have the major problem of being true, but only for that person! Testimonials or personal events can be 100% accurate, and yet not applicable to anyone outside of that specific context or story. Again, they are subjective and biased toward the individual's interpretation of events.

Appeals to emotion: These present us with emotionally charged or emotionally manipulative information. There is a notable lack of factual evidence in the appeal, as the goal is to derail logical thought by enhancing emotional impact. Appeals to emotion can also use gaslighting to make people think they are crazy or abusive for following the science.

Gaslighting: This occurs when communication directed at us causes us to doubt our understanding of the world or even our own sanity. Gaslighting may cause feelings of confusion or powerlessness, especially in the face of an emotional appeal.

Kernel of truth: This technique uses just enough parts of the truth to establish status but then adds on the untruth or veers away from known fact. Pseudoscience can have a "selective relationship to science"—it can use some scientific results, but not in a valid way or erroneously applies "results" that don't actually apply to the topic at hand.

Cherry picking: A hallmark of pseudoscience, cherry picking occurs when the narrative only acknowledges or uses information that conforms to an idea or belief or claim and ignores everything else.

Extraordinary claims: The product of the need for authority and influence that is endemic in pseudoscience. Pseudoscience almost always makes extraordinary claims, such as a vaccine that makes you magnetic or the earth is flat or that there is a diet or a treatment that cures everything—cancer, ADHD, Crohn's disease, and eczema—all in one.

Word of mouth: This effect occurs because we tend to believe things that we hear repeated often. This is why information silos such as Facebook groups, political groups, or listening to one single news channel are so dangerous; we hear the same rhetoric, theories, and ideology repeated to us by different voices, we cease to question it, and, ultimately, become polarized in our beliefs.

Types of Cognitive Biases and Logical Fallacies

Because pseudoscience plays on our cognitive biases, we will review some of the cognitive biases and logical fallacies that are most related to pseudoscience acceptance. This is a selection of possible biases, by no means the only ones that could occur. Everyone needs to know about these so they can analyze their own thinking and logical processes to see where they might be vulnerable to some of these cognitive biases and to work to guard against them.

Confirmation bias is when we tend to search for, pay attention to, and remember information that confirms our already established beliefs. We see and retain the information that matches what we believe to be true, but we ignore and filter out any information that contradicts our beliefs. Science works in an opposite way…it seeks to be disproven rather than to prove anything.

Selection bias has many faces, but one form of this is when we favor what we learn from things that happen to us or to someone close to us. That's why we pay attention to what our mothers, our Facebook groups, or friends tell us about certain products, beliefs, or ideas.

The appeal to authority fallacy occurs when we accept something only because we perceive the person saying it to be smart, powerful, popular, or an expert. In response to questions, a real authority will provide you with evidence and will be honest about what they don't know.

The appeal to nature is the fallacy that if it is natural, it is good for you, and that if it is the result of a scientific process, it is unnatural and not good for you. The problem, of course, is that death, illness, sharks, and poison are "natural," as are many things that are "bad" for us. In contrast, the products of science in healthcare have generally been a trend for good, resulting in longer, healthier lives for more people over time.

The appeal to tradition happens when we call something good because it is traditional, ancient, old, or "the way our grandparents did it." Any time you see that something is from an "ancient secret" or "native tradition" or "opened in 1800," this is telling you that the old way of doing things is best, and the new ways are suspicious.

A false analogy fallacy is assuming that similarity in one respect means that things are similar in all respects. Simply drawing an analogy between two things doesn't mean that you have proven they are the same in critical aspects. For example, an argument was made against contact tracing for COVID-19 that stated that diabetes and COVID-19 are both diseases, but we don't contact trace for diabetes. This, of course, ignores the difference between the two diseases—one is contagious and the other is not.

The Wellness Industry and Pseudoscience

The wellness industry is particularly susceptible to pseudoscience, as it is often poorly regulated and has lots of money associated with it. This is an example of some of the things you see in a pseudoscience advertisement:

…it's a miracle

…it's 100% natural

…it shows a person who KNOWS it works, because it did for them

...it's guaranteed to work

...it's ancient wisdom—people used to know better and conventional medicine can't be trusted

It's no mystery why pseudoscience targets those aspects of wellness that people care the most about and that have the most impact on their lives and functioning, as there is money, fame, and influence to be found in this space. A common target for pseudoscientific products and marketing is weight loss. Fad diets, weight loss schemes, and weight loss supplements are a multi-billion dollar business, but most do not live up to their claims. "Detoxes" and "cleanses" say they will rid the body of toxins, "rebalance" the digestive system, and produce weight loss. A 2014 review of these approaches found that these claims have little support, and that the evidence surrounding these techniques comes from a few small, flawed studies (Klein & Kiat, 2015).

On their face, detox diets are an interesting phenomenon, as the human body has a very highly developed detoxification system of its own via the kidneys and liver. Keeping hydrated, eating a balanced diet, and avoiding smoking, excessive alcohol use, and drug use keep us more "detoxified" than any cleanse could and with fewer side effects. In fact, side effects are common with cleanses and detox diets, and may include diarrhea or constipation, fatigue, nausea, dehydration, and headaches. These negative side effects are reframed as beneficial by wellness gurus, stating that they are "proof" that the detox is "releasing toxins from the body," whereas in reality, your body is telling you that what you are doing is hurting, not helping. Like many aspects of the wellness space, detox diets sound good and make us think we are doing something proactive for our health, but their outcomes are based more on belief and marketing than actual results. Again, you can support your body to detox itself by staying hydrated, avoiding substances like alcohol and nicotine, eating a balanced diet, and exercising regularly.

Homeopathy and Pseudoscience

Homeopathy is based on the idea that "like cures like"—in other words, you would use a small amount of the thing that causes the illness, symptom or disease in a sick person to cure it in a healthy person. One simple example is using a minute amount of coffee to cure insomnia. The actual agent is diluted and agitated in order, supposedly, to train the body to heal itself with an infinitesimal amount of the offending agent. In other words, the original agent is diluted multiple times until it is, for all intents and purposes, water. Since there is essentially no active ingredient in a full homeopathic treatment, the primary function of a homeopathic intervention is as a placebo. To be clear, there is no homeopathic product that is any different from a placebo in actual practice. In regard to severe illness, like cancer or MS, there is no evidence that homeopathic products have any effect when they replace conventional treatments. In fact, they can be deadly when they replace or postpone real medical treatment.

Social Media and Pseudoscience

Everywhere we visit online and all the social media posts we interact with, create a "map" for us online. Computers track the content we view online, and this tracking allows artificial intelligence to use algorithms to target our interests. As we view specific political news outlets, the algorithm created for us focuses on feeding us related news content. In essence, we end up in an echo chamber where what we see aligns with previous news stories we've read. If we are viewing material related to diet fads, the algorithm pushes diet-related content to us. People do not tend to mind this personalized news feed, possibly because algorithm-based information keeps us in our comfort zone and aligns with our current values and biases. However, the algorithm also feeds our searches, preferences, and online tendencies into business enterprises that actively market products to us that can be costly, untested for safety, and of dubious effectiveness.

Most people have searched for health and wellness information online at some point; we search for diagnoses, treatments, advice, terminology, and prevention measures, often before consulting a medical professional for such information. It is increasingly popular to use social media as an authoritative source of information on health issues of all kinds. This was especially true during the COVID-19 pandemic, when social media served as the primary source of information regarding the virus (Zhong et al., 2021). There are numerous problems with relying on social media and other online sources for health information. Many people tend to ignore the credibility of the websites or source where they find the health information. For many of us, as long as the information is congruent with what we want to believe, we accept it (another example of confirmation bias!).

Another issue with online information is that people tend to find anecdotal stories more compelling than statistical data. Reading about someone's change in health after consuming only high protein diets, or how colon cleansing improved a colleague's gut health, or how a new hormone balancing technique really changed a friend's life can be quite astonishing. The data, however, do not support these miraculous changes. Data can be overwhelming at times, and we may get "lost" in all the numbers. Stories are easy to follow, often pull us in emotionally, and leave a lasting impression on us. These anecdotes are not grounded in data or scientific research and are not generalizable to other people. Similarly, popular and trending takes on wellness easily catch our eye and appear to be valid because many people believe in them. In modern society, information is omnipresent and simple to manipulate. The increased saturation of AI into all aspects of our lives makes "truth" even more difficult to ascertain with any degree of certainty, since we can no longer trust our "trusted sources" or even what we see and hear. One way to push back on popular or trending pseudoscience is to develop and nurture intellectual autonomy. Intellectual autonomy is not only "thinking for yourself," it is the ability to independently assess, reflect on, and think critically about all information that you receive. This requires diligence and a purposeful mindset about the value of self-directed information gathering, evaluation, and interpretation. Intellectual autonomy is an active and rational process that underpins a sensible and well-reasoned approach to wellness-related information, products, interventions, and services.

All of these issues are impacted by the way search algorithms are designed. Algorithms utilize our search history and websites we access to understand how to "market" to us better. Marketing efforts then are tailored to our interests and attitudes. This creates a bubble where our prejudices and preexisting beliefs are reinforced (Sinatra & Hofer, 2021). Understanding how this works requires algorithmic literacy. Algorithmic literacy is an understanding of how algorithms are used by online services and, as a result, being able to critically evaluate the information we encounter. Once the algorithm knows what we "want to see," it promotes this information, regardless of its accuracy and truthfulness. As algorithmic literacy develops, we pay attention to the quality of the information we encounter online and reject anything that is not accurate or supported by research. After all, just because something is on the internet doesn't mean it is true.

The Risks of Pseudoscience

Belief in pseudoscience has consequences, many of which can be harmful to us if we believe and act on pseudoscientific claims or to others who we might tell about or try to convince to use a product or "treatment" based in pseudoscience. Pseudoscience is a threat to good outcomes for patients and for the ability of medical professionals to do the right thing for their patients because it:

- Reduces people's belief in the products of science and the scientific method. People no longer ascribe to the best practices that have scientific evidence but rather turn to word of mouth, family and friends, social media, and anecdotal evidence for health and wellness advice.
- Reduces faith in traditional medicine to provide treatments that work and are necessary to address disease and disability. Doctors are seen as "mouthpieces" of big pharma or insurance companies, and their expertise and years of rigorous training are minimized or dismissed.
- Increases actual, real-world risk to people who partake in two ways—by using the pseudoscientific product or treatment and by *not* using a tested and regulated treatment.

Cancer Treatment and Pseudoscience

Cancer treatment is frequently the topic of pseudoscientific claims. This is because cancer itself and many of the treatments can be difficult to endure and cause much suffering. However, the idea that you get cancer from being unhappy, stressed, or out of harmony or that you can cure cancer with homeopathy, vitamins, or a detox are dangerous claims that have themselves resulted in significant human suffering and painful deaths. The problem, of course, is when patients are convinced to stop science-based medical treatments for cancer and replace them with alternative, pseudoscientific treatments. When patients do this, they lose—the only way to rationally approach additional, nonscientific treatments are to consult your doctor about whether it is safe to use the product *in conjunction* with your science-based treatment. It's important that everyone knows that some pseudoscientific treatments for cancer can interfere with or alter the effectiveness of actual cancer treatment. Following the advice of a healthcare professional regarding treatment and treatment supplements will increase the probability of a positive outcome.

The number of products we are being sold every day to address our fears, our desires to be loved and to be found beautiful, and to feel youthful are truly mind-boggling. We want to be happy, for our children to be successful and popular, to have good sex, and for us to feel and look young and fit, and there are hundreds of companies willing to take our money for products they say can help. It seems like it should be easy to discern what is a beneficial and safe product, but it is not. The good news is that science can help us identify what really works for our health and wellness and what does not. Science-mindedness in the wellness space can help us all be discerning consumers, which in turn aids us in our quest for a more healthful and fulfilling life.

Criticisms of a Wellness Approach

As we are learning here, some of the wellness products, programs, and beliefs are pseudoscientific, but others are not—we must practice discernment in the choices we make in the wellness space. The pursuit of wellness in the context of today's social media-consumed, anti-medicine, and health-conscious society can lead to wellness perfectionism and a preoccupation with wellness that, for some, may verge on obsessive behavior. The focus on wellness perfectionism, particularly in eating and fitness, can cause us to be self-blaming, anxious, and critical of others who we perceive are interfering with our wellness or who are imperfectly well themselves. This is the opposite of a growth mindset in that when we set unattainable standards of physical and mental perfection, we restrict our psychological flexibility and short-circuit our coping mechanisms. Wellness culture can be harsh and exclusionary; if you don't look the right way, eat the right things, and have the right opinions, you are subject to derogatory messages, insults to your intelligence, and exclusion.

These aspects of wellness culture can make us less well and more sick by having detrimental effects on our mental and physical health. Wellness perfectionism can result in disordered eating, over exercising, gastrointestinal problems, stress headaches/migraines, anxiety disorders, and even missed diagnoses based on an overfocus on nonspecific symptoms or symptoms that result from the wellness products themselves. The wellness judgment and criticism that is part of wellness culture is, itself, a kind of discrimination, particularly against those with disabilities and those who choose to have their chronic health issues treated with conventional medicine (even if alongside nontraditional approaches). For example, workplace wellness programs can penalize employees with health problems and can even be closed to them; further, it is not unusual for workers to avoid these programs for fear of punishment or even shaming from their coworkers or bosses.

There is also a discouraging link between wellness and wealth. Wellness has been commodified, and it is an industry that is increasingly focused on profit, fame, catchy sound bites, and fearmongering. Wellness supplements, for example, can cost hundreds of dollars or more every month. Practitioners who "prescribe" them often base their recommendations on costly "wellness panels" (typically blood and/or urine or other bodily products) that combine traditional bloodwork with lab-developed tests of dubious worth. These may or may not be covered by insurance, and the out-of-pocket testing expenses can be high. Such practitioners can use nontraditional, untested ranges for optimal blood levels—in other words, they have "customized" ranges for serum levels of vitamins, minerals, and biomarkers that routinely suggest that everyone is deficient in something. This leads to a never-ending cycle in which the client is constantly being tested and found "deficient" in some wellness marker, leading to the addition of yet another costly supplement. The financial stress of this can be substantial and, when added to the stress of wellness perfectionism, can itself lead to stress-related illness.

Seeking wellness can be motivating, invigorating, and pleasurable; feeling well is a worthy, life-affirming, and peaceful way to be. Like all aspects of life, the key is in balancing priorities and maintaining a positive approach; don't get caught up in a culture that causes you to be anxious, self-doubting, and punishing of self and others. Instead, work *with* various wellness approaches that are working *for* you within your financial, physical, and mental capacities, and follow the science closely so that you are not actively endangering your physical and mental health.

Wellness Tip: Intentional Gratitude

Giving thanks, being thankful, and gratitude infuse our societal, cultural, and religious norms. We are exhorted to "be thankful for what you have," and we rigorously teach our children to say "thank you" because ingrates are seen as rude, thoughtless, and privileged. Did you know that there is good scientific evidence that practicing gratitude increases your happiness and feelings of well-being? You might think of gratitude as a spontaneous emotion when someone does something nice for you. As a wellness practice, it is more purposeful and intentional, involving: (1) Telling people that you are grateful for their role in your life, (2) Thanking people specifically and with emotion for the nice things they've done, and (3) Expressing (saying out loud, writing down, creating) appreciation for the joys, pleasures, benefits, privileges, and gifts we have in our lives. Observing, noting, and expressing our gratitude strengthens relationships, protects us from negative emotions, and enhances our positive outlook.

In fact, years of research in the area indicate that regular and purposeful gratitude has positive effects in almost every area of our lives. In a study of almost 300 people seeking mental health counseling at a university, researchers found beneficial effects of adding written expressions of gratitude to psychotherapy (Wong et al., 2018). Participants were randomly assigned to one of three groups—psychotherapy only, psychotherapy and expressive writing (writing about your feelings), and psychotherapy and gratitude writing. At 4 weeks and 12 weeks post-therapy, people in the gratitude writing group self-reported significantly better mental wellness than did those in the other two groups. Robert Emmons, a prominent gratitude researcher, emphasizes the transformative nature of gratitude, in that it inspires an "upward spiral" of positive emotions, while not disregarding negative emotions (e.g., Emmons & McCullough, 2003).

Try it today…Thank each and every person who does something for you, even if it is their job to do so. Look them in the face, smile, and thank them specifically for what they did. Start a gratitude journal in which you write down something you are thankful for every day. You could also start a "three good things" journal, in which you count your blessings each day. Last, but definitely not least, call your mom, dad, sister, brother, grandma, granddad, and/or your best friend and tell them you are thankful they are in your life. When you do, their smile will become your smile!

References

Emmons, R. A., & McCullough, M. E. (2003). Counting blessings versus burdens: An experimental investigation of gratitude and subjective Well-being in daily life. *Journal of Personality and Social Psychology, 84*(2), 377–389. https://doi.org/10.1037/0022-3514.84.2.377

Klein, A. V., & Kiat, H. (2015). Detox diets for toxin elimination and weight management: A critical review of the evidence. *Journal of Human Nutrition and Dietetics, 28*(6), 675–686. https://doi.org/10.1111/jhn.12286

Morris, Z. S., Wooding, S., & Grant, J. (2011). The answer is 17 years, what is the question: Understanding time lags in translational research. *Journal of the Royal Society of Medicine, 104*(12), 510–520. https://doi.org/10.1258/jrsm.2011.110180

Sinatra, G. M., & Hofer, B. K. (2021). *Science denial: Why it happens and what to do about it*. Oxford University Press.

Wong, Y. J., Owen, J., Gabana, N. T., Brown, J. W., McInnis, S., Toth, P., & Gilman, L. (2018). Does gratitude writing improve the mental health of psychotherapy clients? Evidence from a randomized controlled trial. *Psychotherapy Research, 28*(2), 192–202. https://doi.org/10.1080/10503307.2016.1169332

Zhong, Y., Liu, W., Lee, T.-Y., Zhao, H., & Ji, J. (2021). Risk perception, knowledge, information sources and emotional states among COVID-19 patients in Wuhan, China. *Nursing Outlook, 69*(1), 13–21. https://doi.org/10.1016/j.outlook.2020.08.005

Chapter 3
What Is Wellness?

Wellness is experienced when we are in mental, social, and physical good health. It is not only the absence of illness and disability but also when we perceive ourselves to be thriving and well. Wellness involves the whole person, both inside and out…it is holistic and multidimensional. You may have heard both of the terms wellness and well-being (indeed, we use both in this book!); the difference between them is subtle, and the terms are often used interchangeably. Wellness as a behavior or practice is a proactive approach that involves striving for well-being across the lifespan, and which rests on human agency and purposefulness. Wellness is active and self-directed—it is an approach to life, whereas well-being is a state of positive health, satisfaction, and functioning. In other words, one can look at wellness as the personal processes, decisions, and behaviors involved in achieving a state of well-being.

Mind/body wellness is a discipline within the wellness movement. Mind/body wellness emphasizes wholeness of being, balance between the mind and body, and gives us information on ways to live a fulfilling life. Just like wellness as a whole, mind/body wellness is an approach to life—a way of moving toward a goal of abundance, breadth, and depth of well-being via the integration of our mind and body. In this book, we will use the terms "wellness" and "well-being" often with the understanding that we are talking about a mind/body approach to wellness.

Physical health is certainly important to our sense of wellness in that feeling ill and in poor health challenges our perceptions of our vitality, vigor, and physical fitness. On the other hand, having good physical health can be seen as a gateway or springboard to other types of wellness. This implies that wellness is not only about objective measures of health, like blood pressure, cancer diagnosis, or diabetes, but also about subjective well-being.

Subjective well-being includes a preponderance of positive emotions (i.e., joy, happiness, contentment) over negative emotions (i.e., anger, depression, anxiety), a feeling of meaning and purpose, and a positive assessment of life satisfaction. There are several types of subjective well-being, and these types have various lifestyle, behavioral, and psychological correlates (National Center for Complimentary and

S. M. Henney, J. D. Hackett, *Mind-Body Wellness*,
https://doi.org/10.1007/978-3-031-91611-3_3

Integrative Health (NCCIH), 2018). One type of subjective well-being is broadly how we "feel" about our lives in terms of whether we are happy or sad or depressed or joyful—this can be called hedonic well-being (the word hedonic means pleasurable behaviors, activities, and sensations). This is encompassed by the question, "How am I feeling (both right now and over time)?" Another type of subjective well-being is how we judge or evaluate our own satisfaction with our lives and with how and who we are—this can be called "evaluative well-being." This is the answer to the question, "How satisfied am I with my life right now?" A final type of subjective well-being is called eudaimonic well-being, which occurs when we find meaning and purpose in our lives and also when we embrace positive change and personal growth. Eudaimonic well-being can be assessed via the question, "Is what I am doing with my life worthwhile?"

Another way to understand wellness is to conceive of it as a continuum that covers the range from ill health to optimal wellness, as shown in Fig. 3.1 (Travis & Ryan, 2004). The end of the continuum that signifies illness tends to follow the medical model in that when we start to feel significantly ill or disabled, we tend to engage with the medical system for treatment. The other pole of the continuum is the wellness approach we will learn about in this chapter, where people are actively invested in their own growth, a meaningful life, personal and relationship satisfaction, and a sense of well-being. The middle portion of the continuum is sometimes called *false wellness* or the *comfort zone* of wellness. In this space, we don't feel sick, but we are not as well as we could be; it is possible that we don't know what it feels like to feel the very best we could feel because we have never experienced it. Where we are on this continuum can change over our lifetimes or even on a day-to-day basis, and it can also change as we grow in knowledge and autonomy.

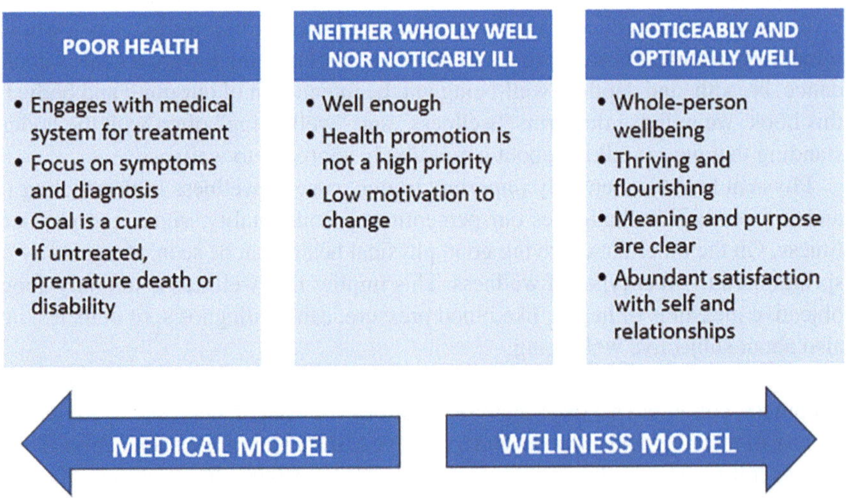

Fig. 3.1 The wellness continuum

The Goals of a Wellness Approach

People are motivated to behave in certain ways and to make specific choices when it benefits them and/or the people around them to do so. They feel better mentally and physically, enjoy health throughout their lifespan, are able to pursue their dreams and desires with purpose and vigor, use their agency to pursue the things that make them feel satisfied and content with their lives, and enjoy meaningful relationships and community involvement. The goals of a personal wellness approach typically include:

- To thrive in all dimensions of living.
- To experience a long, healthful, and fulfilling life.
- To pursue essential goals and to have the vitality to fulfill needs and wants.
- To cultivate and maintain meaningful connections with others.
- To empower people to be active, conscious, and self-directed in pursuing life-long health.
- To work with and maximize people's natural motivation to pursue and maintain wellness.

The Philosophy of Wellness

Underpinning the goals of a wellness approach is a philosophy that is designed to guide people's attitudes, beliefs, and behaviors. Components of a holistic philosophy of wellness include:

- *Emphasizes health, not disease.*
- *Is outside of the "medical model," but complimentary to it.*
- *Is not reductive to biological processes and individual organ systems.*
- *Wellness is disease prevention ("If we don't make time for our wellness, we will be forced to make time for our illness").*
- *Is holistic, valuing the dynamic whole person.*
- *Assumes the importance of health symmetry and health balance.*
- *All of the dimensions of wellness contribute equivalently to health.*
- *Wellness is personal..."one size" does not fit all.*
- *Centers human agency, emphasizing a proactive approach to health.*
- *Health-promoting behaviors are developed and maintained.*
- *Pursuit of wellness is thoughtful and purposeful.*
- *Requires learning and adjustment of behavior as we age and/or change environment.*

Importance of a Personal Philosophy of Wellness

It is critical to not only know the components of a general philosophy of wellness but also to adopt it as personally significant, relevant, and compelling. Behaviors and attitudes that promote and emphasize wellness derive from a personal philosophy that centers them. It is important to adopt the belief that each of us, personally, can benefit from healthy choices, health-promoting activities, and avoiding risky behaviors. If we believe that we can benefit, then we are more likely to be motivated to engage with the process. Our personal needs, beliefs, and goals become the centerpiece of action. When we prioritize wellness, we realize that wellness is the sum of specific choices made each and every day over our lifespan.

This is important because in countries with developed public health systems, most of the major causes of mortality and disability are not related to communicable diseases, but rather to factors over which we have more control, like diet, activity level, smoking, and weight (Khaw et al., 2008). Lifestyle factors matter, and we typically have some control over one or more of these key factors. If we have less control over one factor (i.e., diet), this doesn't mean that we have to have unhealthy behaviors in other important areas (Alosaimi et al., 2023). For example, even if we live in a healthy food desert, making it difficult to regularly acquire nutritious food, we can still avoid smoking or quit if we've started. This highlights the fact that a personal philosophy of wellness doesn't have to be perfectly visioned or perfectly executed. Indeed, it must specifically fit us…our personality, circumstances, motivations, and abilities. When it doesn't, it can feel like continuous failure, which is related in turn to lack of persistence and motivation; when it does fit us, it will lead to achievements of wellness that fit our life and associated feelings of success and continuous motivation.

The Dimensions of Wellness

The dimensions of wellness are often described by the acronym "SPECIES"—Social, Physical, Emotional, Career, Intellectual, Environmental, Spiritual. We will add "financial wellness" as an eighth dimension to this list because of the relative importance of financial security to a person's sense of well-being (see Fig. 3.2).

Social Wellness

Social wellness starts with a sense of belonging and can encompass all aspects of the social world, but especially friends, family, and romantic or sexual partners. In order to feel like we are an active participant in the social world, we must feel like we connect with others and that we belong in relationships with them. We want

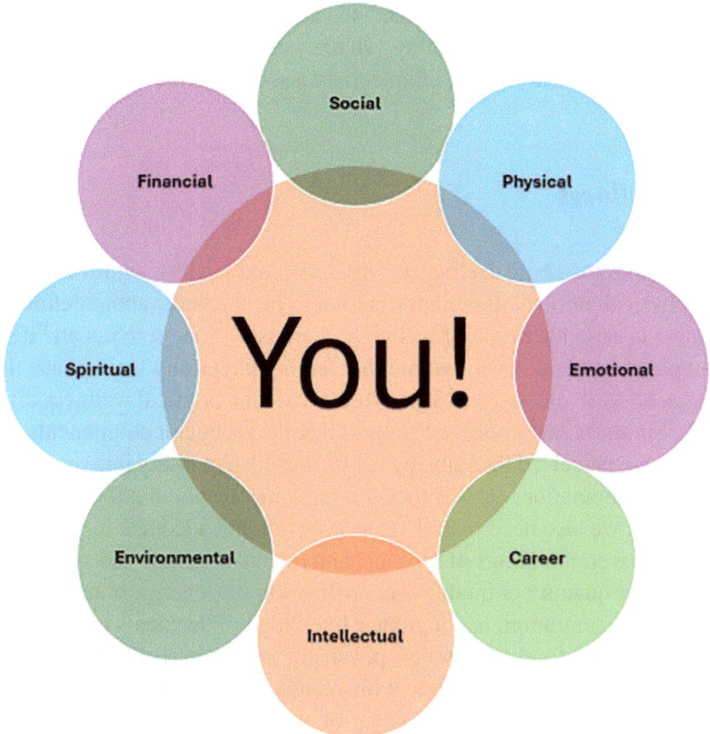

Fig. 3.2 Dimensions of wellness

these relationships to be warm and welcoming, not cold and distant. For example, it is important to have both a desired frequency of interactions with our friends as well as to have positive, satisfying interactions with friends, as these qualities of friendships are related to greater life satisfaction (Amati et al., 2018).

We also seek to develop relationships where we can be our authentic selves—it is exhausting and demeaning to feel like we need to hide who we are from those closest to us. Everyone has experiences of stress and adversity, and one of the best things about social wellness is that our relationships serve as sources of support, stability, and emotional uplift. It's also important to understand how our social world affects our wellness behaviors. When we are children, we are typically exposed to those healthy—and unhealthy—behaviors that our parents and our schools allow us to experience. As we mature, we have more choices and autonomy, but we continue to both influence and be influenced by, those we are in relationships with. We maintain ties to those with similar behaviors and attitudes around healthy eating, exercising, smoking, and a host of other lifestyle behaviors. Finally, giving of oneself through meaningful engagement in our community or volunteerism is a great way of growing and thriving in the social sphere. Volunteerism is strongly related to lowered depression, increased life satisfaction, improved self-esteem and self-efficacy, feelings of connection and social support, increased physical activity, and, importantly, decreased mortality (Henney & Hackett, 2019; Jenkinson et al., 2013). These factors truly make volunteerism a social wellness activity.

Physical Wellness

Physical wellness is about feeling fit, vigorous, and healthy within the context of our own physical abilities. It is important not to be absolutist about defining physical wellness or any other type of wellness; there is no "one size fits all" definition. For example, we would never assume that feeling physically well means the same thing for an 80-year-old and an 18-year-old; we define physical wellness differently as we age. Similarly, we would not suggest that the feeling or components of physical wellness are perceived the same by someone with a mobility impairment (wheelchair, walker, amputation, etc.) as they are for someone without these challenges.

To feel well we also need restful sleep in an amount adequate for our age. Sleep contributes to overall feelings of physical and mental alertness and vitality. Lack of sleep—in either quantity or quality—contributes to low energy, brain fog, impaired memory and concentration, and a greater likelihood of accidents and mistakes. We also need nutritious food to function physically at our best. Eating well does not require an elaborate diet or even one with a name, but eating nutritious foods in the right amounts does require a knowledge of the major food groups, some understanding of the calorie content of food, and the ability to afford and source nutritious food. Also, don't forget that check-ups with a healthcare professional are a way of maintaining physical wellness by catching problems early and managing chronic conditions.

Emotional Wellness

Emotional wellness is concerned with how we understand, experience, and express our feelings. Our emotional wellness improves when we are able to look realistically at our feelings, accept them as an important part of our human experience, and express those emotions in a way that is appropriate both personally and within our social context. This doesn't mean we always like what we see when we look inside, and part of emotional wellness is having reliable ways that we can cope with intense, uncomfortable, or distressing emotions. We will all encounter situations and events that challenge our emotional wellness, and strong, reliable coping mechanisms and resources will help us to work through these challenges in ways that are not damaging to us or our relationships. Emotional wellness is often confused with happiness, but Seligman (2011) notes that happiness is commonly understood as requiring cheerfulness and being upbeat. Although positive emotions are clearly part of emotional wellness, happiness per se is not synonymous with emotional wellness.

We can build our emotional wellness in many ways, and some of our tactics and coping measures will be unique to our preferences and environment. Managing our stress is one clear way that we can improve our emotional wellness, and we can influence situational or daily stress by practicing ways to better manage our time, improve our organization, handle our commute to school or work, and plan and implement self-care into our days. We can also have practices or habits that continuously support to our emotional wellness, such as mindfulness, yoga, cultivating a positive mindset, and engaging in both the attitude and behaviors of gratitude. One of the more consistent ways we can improve our emotional balance, reduce distress, and cope with symptoms such as anxiety or depression is to participate in regular exercise. It appears that all forms of exercise can have some emotional benefits, including walking, aerobic exercise, and resistance training (e.g., LeBouthillier & Asmundson, 2017).

Career/Occupational Wellness

Career wellness is characterized by engaging in work that is meaningful to us and is aligned with our personal goals, identity, and values. Our career should, in essence, be a "good fit" for us as a whole person. Work can enhance our life, providing enrichment, intellectual stimulation, social opportunities, and financial security. Work, even enjoyable work, is not without stress, and many people have not yet found jobs that they enjoy or are "stuck" by life circumstances in jobs that they do not like. The American Psychological Association's 2021 Work and Well-being Survey found that an incredible three-fourths of workers surveyed had recently felt work-related stress, and that they reported a range of negative results, such as low levels of motivation and high levels of tiredness and emotional exhaustion (Abramson, 2022).

Career well-being is influenced by many factors, both personal and organizational. Fulfilling and satisfying career paths can be found by capitalizing on our strengths and discovering our passions. Even when we have found our preferred career path, we can have workplaces that fulfill our needs or ones that are not a good fit. Workplaces matter to career wellness, including leadership and management, how well we align with the work culture and company values, as well as workload and intrusions on personal time. It is important to not settle and to not stay stuck in an unhappy work situation; this increases our potential for chronic stress and the related health consequences. Rather, we must keep moving toward our goals and re-tool our skills or gain further training if needed.

Intellectual Wellness

Intellectual wellness sounds like something that would be found particularly in a college environment, and for many people it is, but it is not *only* to be found in academic institutions. Anyone who is open to learning, actively pursues knowledge, cultivates their own curiosity about the world, and thinks critically about their internal and external worlds has the foundation of intellectual wellness. It is the experiences of life that provide the content for our intellect; if we are open to new experiences and to the knowledge and challenges they provide, we can improve our intellectual wellness through the very act of living.

Many of the activities that contribute to intellectual wellness have crossover impacts on other types of wellness. For example, reading supports intellectual development via engagement of language, learning, and imagination, while also having stress reduction and physical and mental health benefits. Even a small amount of reading can relieve stress relatively quickly and reliably, and it can also help to improve sleep (Levine et al., 2020). Our hobbies and recreational activities can also contribute to intellectual wellness and, for example, physical wellness. Play is a great example of this, as both structured play, such as sports, and unstructured play, such as hanging out at the beach with friends or hopping on a swing, let our minds run free while engaging our bodies in physical activity.

Environmental Wellness

The environment that surrounds us should support our health and well-being by being safe, nontoxic, stimulating, and health-enhancing. Most people would like to live and work in peaceful, safe, and healthful places, and most would like to enjoy healthy food, green spaces, and a variety of recreational options. We tend to place a high value on our personal safety and will actively avoid danger if we can accurately foresee it. Paying attention to the health of our planet and the natural world is another important facet of environmental wellness, as we all require clean air, water, and land to thrive. Additionally, environmental components like exposure to infectious disease, noise and light pollution, traffic, consumer product safety, timely and affordable access to needed healthcare, and many more impact us throughout our lives in ways that are often dependent on geographical location, socioeconomic status, and political climate.

There are many ways that we can enhance our environmental wellness, and although our ability to access wellness-enhancing settings can be related to socioeconomic and geographic factors, there are some low-cost ways to do so. For example, we can educate ourselves about ways to enhance our personal safety, such as being situationally aware, minimizing sources of accidental injury in our homes, and practicing firearm safety. We can also be advocates for safer communities, clean air and water, safe roads, public transportation, and good schools. We can improve our environmental wellness through simple behaviors, our voice, and our vote.

Spiritual Wellness

Perhaps more than any other dimension of wellness, spiritual wellness means different things to different people. Many people equate spiritual wellness with consistent, devoted, and faithful adherence to and practice of the beliefs of a certain religion. Other people equate spirituality with the natural world, and their immersion in it and respect for it. Still others find spirituality in relationships, with compassion, empathy, and interconnectedness characterizing their sense of spirituality. Overall, most people equate spirituality with meaning, allowing one to find joy, awe, purpose, and deep emotion in the experiences of everyday life. Spirituality can provide a framework for values and morals, upon which people act to better themselves, their families, and their communities. There is evidence that people who are spiritual, and particularly those who attend church regularly, may have lower mortality risk, but there is more research to be done in this area (Chida et al., 2009; Lindström & Pirouzifard, 2023).

Spiritual practices can be individual, private activities, but they are often done within a community of like-minded people. In fact, building community and common purpose represent strengths of many spiritual practices and the hallmark of many religions' services, rituals, and rites. Religious marriage ceremonies can, of course, be conducted in private with just the couple, officiant, and witness, but the overwhelming majority of religious marriage ceremonies are purposefully conducted with many family, friends, and guests in attendance. The relational community of the couple witnesses the marriage rites with an implied or overt charge to support the marriage and the couple's family journey.

Financial Wellness

Financial wellness does not imply that we must be rich or well-off or have many physical possessions. Rather, financial wellness is achieved when we are satisfied with our current and potential financial situation, we feel secure with our finances, and we have comfortable and realistic financial goals. Furthermore, our finances should be such that we have freedom of choice in living situations, our must-have needs are met, and we can afford our desired leisure activities. Financial wellness also includes having a "rainy day fund" that will allow one to deal with emergencies and unexpected expenditures. For example, cars do break down and being able to get on the road again so one can get to work is essential to meet one's work obligations.

It's also important to have an understanding of our (and our partner's, if applicable) values related to money, as our financial values drive our decision-making and behavior. Before we can make financial goals or even a simple budget, we must understand how we spend money, what we spend it on, and why we do these things. Some people value a simple lifestyle with more time for lower-cost leisure activities (like gaming or reading), while others value an experience-oriented lifestyle with ample opportunities for eating out, nightlife, and travel. These choices drive our financial decisions, as do our attitudes toward spending versus saving and buying with cash versus buying on credit. Once we understand these things about ourselves (and our partners), it is much more likely that we will develop financial goals and plans that we can commit to and succeed with.

The PERMA Model

The PERMA model of well-being, as developed by the positive psychology pioneer Seligman (2011), defines five measurable concepts that contribute to a person's well-being throughout the lifespan. Seligman describes the five PERMA elements as the "building blocks of well-being," indicating that they are part of the process of developing well-being, rather than defining a fixed model of well-being (Seligman, 2018). These five elements are intrinsically motivating to us, meaning we don't have to be reinforced or persuaded to pursue them, and each is characterized by both hedonic and eudaimonic aspects. The PERMA elements contribute to what Seligman calls "flourishing" and what others call "thriving" (see the Wellness Tip for this chapter).

The five PERMA elements of well-being are:

Positive emotions (P): This is the "feel good" element of the theory and includes the emotions we like experiencing, such as happiness, joy, satisfaction, and gratitude.

Engagement (E): Engagement occurs when we have successfully identified and fully involved ourselves in things we care passionately about. When we engage fully, we enter a state where we are completely in the moment, neither feeling nor thinking, but rather totally present in the activity. This is also called "flow," although many people would also call it being "in the zone" or "on a roll" (Csikszentmihalyi, 1990).

Relationships (R): We are inherently social people, and building relationships with others—family, friends, coworkers, romantic partners—is an essential part of being well. When we share the fruits of our well-being with others, we elevate our own wellness and support theirs as well.

Meaning (M): Creativity, purpose, giving back, spiritual fulfillment—these and similar concepts tap into the human search for meaning and significance in life. We search successfully for meaning when we have identified the behaviors and activities that make us "more ourselves," in other words, that are an expression of our true self.

Accomplishment (A): Investing in the successful pursuit of our goals through attaining mastery of our craft is the essence of achievement. This concept is not about status, power, money, or possessions; rather, it is about being confident that we have the skills to attain our goals, achieving them, and then savoring a job well done.

The Concept of Flow

Hungarian psychologist Csikszentmihalyi (1990) introduced us to the concept of flow, which is now an important concept in positive psychology, the study of creativity, and in sports psychology. Flow is a mental state in which we are motivated, focused, and fully engulfed in the moment. Flow is intense! It is a full commitment to the process of what we are doing, and, for some, this is so engrossing that there is a loss of awareness of self and surroundings. In his book on flow in endurance athletes, Kotler (2014) states that flow occurs when we are, "…so focused on the task at hand that everything else falls away. Action and awareness merge. Time flies. Self-vanishes. Performance goes through the roof." Flow is associated with greater happiness and satisfaction, which is what makes it intriguing from a wellness perspective.

Flow is not necessarily about the outcome; in fact, many people who experience flow don't pay attention to the final "product"—They are consumed by the process. Typically, flow is most likely to occur when ability or skill level matches the challenge; if one is very skilled at a task (like a master painter), flow can be best achieved by undertaking one's most challenging portrait to date. Flow can be seen in a chess grand master's laser intensity, in a pianist's complete absorption in the music, and in a professional rock climber's relentless drive to the top of the cliff. One of the most famous F1 drivers of all time, Ayrton Senna describes his experiences of flow, "and suddenly I realized that I was no longer driving the car consciously. I was driving it by a kind of instinct, only I was in a different dimension."

Csikszentmihalyi is also careful to say that flow can be achieved by anyone who is working on a task or activity in which they want to achieve their highest level of performance. Even if we are not professional athletes or master painters or grand masters, we can achieve flow by pushing ourselves to our highest peak of execution in the activity we are doing. People everywhere have found flow in yoga or running or writing or cooking or woodworking—We are each able to find that activity that uniquely capitalizes on our ability to become wholly and fully immersed and absorbed in the task. Then we can experience the benefits of flow.

Further research into the PERMA approach has suggested that other elements of wellness could be usefully and beneficially added to the original five elements, and the result is sometimes referred to as the "PERMA+" model (e.g., Donaldson et al.,

2021; Madeson, 2017). The PERMA+ model can include one or more of the following elements:

Vitality: An aspect of physical health, this element includes both physiological and functional health. In this category, we not only are objectively healthy by the medical model, but we also feel physically well, and we can use our physical selves to achieve the tasks we want and need to do to thrive in our lives.

Mindset: As we learned from the "Wellness Tip" in Chap. 1, a growth mindset is maintaining a positive and optimistic outlook on life, with plenty of flexibility, willingness to challenge oneself, and the search for self-improvement. This mindset allows us—even motivates us—to capitalize on the opportunities of life, including opportunities to enhance our wellness.

Economic Security. There is a considerable personal and familial cost to being or feeling financially insecure. Economic security means that we can meet our needs and some of our wants in a consistent, sustainable, and reliable way.

Work Environment, Sleep, Nutrition, Optimism (separate from mindset), Culture, and Autonomy have each also been suggested as additions to the PERMA+ model.

Each of the five+ PERMA categories supports the others; they are interdependent and interactive. For example, improving positive emotions (P), including self-valuing and obtaining positive self-esteem, will often result in a greater motivation to engage in the world and confidence to explore our passions (E), which in turn opens the door to more profound search for meaning and purpose (M). However, the most important thing to know about the PERMA model is that it is meant to be used in real life. Anyone can assess their own abilities and make a plan for growth in each of the PERMA categories. The key is to be purposeful, goal-oriented, and realistic. Remember that deep and sustained changes in well-being do not happen overnight; it takes planning, persistence, and commitment to make our wellness goals take shape.

Dunn's Model of Wellness

Often called the "father" of the wellness movement, Dunn's (1959) model portrays wellness from a person-in-context perspective. This model is portrayed visually in Fig. 3.3 as a grid in which we can see the relationship between optimal environment and optimal wellness for humans, meaning we cannot have one without the other. The horizontal axis is health and wellness spanning from optimal wellness to death, with the vertical axis representing the environment spanning from unfavorable environment to very favorable environment. Quadrant A represents the convergence of peak wellness and favorable environment. In this quadrant, a person enjoys good health and a healthy lifestyle, with an environment that supports and maximizes opportunities for wellness. In quadrant B, we see the conditions of poor health in a favorable environment. This occurs when someone is sick but has a supportive healthcare environment and can find treatment within the care system. This person

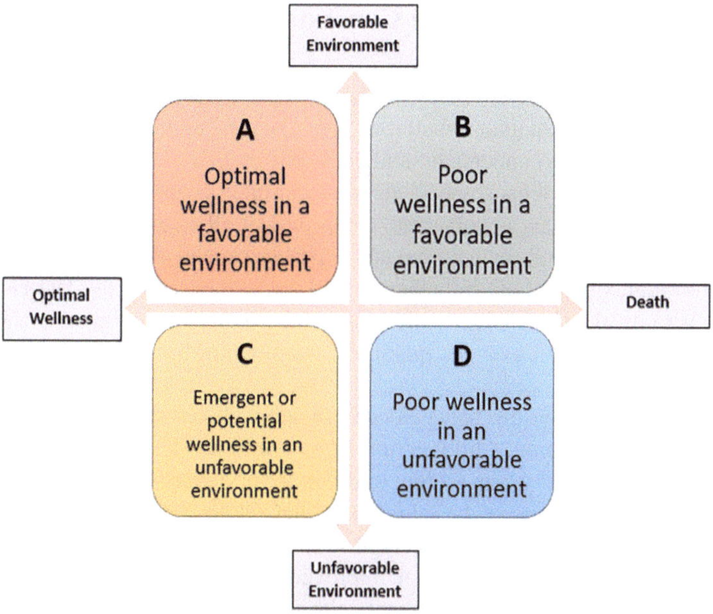

Fig. 3.3 Dunn's high-level wellness grid

could move from quadrant B to A if they recovered from their illness (or, alternatively, someone could move from A to B if they became significantly ill). Below the horizontal line in quadrant C is the convergence of good health and poor environment. Here, the person knows what to do to live a healthy lifestyle or desires to live a healthy lifestyle, but there is a lack of environmental support or a preponderance of environmental barriers to wellness. An example would be someone who would love to exercise in order to increase wellness, but they live with many people in a small apartment in a dangerous housing complex. Quadrant D represents the highest risk for chronic disease, disability, and death—someone in poor health who is also in an environment that has many barriers to wellness and few positive supports. This is exemplified by a diabetic struggling with obesity and illness who wishes to eat a healthful and nutritious diet, but they live in a healthy food desert and have few resources to obtain or afford healthy food options.

Dunn's model suggests that optimal wellness is unlikely to exist within an unfavorable environment, although the seeds can be there. The practical implication of this is that "if we want to change ourselves, change our environment." We can see this play out in practice if we look at addiction, criminality, or juvenile delinquency, to name a few. If, say, an addict or a gang member gets out of treatment or jail and returns to the exact same environment—same drinking/drugging buddies, same gang, same lack of opportunities or education—then how can the person change? The environment effectively locks the person into who they were, instead of who they could be.

Bioecological Model: Nested Contexts of Wellness

We will finish our overview of wellness concepts by discussing the contexts in which we pursue and maintain wellness. It is always important for us to consider context when we try to understand and grow our own or someone else's wellness factors. Figure 3.4 presents some of the most common contexts that surround individuals. The first context is ourselves, comprised of all of our personal assets and disadvantages and all of our accumulated experiences, and our "self" is nested in a variety of contexts that both influence us and are influenced by us. The closer the context is to us, the more it can impact us and the more we can impact it; we have more individual control over the quality of our relationships than we do over the quality of our air.

To make the relationship between context and wellness clear, we will examine the example of education. Children and teens spend much of their day in educational settings, many of which feature traditional "sit, listen, and learn" educational approaches for large parts of the school day. McCallum and Price (2016) point out that children who experience educational settings that feature purposeful efforts to improve student wellness also foster improved academic achievement, decreased behavior issues, and more engagement with school tasks. In fact, these authors argue that things like hope, optimism, and resilience (personal level), belongingness and supportive faculty/staff (relational level), and engaging curriculum, a peaceable space, and reasonable policies and expectations (community level) are all related to

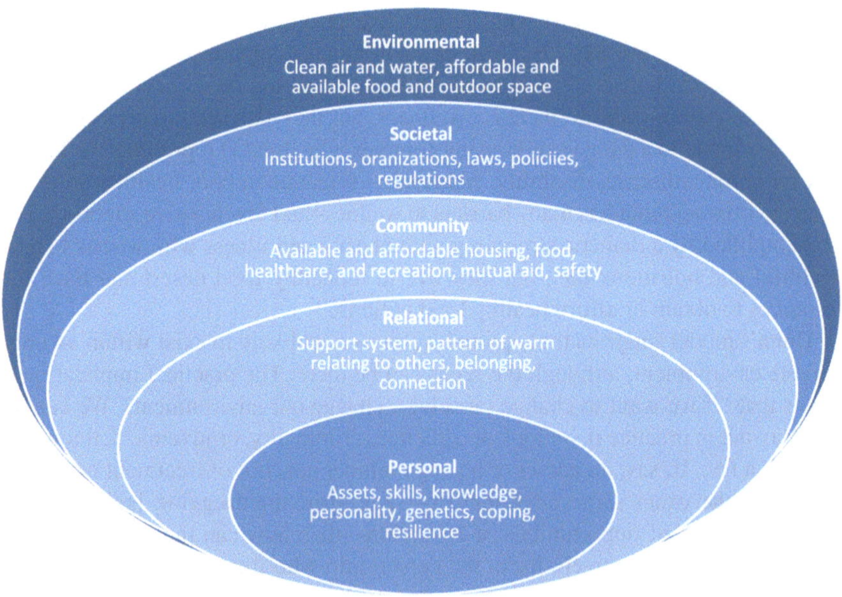

Fig. 3.4 Nested contexts for wellness

the outcomes we want for children, like productivity, motivation to achieve, and pro-social attitudes and behaviors.

Through focusing on programs, policies, activities, and expectations that prioritize well-being for students, faculty, and staff, schools create a well-being-enhancing positive school ecology.

When we allow students to revise work to improve their grade, for example, this is a way to use reasonable policies (community level) to encourage optimism and resilience regarding their grades (personal level). Similarly, when school faculty feel empowered by district policy to raise concerns about their own and students' wellness (societal level), they also are more comfortable facilitating positive change in their schools and classrooms (community and relational levels). Regarding school programming, Schonert-Reichl et al. (2015) found that a school program featuring mindfulness (community level) was associated with improved socioemotional functioning among participating students, like greater emotional regulation (personal level) and more peer acceptance and prosocial interactions (relational level). It is only by examining the various levels of context that can we assess, which wellness practices actually work to improve outcomes for students and to planfully include them at the right type, timing, and level to affect students' lived experiences.

When we fail to consider context, we also fail to implement interventions, programs, and policies that accurately match what people can accomplish. For example, if someone says to a domestic violence victim, "you should just leave," this makes a host of assumptions about context—that the person has somewhere to go or the resources to find somewhere to go and, importantly, that the person can overcome fear of failure, fear of homelessness, hunger, and lack for self and perhaps children, and fear of the abuser in order to even try. If someone says to another who is struggling with obesity, "you should eat better and exercise," again, this makes many assumptions about context, like healthy food knowledge, healthy food availability, and wealth while simultaneously imposing the societal idea that obesity is a personal failure. The take-away here is that we can only facilitate and support wellness in people when we, first, understand context and its implications for individual behavior and, second, are able to fully account for it when we offer advice, interventions, programs, and policies.

Wellness Tip: What Does It Mean to Thrive?

Thriving is a key process that contributes to lifelong wellness. Su et al. (2014, p. 256) define thriving simply as, "The state of positive functioning at its fullest range—mentally, physically, and socially." In practice, thriving encompasses so much more depth and richness of our lives. Thriving is what we experience when we are fulfilled, creative, happy, prosperous, productive, resilient, and giving and receiving love and affection. When we do these things, we are flourishing in all of the ways that make us feel "more like ourselves" and comfortable in our own minds and bodies.

Thriving can occur after trauma, stress, and hard times or it can occur after growth and opportunity. There is no general "way to thrive" that works for everyone—it is personal to who *you* are and can only be described within your own personhood, environment, and relationships (e.g., Brown et al., 2017). Nonetheless, Fig. 3.5 illustrates some of the personal and environmental characteristics that may make each of us more likely to thrive. If we don't currently have these or the ability to obtain them in our lives, then goal-directed behavior becomes important—we can always strive toward thriving and flourishing through planful effort, adaptation, and growth.

How do you convert these characteristics of thriving into an action plan for well-being?

Be...

Yourself
Kind to yourself and others
Compassionate
Flexible and adaptable

Invest in...

Better relationships through attention, consistent communication, respect, trust, and intimacy
Meaningful goals and purpose
Others through volunteerism
Your self-worth
Creativity

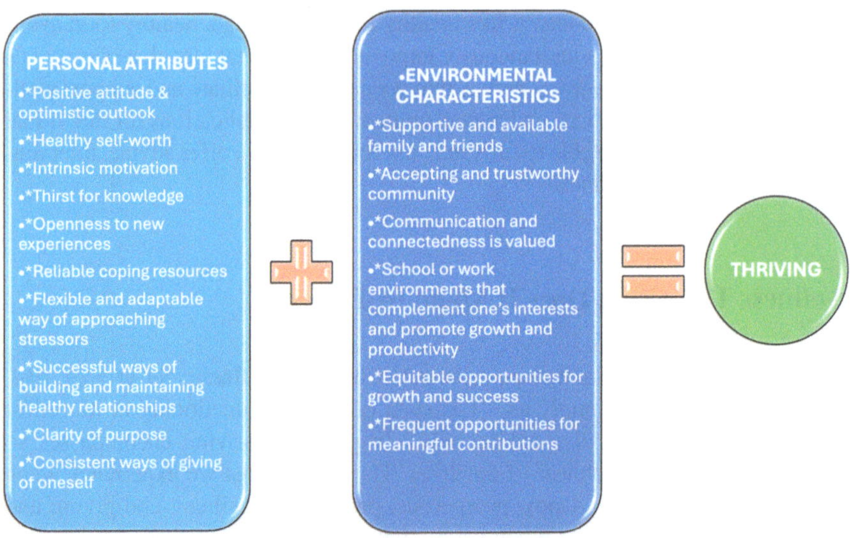

Fig. 3.5 Personal and environmental contributions to thriving

Fairness and equity
Self-care

Savor...

Experiences
Learning
Laughter
Love and affection
Change

References

Abramson, A. (2022). Burnout and stress are everywhere. *Monitor on Psychology, 53*(1), 72. Retrieved from https://www.apa.org/monitor/2022/01/special-burnout-stress

Alosaimi, N., Sherar, L. B., Griffiths, P., & Pearson, N. (2023). Clustering of diet, physical activity and sedentary behaviour and related physical and mental health outcomes: A systematic review. *BMC Public Health, 23*(1), 1572. https://doi.org/10.1186/s12889-023-16372-6

Amati, V., Meggiolaro, S., Rivellini, G., & Zaccarin, S. (2018). Social relations and life satisfaction: The role of friends. *Genus, 74*(1), 7. https://doi.org/10.1186/s41118-018-0032-z

Brown, D. J., Arnold, R., Fletcher, D., & Standage, M. (2017). Human thriving: A conceptual debate and literature review. *European Psychologist, 22*(3), 167–179. https://doi.org/10.1027/1016-9040/a000294

Chida, Y., Steptoe, A., & Powell, L. H. (2009). Religiosity/spirituality and mortality. A systematic quantitative review. *Psychotherapy and Psychosomatics, 78*(2), 81–90. https://doi.org/10.1159/000190791

Csikszentmihalyi, M. (1990). *Flow: The psychology of optimal experience*. Harper Collins.

Donaldson, S. I., Heshmati, S., Lee, J. Y., & Donaldson, S. I. (2021). Examining building blocks of well-being beyond PERMA and self-report bias. *The Journal of Positive Psychology, 16*(6), 811–818. https://doi.org/10.1080/17439760.2020.1818813

Dunn, H. L. (1959). High-level wellness for man and society. *American Journal of Public Health and the Nation's Health, 49*(6), 786–792. https://doi.org/10.2105/AJPH.49.6.786

Henney, S. M., & Hackett, J. D. (2019). *The development of community engagement from infancy to adulthood.* Routledge. https://doi.org/10.4324/9781315122823

Jenkinson, C. E., Dickens, A. P., Jones, K., Thompson-Coon, J., Taylor, R. S., Rogers, M., Bambra, C. L., Lang, I., & Richards, S. H. (2013). Is volunteering a public health intervention? A systematic review and meta-analysis of the health and survival of volunteers. *BMC Public Health, 13*, 773. https://doi.org/10.1186/1471-2458-13-773

Khaw, K. T., Wareham, N., Bingham, S., Welch, A., Luben, R., & Day, N. (2008). Combined impact of health behaviours and mortality in men and women: The EPIC-Norfolk prospective population study. *PLoS Medicine, 5*(1), e12. https://doi.org/10.1371/journal.pmed.0050012

Kotler, S. (2014). *The rise of superman: Decoding the science of ultimate human performance.* New Harvest/Houghton Mifflin Harcourt.

LeBouthillier, D. M., & Asmundson, G. J. G. (2017). The efficacy of aerobic exercise and resistance training as transdiagnostic interventions for anxiety-related disorders and constructs: A randomized controlled trial. *Journal of Anxiety Disorders, 52*, 43–52. https://doi.org/10.1016/j.janxdis.2017.09.005

Levine, S. L., Cherrier, S., Holding, A. C., & Koestner, R. (2020). For the love of reading: Recreational reading reduces psychological distress in college students and autonomous motivation is the key. *Journal of American College Health, 70*(1), 158–164. https://doi.org/10.1080/07448481.2020.1728280

Lindström, M., & Pirouzifard, M. (2023). Religious service attendance and mortality: A population-based prospective cohort study in southern Sweden. *SSM - Population Health, 23*, 101492. https://doi.org/10.1016/j.ssmph.2023.101492

Madeson, M. (2017). *Seligman's PERMA+ model explained: A theory of wellbeing*. Positive Psychology. Retrieved from https://positivepsychology.com/perma-model/

McCallum, F., & Price, D. (2016). *Nurturing wellbeing development in education: From little things, big things grow*. Routledge. https://doi.org/10.4324/9781315760834

National Center for Complimentary and Integrative Health (NCCIH). (2018). *Emotional well-being: Emerging insights and questions for future research*. NCCIH. Retrieved from https://www.nccih.nih.gov/research/emotional-well-being-emerging-insights-and-questions-for-future-research

Schonert-Reichl, K. A., Oberle, E., Lawlor, M. S., Abbott, D., Thomson, K., Oberlander, T. F., & Diamond, A. (2015). Enhancing cognitive and social-emotional development through a simple-to-administer mindfulness-based school program for elementary school children: A randomized controlled trial. *Developmental Psychology, 51*(1), 52–66. https://doi.org/10.1037/a0038454

Seligman, M. (2018). PERMA and the building blocks of well-being. *The Journal of Positive Psychology, 13*(4), 333–335. https://doi.org/10.1080/17439760.2018.1437466

Seligman, M. E. P. (2011). *Flourish: A visionary new understanding of happiness and well-being*. Free Press.

Su, R., Tay, L., & Diener, E. (2014). The development and validation of the comprehensive inventory of thriving (CIT) and the brief inventory of thriving (BIT). *Applied Psychology: Health and WellBeing, 6*, 251–279. https://doi.org/10.1111/aphw.12027

Travis, J. W., & Ryan, S. R. (2004). *Wellness index* (3rd ed.). Clarkson Potter/Ten Speed.

Chapter 4
Planning for Wellness in Mind and Body

Why is it important to have a plan for wellness? It seems like "being well" should be natural and easy—nothing that needs to be planned for. However, it is clear that our decision-making about wellness is increasingly complicated by pseudoscience, misinformation, disinformation, uneven health literacy, and an overwhelming array of choices. A personal wellness plan is a guide to setting goals, identifying relevant and accurate health information, and tracking progress toward optimal wellness outcomes.

Wellness does not entail just one goal or one part of our life. We are complete, whole beings, and wellness touches on every aspect of what makes you, "you!" The most straightforward way to goal-set for a wellness plan is to use the dimensions of wellness that we discussed in Chap. 3. Recall that there are eight dimensions of wellness: social, physical, emotional/mental, career, intellectual, environmental, spiritual, and financial. To be clear, few people need a wellness plan for *every* dimension of wellness and even fewer for every part of every dimension—this would be overwhelming and exhausting. Rather, most people have dimensions where they already feel well and others where they desire to improve their wellness ("I love my job and am fulfilled in my career, but I'm worried about my relationship because my partner and I argue all the time."). It is very common to have problems in one dimension of wellness impact our well-being in another dimension or multiple dimensions ("I have no money by the second week of the month, and I worry all the time how I will feed my kids."). Many people also have varying degrees of wellness within one dimension ("I eat right, work out, and sleep well, but my asthma keeps flaring up!"). It should be clear that the first thing we must do is take stock of our wellness-related strengths and needs across and within the eight dimensions of wellness.

S. M. Henney, J. D. Hackett, *Mind-Body Wellness*,
https://doi.org/10.1007/978-3-031-91611-3_4

Wellness Self-Inventory

The first step in any plan designed to decrease stress and increase wellness is a self-assessment or an inventory of our assets and needs across the dimensions of well-being. Our self-assessment should be holistic at first, looking at as many aspects of personal wellness as are relevant. For example, look at the wellness diagram in Fig. 4.1—the bigger circles represent what is most prominent in our personal wellness picture (in other words, if you are doing this for your own wellness self-assessment, you would switch around the labels so that the bigger circles represent what is most important to your personal well-being). Then look at how far the smaller circles are from the largest circle—farther circles should represent those dimensions that are less pressing at the current time. This is not to say these aspects are less important, but rather that they are where there are current feelings of well-being, where there is not currently a high level of control, or that are not highly relevant to current well-being.

For each aspect that is identified as most relevant (perhaps the three or four largest circles), write down one strength, one stressor, one goal, and what the outcome will be if the goal is achieved. Here is an example for the social dimension:

One strength: "I have good friends who I enjoy spending time with and who support me when I need it."
One stressor: "My relationship with my partner is not great, and they put me down a lot."
One goal: "I want to make a boundary with my partner about criticizing me."
What the outcome will most likely be: "I think that if I clearly communicate with my partner that putting me down must stop, then there will be more positivity in my relationship, or it will become clear that I need to leave the relationship."

The purpose here is to be intentional about what we want to change and what the expected outcome is from the change. A solid and methodical assessment will be more likely to produce goals that we can clearly articulate, are relevant and important, and for which we can foresee the possible outcome(s) that we can reasonably

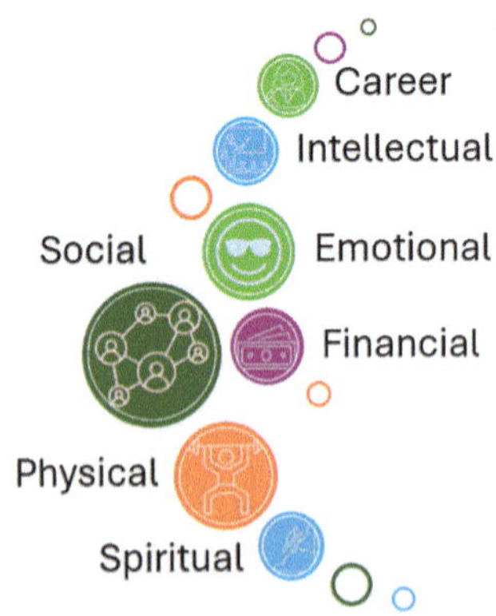

Fig. 4.1 Personal dimensions of wellness

expect to achieve. Interestingly, most people are actually pretty good at identifying areas of their life that they wish to improve. They can name big goals like saving money for the down payment on a house, or smaller goals like reducing the number of cups of coffee they drink each day. In other words, we don't necessarily lack vision on what we would like to do and be and achieve, but rather we lack either a plan for, or knowledge about, how to engage in behaviors that allow us to reach our goals.

Goal Setting

Goals are *part* of an overall wellness plan. One goal is not a plan, but rather a system of interrelated goals that makes up a plan. Being more planful and less reactive means that we will have clarity in both thought and action, be able to actively improve our own wellness, and be able to handle stress better. Every plan must start with a foundation of goals, and this is where learning how to set SMART goals comes in. SMART is an acronym for specific, measurable, achievable, relevant, and time-bound goals, and these components are defined as follows:

Specific: Goals must be specific because we are much more likely to achieve specific, definitive goals than general ones. Specific goals have clarity and precision; they require a clear definition of the goal, what the steps are to accomplish it, when it will be accomplished, and where it will be accomplished. We should always try to state our SMART goal positively by stating what we are going to do and what we are going to achieve rather than what we are not going to do.

Measurable: We can't tell if we've achieved a goal unless we can clearly state how the goal is measured. We must quantify or name both what progress looks like and how we will know if the goal has been achieved. In other words, if we can't quantify or name what achievement of the goal is, then it is not a measurable goal. This measurement of progress or success could be a concrete attainment, like an award, graduation, or promotion, or it could be a percent change, something that increases or decreases, or some other way of measuring the event. For example, if we want to work on sleep habits so that we are less tired during the day, a measurable goal is going to bed 30 min earlier every day this week than we did last week. Thus, if we went to bed last week at an average of 11:00 pm, we could track and measure whether we go to bed this week every night at 10:30 pm.

Achievable: Goals are only attainable within the context of our current life situation. Achieving a goal doesn't have to be easy, but it also should not be impossible. It is often positive to dream big, but the first steps toward the big dream must be attainable in the context of our personal assets and responsibilities. One way to make a big goal more achievable is to take the larger goal and break it down into smaller, more possible goals. This not only makes it more achievable but also makes it less stressful and overwhelming. Bigger goals can seem very far off in the future, but setting smaller and more immediate goals or middle-term milestones enables us to focus on them and make them a priority. We can also set stretch goals for ourselves, which motivate us to reach beyond what we think we can do.

Relevant: Goals must be meaningful and significant to us in some way, or why invest in them? We must care about the goal enough to devote our effort to it through to the end. The meaning behind the goal enables us to persist through roadblocks and detours that can inhibit goal achievement. It very much helps if we can envision ourselves working toward and achieving the goal. By engaging in this process, we give energy to a success mindset and can feel how fulfilling and pleasurable it will be to achieve the goal. If we can't envision ourselves working toward a goal, then it's hard to imagine how we could commit to achieving it. Thus, envisioning a goal, caring about it, evaluating its meaningfulness, and committing to it are all part of *one* process.

Time-Bound: SMART goals require a timeline for goal achievement, which has the benefit of keeping us accountable for our progress toward the goal. Both interim/milestone target dates and an outcome target date are important for tracking goal attainment. Interim or milestone target dates define some mid-process, measurable events that allow us to track our progress, and these can be very motivational if the ultimate goal is far in the future. Also, there's good research to show that sharing our goals and goal timeline with someone who we respect and whose opinion we value will increase our ability to meet goals (Klein et al., 2020). This is called having an accountability partner, and this person can remind us, work with us, provide a listening ear, support us, and celebrate our accomplishments.

Aligned: Finally, although it's not part of the SMART acronym, some experts add the term aligned to the SMART goal concept. Alignment of goals means that they are compatible and work together harmoniously in the context of an overall wellness strategy. If goals are not aligned, we risk actively pitting one goal against another and creating conflict between goals, which increases stress and can hinder or block goal achievement. For example, spending money on one goal (say, an expensive gym membership or meal kit delivery service) may not be aligned with another goal of saving money for a down-payment on a house.

Stretch Goals and Visualizing

Stretch goals are goals that we set for ourselves that are beyond our current capabilities, but we deliberately and purposefully challenge ourselves to achieve them. Stretch goals are not easily attained, but they have a larger meaning or purpose for us. Examples of stretch goals might be running our first marathon, achieving a straight-A semester, or building and selling a new fitness app in the next 12 months. Stretch goals can really be any goal that challenges us to be more than we are, to grow, to change, and to achieve.

Our chances of successfully reaching our goals increase significantly if we can envision both goal attainment *and* the steps to get there. In other words, to picture ourselves getting the job, buying our dream house, winning a game, or finding a romantic partner and to walk ourselves through the steps we need to take to achieve these things. Visualization sounds like it should only use our "mind's eye," but it really should engage all our senses. By feeling what it's like to proceed successfully toward an outcome, we can learn how.

Katie Ladecky, one of the best female swimmers of all time, documents how she sets and reaches goals in her book *Just Add Water: My Swimming Life* (2024). ALL of her goals are stretch goals in that she embraces the goals that challenge and "scare" her (in a good, high-motivation way). She visualizes not only winning, but how her stroke feels, how the water feels when she is at her best, and how it feels to reach for the wall. She is an active visualizer—envisioning each part of a successful swim—rather than a static visualizer—focusing narrowly on "winning" as a singular event. This highlights the fact that success is a whole-person endeavor, requiring mind, body, emotions, and spirit to be aligned and working in concert toward an outcome. She identifies the transcendent place where wholeness of mind and body contributes to success as, "the space where your mind can run quiet, and your body can try hard."

It can be challenging to take a desire or idea for self-improvement and transform it into a SMART goal. A very simple template for setting goals is to first make a goal statement, such as, "In order to do X, I will do Y this many times (or by this date)." Then we can take the simple goal statement and make sure that all of the SMART elements are expressed in ways that we can track. Table 4.1 shows how to take common self-improvement ideas and transform them into SMART goals.

Table 4.1 Making goals SMART

Not SMART	SMART
I want to be in shape, so I will exercise more	To improve my overall fitness, my wellness goal is to exercise four times a week (Monday to Sunday) in the evening for a minimum of 20 min of cardio and 20 min of weight training each time
I will do better in school	My goal is to improve my GPA by the end of this semester, so I will study 5 days a week by reading, taking notes, and reviewing lecture notes for at least 2 hours
I will get out of debt	To pay off my credit card debt, I will order delivery food only once a week instead of three or four times, and I will put the savings of $50 per week in a separate savings account
I will eat better	Each Sunday I will make a menu plan for the next week, shop only for the food items relevant to the menu, and meal prep for lunches

Practice Developing SMART Goals

It is common to struggle at first in making our goals and aspirations SMART. We are very used to being general and nonspecific in our goals ("I want a degree" or "I want to be rich"), and it is a new skill set to be purposeful, clear, and specific in defining our goals. Here are some tips for getting started.

First, think about a way you are actively stressed or dissatisfied in one of these categories:

Daily routines
Sleep
Nutrition/eating
Physical wellness/exercise
Relationship/social wellness
Mental health
School/education
Alcohol management or smoking cessation
Work/career

You might have things you want to change in several of these categories—Most people do. However, to begin with, pick the one that you most want to address, the one that you can set a SMART goal for and think you can commit to. Thinking about that one item, write down:

- What is the thing you want to change or do?
- Why is it meaningful and important to you, and how will it increase your wellness?
- Can it be measured? If so, how?
- Considering your life circumstances, can you take the steps to change this? Is it realistic for you to commit to it?
- What would be a reasonable time frame for achieving the goal or an intermediate step toward the goal?

These answers are essential to your goal-setting process. If you can't answer all of these questions, then you should think about a different goal for now. Once you have written down your responses to these items, you are ready to develop your SMART goal. It should be no more than one to two sentences long, and you should be able to point out each SMART characteristic in your goal statement. A good format to start out in is:

"In order to improve/change/stop/start (doing X), I will do Y (this many) times a day/week at (this time/times)" or "to achieve X (a skill, award, achievement, or benefit), I will do Y (the specific behaviors and actions required) for (this amount of time or by X date)."

An example is: "To achieve a promotion to district manager, this quarter I will improve my total sales figures by 20%, complete all personnel reviews on time, and meet my personnel hiring metrics at an "exceeds" level."

Finally, write your goal down in a place you can see it regularly (next to your coffee machine or toothbrush) and set it as a regular reminder or even as wallpaper on your phone.

Goal Tracking

Tracking progress is key to successful achievement of goals. Goal tracking helps us to stay motivated, enables us to see that we are making progress, helps identify roadblocks, and keeps us accountable. Tracking can be done in low-tech ways, such as lists, reminder sticky notes, or a physical calendar with interim and final deadlines. Bullet journaling is also a highly popular analog method of tracking goals, as is using a whiteboard. The benefits of whiteboards and physical calendars are that they can be used by teams or in families to make sure that everyone is aware of goals and timelines. This type of tracking may seem clunky and old-fashioned, but it works really well for people who like tangible reminders, are best motivated or reminded visually, and are inspired by physically crossing accomplishments off of lists.

Tracking can also be done in medium- to higher-tech ways, such as using a spreadsheet, smartphone, or tracking app. It is easy to use our phone both to track progress and for reminders—a reminder to "run for 30 min after work" can come from the phone calendar, and we can also track progress on the phone after completion. There is a multitude of tracking apps available for every type of tracking that one can imagine, but here is a convenient way to break them down (listing of apps does not constitute an endorsement of any kind, just items to explore):

Goal tracker (general): Todoist, Strides; Success Coach; Goal Setting Tracker Planner.
Habit tracker: Fabulous; Productive; Habit Rabbit; Way of Life; Habitica.
Self-Care: Tangerine; Daylio; Finch.
Fitness: MyFitnessPal; Fitlist; STRONG Workout Tracker.

Some people use different apps for different goals, and some people track the same goals in several ways. For example, we can use one page, list, or app for short-term goals, such as what we will accomplish this week or this month, and a different one for long-term goals, such as saving for a down-payment on a house or planning for weight management.

Goal Keeping

The Role of Motivation

Motivation can be seen as the single most important factor in predicting whether people will respond to any new behaviors or changes, such as engaging in mental health counseling, adopting a new approach to food, exercising, setting a budget, or anything that means a person will have to think or act in a new or different way (e.g., Simpson & Balsam, 2016). Motivation is a very tricky issue overall—for example, there are times when a person might be "required" to change (i.e., court-ordered substance abuse treatment after a DUI) and their motivation is almost entirely external, but they still achieve the outcome. Other people may be very motivated to change one thing about their problems (i.e., they will stay on an antidepressant to help control their depression), but they will be unmotivated to quit heavy drinking (which, of course, contributes to their depression). Still others might be powerfully motivated to strive ahead in one area, say their career, and sacrifice other parts of their wellness to achieve in that one area.

When people are asked what the best way is to motivate another person to change, they often say to "praise them" or "reward them." It is common for parents, for example, to give their children rewards for good behavior, such as candy/food, money, screen time, or many other desirable things. Is this effective to increase motivation? Motivation is a complicated matter—research has found that money can reduce intrinsic motivation (the kind of motivation that produces lasting behaviors) in some circumstances, but that rewards that are specifically linked to performance and those that are immediate and frequent can improve intrinsic motivation (e.g., Cameron et al., 2001; Woolley & Fishbach, 2018). However, even in situations where motivation might be reduced or stifled by rewards, goals (or a clear reason behind the work) can instead be quite motivating. Motivation relies on:

1. Positive self-assessment of individual effort and autonomy.
2. Knowing the purpose of the task and understanding the goal.
3. Valuing the expected outcome.
4. Understanding the task itself.
5. Knowing one has the skills/ability to actually perform the tasks and behaviors necessary to reach the goal.

For creative tasks, in particular, some researchers argue that rewards reduce investment in the task, impair performance, and reduce satisfaction, particularly rewards that focus only on completion of the project or an arbitrary performance level (c.f., Baer et al., 2003; Byron & Khazanchi, 2012). The problem with rewards is that they can, in some circumstances:

1. Impair judgment, innovation, and creativity.
2. Reduce processing speed.
3. Reduce perceptions of self-efficacy.
4. Remove our feelings of responsibility for the task and our personal autonomy by making the incentive external (there is a subtle, but important, difference between "getting an award" and "earning an award").

Thus, it pays to be very careful about motivation, both motivating ourselves and motivating someone else. When we are trying to improve our own wellness, we should try to shut out the expectations of others and whether they approve of our actions. Instead, focusing on our own goals and how great it feels to make even small steps toward these goals will help us to stay intrinsically motivated. Also, we shouldn't be afraid to treat ourselves when we succeed; small, consistent rewards for meeting specific goals can help us move forward positively and to feel good about ourselves while doing it.

Wellness Programs

One of the main ways that people incorporate planful wellness activities into their daily lives is through wellness programming. Wellness programs are an organizational or systemic way to help people improve their health and wellness and can include programs focusing on weight management, smoking cessation, diabetes management, vaccination clinics, and mindfulness, just to name a few. Wellness programming has traditionally been offered primarily through workplace wellness programs, insurance companies, and local or state government programs. These programs are typically low- or no-cost and are often incentive-based. Incentives for participation can include gift cards, cash rewards, premium discounts, swag, gym memberships, or even time off.

About half of US employers offer some form of workplace wellness program, and this number goes up for very large employers and down for small businesses (Centers for Disease Control and Prevention, 2018). Investment in wellness programming by both employers and the government has been significant; companies can spend hundreds or thousands of dollars per employee on wellness initiatives. The common understanding of these programs is that they are not only attractive benefits to workers, but that they decrease absences, improve worker productivity, increase worker well-being and work-life balance, and reduce turnover. They also were initially found to have a positive return on investment for companies, with about a \$2–\$3 reduction in both health care costs and absenteeism for every dollar spent on wellness (Baicker et al., 2010). However, two very large studies, one in the UK and one in the United States, indicate that there is some question about whether these programs produce the desired positive outcomes for workers or companies. Song and Baicker (2019) conducted a randomized trial of more than 30,000 employees working for a large US company that offered a substantial multifaceted wellness program. The results indicated that a greater percentage of participating employees exercised regularly and watched their weight, but this did not translate into improved biomarkers of health, reduced healthcare costs, or job-related gains, such as reduced absenteeism or improved performance. Fleming (2024) surveyed more than 45,000 British workers across 233 companies and compared those who participated in wellness programs, such as mindfulness and wellness apps, and those who did not. There was no significant difference between participants and nonparticipants on a variety of measures of subjective well-being, such as psychological distress, job satisfaction, life satisfaction, and others. Thus, the picture on wellness programming is cloudier than we first imagined—participating in something "to improve wellness" doesn't guarantee that well-being will improve in any measurable way, and there is much research still to be done on what works and what does not in wellness programming.

Wellness Tip: Aging and Wellness

We all want to have the best quality of life possible as we age, with the vigor and health needed to take part in life to the fullest. People also want to live long lives, with the mental and physical ability to work, travel, play with grandkids, and engage in hobbies. However, when people say they want to age well, it doesn't only mean living as long as possible or being able to tackle the activities of daily living—for many people, healthy aging means maintaining their appearance as they age. People invest significant time, money, and resources into anti-aging products and programs, sometimes with the goal of feeling good, but often with the goal of looking good.

This sector covers a wide range of products, programs, and services. Anti-aging supplements abound, claiming to promote skin health and elasticity, joint health, metabolic functioning, and boost the immune system, as well as reducing general stress and oxidative stress. However, the anti-aging sector is dominated by skincare, including preparations containing antioxidants, retinoids, hyaluronic or salicylic acid, sunscreen, cleansers, and red-light therapy. However, more invasive procedures targeting aging skin are also common, including Botox, dermal fillers, chemical peels, laser treatments, microdermabrasion/microneedling, fat transfer, and face/neck/brow lifts. Indeed, if you search the internet for "anti-aging treatments," you will find that almost all focus on the skin—the visible results of aging that we see in the mirror.

Like many wellness sectors, the anti-aging domain is a blend of science, pseudoscience, and marketing. There are many concerns over unregulated products and unverified claims, and the anti-aging industry is rife with money-making schemes packaged as wellness approaches. One problem is that the "innovations" in this sector far outpace the science that examines them for safety and efficacy. Red light therapy is a good example of this, as it is very popular on social media, makes wildly exaggerated claims about outcomes ("repairs damaged skin," "dramatically reduces wrinkles," and "relieves joint pain"), and has many products popping up—from inexpensive face masks and wands to blankets, light panels, and even full-coverage red light beds. It is possible that red light therapy might reduce inflammation and increase elastin and collagen, but we don't know if the mask, wand, or bed that *you* are looking at or using does so.

More than 80 years ago, the Harvard Study of Adult Development began studying the adult lives and aging processes of a cohort of Harvard men and then, later, their children and wives. In his book *Aging Well*, Vaillant (2008) describes the six features of healthy aging: (1) consistent physical activity, (2) avoidance of unhealthy habits, like alcohol and drug use, (3) reliable methods of coping with hardships, (4) maintaining a healthy weight, and (5) enjoying stable and positive relationships. Similarly, the Rowe and Kahn (1997) perspective on successful aging identifies three main components of healthy aging: (1) avoiding disease and disability, (2) staying active both cognitively and physically, and (3) continuous engagement in social life, relationships, and productive pursuits.

The moral of the story? *Nurture your relationships throughout life* for a healthy and satisfying aging process. Our genetic heritage sets the stage for aging, but it is the lifestyle choices, habits, and practices we develop that make the difference to healthy aging—particularly those having to do with finding, building, and maintaining strong and healthy relationships. Remember, aging is a continuous process—it cannot be stopped or diverted, but it can be done slowly, healthfully, surrounded by people we like and love, and with a positive mindset.

References

Baer, M., Oldham, G. R., & Cummings, A. (2003). Rewarding creativity: When does it really matter? *The Leadership Quarterly, 14*(4–5), 569–586. https://doi.org/10.1016/S1048-9843(03)00052-3

Baicker, K., Cutler, D., & Song, Z. (2010). Workplace wellness programs can generate savings. *Health Affairs, 29*(2), 304–311. https://doi.org/10.1377/hlthaff.2009.0626

Byron, K., & Khazanchi, S. (2012). Rewards and creative performance: A meta-analytic test of theoretically derived hypotheses. *Psychological Bulletin, 138*(4), 809–830. https://doi.org/10.1037/a0027652

Cameron, J., Banko, K. M., & Pierce, W. D. (2001). Pervasive negative effects of rewards on intrinsic motivation: The myth continues. *The Behavior Analyst, 24*(1), 1–44. https://doi.org/10.1007/BF03392017

Centers for Disease Control and Prevention. (2018). *Workplace health in America 2017*. Centers for Disease Control and Prevention, U.S. Department of Health and Human Services. Retrieved from https://www.cdc.gov/workplace-health-promotion/media/pdfs/2024/06/2017-Workplace-Health-in-America-Summary-Report-FINAL-updated-508.pdf

Fleming, W. J. (2024). Employee well-being outcomes from individual-level mental health interventions: Crosssectional evidence from the United Kingdom. *Industrial Relations Journal, 55*, 162–182. https://doi.org/10.1111/irj.12418

Klein, H. J., Lount, R. B., Jr., Park, H. M., & Linford, B. J. (2020). When goals are known: The effects of audience relative status on goal commitment and performance. *Journal of Applied Psychology, 105*(4), 372–389. https://doi.org/10.1037/apl0000441

Ladecky, K. (2024). *Just add water: My swimming life*. Simon & Schuster.

Rowe, J. W., & Kahn, R. L. (1997). Successful aging. *The Gerontologist, 37*(4), 433–440. https://doi.org/10.1093/geront/37.4.433

Simpson, E. H., & Balsam, P. D. (2016). The behavioral neuroscience of motivation: An overview of concepts, measures, and translational applications. *Current Topics in Behavioral Neurosciences, 27*, 1–12. https://doi.org/10.1007/7854_2015_402

Song, Z., & Baicker, K. (2019). Effect of a workplace wellness program on employee health and economic outcomes: A randomized clinical trial. *Journal of the American Medical Association, 321*(15), 1491–1501. https://doi.org/10.1001/jama.2019.3307

Vaillant, G. E. (2008). *Aging well: Surprising guideposts to a happier life from the landmark study of adult development* (1st ed.). Little Brown & Company.

Woolley, K., & Fishbach, A. (2018). It's about time: Earlier rewards increase intrinsic motivation. *Journal of Personality and Social Psychology, 114*(6), 877–890. https://doi.org/10.1037/pspa0000116

Chapter 5
Theories of Change

People can change and do change all the time, and they can even successfully change multiple things at one time. What do we know about how people change? A theory of change describes several aspects of change—not only what changes, but how and why a change occurs within a specific context. This section will provide an overview of several of the theories of behavior change that are most pertinent to the mind-body wellness space.

Health Belief Model (HBM)

The HBM is a framework that helps us to understand how and why people change their health-related behaviors, including their wellness behaviors. The model is based on the (admittedly optimistic) assumption that change is possible if people: (1) want to avoid being and feeling sick or become well if they are currently sick, and (2) believe they have the ability to behave in ways that will prevent sickness or help them recover more quickly. Using the HBM, if we wanted to change something about our wellness, we would ask ourselves the following six questions. Table 5.1 provides examples of how these factors work to distinguish between those who engage with behavior change and those who do not.

How susceptible am I to this problem, and what is my risk of having or acquiring it? This is also called "perceived susceptibility," and it taps into our level of concern about the health issue and how vulnerable we feel about it. For example, a woman might have many close relatives who have been diagnosed with breast cancer, which makes her feel like she is in danger of having it herself. She will engage in preventive measures and get screenings because she feels vulnerable.

How serious will it be if I have or acquire this problem? This is "perceived severity," and it means that we evaluate many types of consequences (medical, work,

S. M. Henney, J. D. Hackett, *Mind-Body Wellness*,
https://doi.org/10.1007/978-3-031-91611-3_5

Table 5.1 The health belief model in action

HBM component	Behavior change	No behavior change
Perceived susceptibility	I am at risk, and I will take action to change my behavior to avoid becoming ill	I am not at risk of getting sick, and there is no need for me to change what I'm doing
Perceived severity	The negative consequences of me becoming sick, such as medical bills, missing work, becoming disabled, or even dying, motivate me to behave it ways to avoid this problem	This is no big deal. Even if I was exposed or became sick, I am sure I will recover easily
Perceived benefits	I can clearly see benefits of this behavior to me, and I value these benefits, so I'm going to start doing this regularly	I don't believe this will help me to feel well or not become sick, so I'm not going to do it
Perceived barriers	There are costs associated with this new behavior, but they are worth it to feel well	The costs to me outweigh any benefits I could have, so it will actively harm me to change
Cue to action	I heard that there is a new treatment for my problem, so I'm going to try that instead of the old one that has lots of side effects	I don't believe that this is as important or as severe as people say, so I don't have any reason to change
Self-efficacy	I know I have the skills and ability to make this change; I just have to start!	I feel helpless to change this, and I just don't have the bandwidth or the resources to address this problem

quality of life, etc.) when we decide how severe a threat something is. For example, some people took the risk of contracting COVID-19 very seriously because they believed that it could cause them great harm, and subsequently engaged in a variety of preventive behaviors like masking, social distancing, and vaccination. However, others judged that it was not a threat to their health or wellness and did not engage in preventative behaviors.

What are the benefits to me of trying to prevent or treat this problem? This factor, called "perceived benefits," is when a person looks at the range of options for preventing or addressing a problem and decides if they believe they will work. For example, some people take supplements (vitamins, minerals, herbs, etc.) because they believe that they will prevent or treat illness, whereas others believe that people who eat a balanced diet don't require supplements.

What is the cost to me of trying to prevent or treat this problem? This is also called "perceived barriers," and it refers to people's assessment of how hard or costly it will be to adopt the new behavior. People take into account whether they can afford a treatment, product, or intervention, how their family and friends will react to it, if it will affect their job or career, how difficult it is to obtain, and many other barriers. For example, people with few financial resources often choose not to treat or even be evaluated for an illness because they can't afford it—behavior change is just too costly for them. This highlights a limitation of this model; people have barriers to change that are real, important, and not easily overcome. The model doesn't directly address poverty, food deserts, racism, or cultural traditions.

What is making me think I need to prevent or treat this problem? This is a "cue to action," which means there is something that prompts or motivates a person to start working on a problem. This sign could be something about the person (e.g., pain, concerning symptoms, anxiety/depression) or something in the social world (e.g., something heard on social media or from a friend/family member). People vary widely in how intense the sign or symptom has to be in order to motivate them to action; for some people, a warning label on a product is enough, but others have to be in severe pain or have an actual test result in order to change their behavior.

Am I confident that I can prevent or treat this problem, even if I want to? This is also called "self-efficacy," and it concerns a person's belief in their own ability to change and to address health and wellness problems. Without belief in one's ability to change in general or in relation to a particular problem, it is close to impossible to change in any meaningful way.

To be clear, HBM does not suggest that all health- or wellness-related behavior change is positive. For example, the "cues to action" can be from credible sources, such as doctors or legitimate research, or non-credible sources, but both types can and do motivate people to adopt new behaviors. There are many sources on social media suggesting "natural" ways of treating diabetes or cancer that have low or no side effects. People struggling with a cancer diagnosis or the side-effects of treatment have been known to drop conventional treatment for the "natural" approach, with disastrous results. Nonetheless, HBM can be used to design wellness education and interventions that meet people where they are in ways relevant to their specific issues, typically by targeting specific aspects of the model. For example, although most smokers know that this behavior is detrimental to their health, they underestimate the risk of continuing smoking, downplay the benefits of quitting, and focus on the barriers, including psychological and physical dependence (Pribadi & Devy, 2020). Any intervention must address these factors straightforwardly, starting with dependence, or there is little chance of the intervention succeeding.

Wellness in the Disabled Community

Disabled people have traditionally been outside of wellness messaging and programming, perhaps because of uneducated perceptions about disability as illness, frailty, and dependence. Disability is not synonymous with being unhealthy but rather encompasses a range of strengths, assets, competencies, as well as needs and obstacles (Centers for Disease Control and Prevention, 2014). It is clear that people can live with a disability and still perceive themselves as well and be motivated to strive toward wellness in their life. They have the capacity to live fulfilled lives full of joy, promise, and wellness.

Disabled people also have the ability to vision and to work on wellness in their lives and, if they cannot do this independently, then their caregivers can help them achieve a level of wellness possible in the context of their disability. This is an example of a point we have made several times in this book—No one has to be perfectly functional in all areas of their life to experience wellness. Disabled persons' quality of life depends, in part, on their perception of their own wellness and how they are included or excluded from both private and public discourse on wellness. In many instances, lack of wellness in the disabled community is related to a lack of access. About 68% of nondisabled women over 40 participate in wellness programs and activities, however, that number decreases to 54% for disabled women. Most wellness programs are profit-driven enterprises, which find the largest market in the able-bodied population.

In terms of marketing of wellness products and services, much of the materials showing people engaging in healthy behaviors are of able-bodied persons. Most fitness apps are entirely designed around the assumption that the user is able-bodied. Additionally, nearly all advice on workouts, diets, supplements, and mental health that does not originate within disabled communities centers on the able-bodied.

Another cause of barriers to wellness for disabled people is that the able-bodied population often doesn't consider the needs of the disabled (Moss, 2005). For example, gym machines are largely built around standard biomechanics and involve sitting in and interacting with them in a way that may be very difficult for a disabled person. Similarly, wellness initiatives are rarely marketed to the disabled. Wellness influencers often attempt to legitimize themselves by using complex language, which may be out of reach to someone with an intellectual disability. Standard instructions for at home care by medical professionals and wellness professionals alike may only exist for those who are capable of two-handed tasks, standing, or other physical tasks that require a degree of dexterity that a disabled person may not be able to achieve.

The US Surgeon General has called for us as a nation to do more to include disabled people into the modern health and wellness sphere and welcome them into a role in shaping the future of the wellness field Office of the Surgeon General (US); Office on Disability (US) (2005). Designing and implementing strategies for finding wellness while disabled is difficult, because the term disabled is a descriptor of a wide variety of unique disorders, disabilities, and challenges that differ in type, scope, and impact. The disabled population is not monolithic, and the wellness interventions will not be, either. Wellness for disabled people must take a personalized approach based on their individual needs and abilities.

Theory of Planned Behavior (TPB)

The TPB provides a model of our intentions to engage in specific behaviors, particularly those over which we have a high level of control. It assumes that people act rationally in their decision-making process, and that eventual behavior is directly

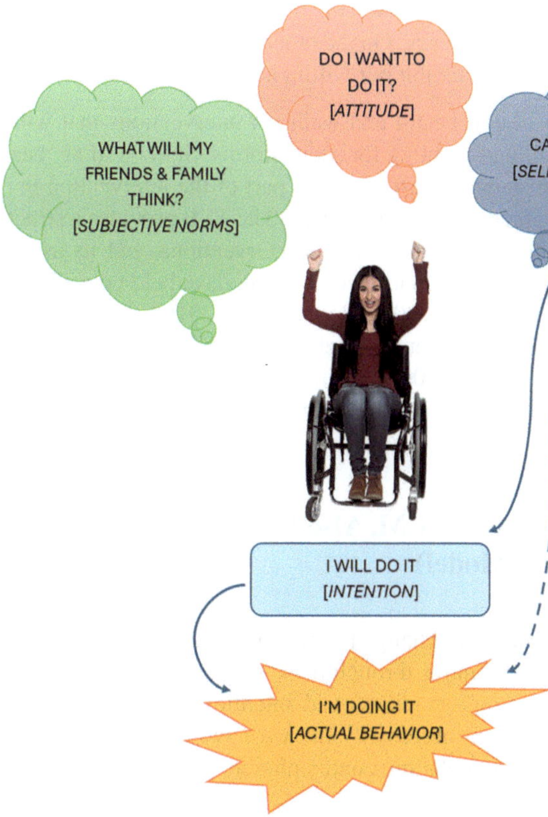

Fig. 5.1 The theory of planned behavior

linked to our intention to enact the behavior, which itself is determined by our attitudes about a behavior, our evaluation of subjective norms surrounding the behavior, and our ability to control/influence this behavior. As presented in Fig. 5.1, these three factors break down as follows:

Attitude—Am I for or against doing it? This factor is composed of all of our thoughts, assumptions, ideas, and knowledge about a particular behavior. We use these to determine if we believe we should behave this way and if it will benefit or hurt us.

Norms—Are my family, friends, and cultural norms supportive of it? This refers to our perception of what other people think about a behavior as well as what they will think about us if we do it.

Perceived control—Do I have the skills, ability, and conviction that I can do it? Here we weigh what we think we can do versus how difficult we think it will be to achieve the outcome or perform the behavior. This is a key factor in transforming intention into action. Even if we are in favor of a behavior or a change and our environment supports it, if we think it is impossible, then we won't even try.

Sometimes we might be unsure if we can do something, and we try it successfully, which builds our confidence. On the other hand, we can also be unsure and be unsuccessful, which can inhibit our willingness to try next time.

The TPB is used to design health and wellness interventions that will change attitudes and beliefs, while accounting for social norms. Skill building, health education, and change management must also be a part of the intervention in order to increase participants' perception of self-efficacy. The TPB provides a structure and a roadmap for designing health and wellness interventions, and its assumptions, particularly around the perceived control component, have held up well in research studies (e.g., Armitage & Conner, 2001; Sheeran et al., 2016). Nonetheless, there is also evidence that the association between behavioral intentions and actual behavior is small (e.g., Webb & Sheeran, 2006). This means what we all know is true—even if we fully intend to change, sometimes we don't actually do it.

Stages of Change Model (SCM, Also Called the Transtheoretical Model)

The SCM identifies the stages of change for health-related behaviors and proposes the process by which people move through these stages. This model assumes that change is based on a person's readiness and intention to change, but that such change is a process that is not necessarily linear or swift. There are six stages of change in the SCM: precontemplation, contemplation, preparation, action, maintenance, and termination.

Precontemplation is when people don't realize they need to change and have no intention to do so any time soon. The challenge here is to build awareness of the need to change.

Contemplation occurs when people are aware they need to change, but they can't/won't commit to doing so. The challenge here is to increase awareness of the benefits of change and decrease the barriers to change.

Preparation is when people have the clear intention to change in the near future and have taken small steps to do so. The challenge is to plan and make goals.

Action is when people have taken positive and real steps to change, and they are exerting the time and energy necessary to adopt the new behavior. The challenge here is to consolidate change and focus on the positives of the new behavior.

Maintenance occurs when people have solidified the new behavior for a period of time and intend to keep the behavior into the future. They have fully integrated the behavior change into their lives and are "living the change" every day. The challenge of this stage is to avoid relapsing into old behaviors.

Termination is the closure phase of behavior change, where people have no desire to return to the old behaviors and have conviction in their changed behavior. This is a very demanding stage to reach with certainty, and many people remain (without harm) in the maintenance stage.

It is very common for people to proceed forward with health and wellness goals and then regress back to an earlier stage. For example, more than half of people who smoke want to quit (preparation), but most who try to do so (action) will relapse back into smoking. People can enter into the SCM and exit at any stage multiple times for the same behavior. The SCM is used to design interventions, programs, and practices that meet people where they are in these stages and provide them with tools to initiate, plan, enact, and maintain change.

The job of the professionals designing these interventions is to make them useful and usable to assist people to engage in change and incorporate it into their lives. These interventions should be matched to the stages in which they will have the most effect. Figure 5.2 illustrates that interventions in the SCM model can be divided into two categories: cognitive-emotional processes and behavioral processes. Cognitive-emotional processes are most useful when they are applied in the Precontemplation and contemplation stages; this is because thinking, feeling, motivation, and planning are most important to these stages. Behavioral interventions are most pertinent to the preparation, action, and maintenance stages, as these stages are when people are actively engaged in change; they must behave differently and so the interventions must target actions. Cognitive and emotional processes include:

Consciousness-raising: Improving awareness of and knowledge about the healthy behavior, typically through health education.
Emotional arousal: Learning to be aware of all emotions, good and bad, and to approach them as useful guides.
Self-reappraisal: Using fresh aspirations and goals to realize that the new behaviors can be part of a better, more positive self-concept.
Environmental reevaluation: Becoming aware of how our behavior affects others and how new behaviors can positively affect those around us.

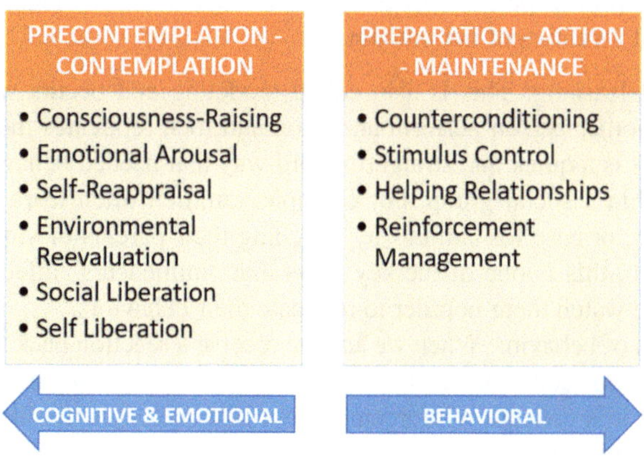

Fig. 5.2 Processes of change in the stages of change model

Social liberation: Realization that life is better when those around us support and value our changed behavior.
Self-liberation: Belief that changes is possible for us as individuals, and it's okay to make well-being a priority.

Behavioral processes include:

Helping relationships: Surrounding ourselves with people who cheer us on toward new behaviors, while distancing ourselves from those who encourage old, harmful behaviors.
Counterconditioning: Habitually replacing unhealthy patterns, thoughts, and behaviors with new ways of being.
Reinforcement management: Commit to situations and experiences that directly reward the new behavior and actively avoid situations that reward old behaviors.
Stimulus control: Eliminate cues and triggers for old behaviors and replace them with reminders and reinforcers of new, healthy behaviors.

Social Cognitive Theory (SCT)

SCT is a theory about how we learn things, so it is particularly useful in the wellness space. SCT proposes that we learn and change through the multidirectional influence of environment, person, and behavior. This is called reciprocal determinism, because each part influences the other. In SCT, the environment is composed of everything "outside" of a person that impacts them in some way, such as reinforcement or punishment, "likes" on social media, social norms, and our influence on our own environment. The "person" in SCT refers to internal factors, like knowledge, cognitive abilities, emotions, temperament, and efficacy beliefs, whereas "behavior" refers to skills, performance, and behavioral choices. One of the implications of this is that we are not passive recipients of wellness promotion; we are embedded in a dynamic network of person, environment, and behavior, in which we are actors, recipients, and inventors of our outcomes.

Observational learning: This is also called modeling and occurs when a person watches another person perform an action and then replicates the action themselves. This is a quick and straightforward way that needed behaviors are transmitted within a social group. For example, children often learn how to cook, repair a car, or care for animals by watching their parents or siblings do these things. Also, this is one of the key ways that "influencers" affect us on social media—we watch them in order to replicate their behaviors.
Consequences of behavior: When we act, we receive a reaction back from our environment. If this feedback increases the likelihood that we will behave in the same way again, it is called a reinforcement, but if it decreases the likelihood of the behavior recurring, it is a punishment. Reinforcements are not necessarily good (sugar is sweet and tasty, which can reinforce us to eat too much of it), and punishments are not necessarily bad (a hangover can teach us not to drink so much

alcohol); they are both an important part of learning. However, reinforcements are more effective than punishments for maintaining desired behaviors.

Self-efficacy: This is our belief that we possess and can use the knowledge, skills, and abilities to perform a particular behavior. Self-efficacy comes, at least in part, from our past successes; the phrase "success breeds success" has some truth here. However, as Fig. 5.3 illustrates, self-efficacy also develops from: (1) vicariously watching others succeed and comparing our abilities with theirs, (2) how effectively we are encouraged (or discouraged) from pursuing a certain behavior, and (3) getting feedback from our own bodies and minds to determine when and if we reach our limits. Self-efficacy is, perhaps, the most important of all the parts of SCT for wellness, because it reliably predicts health- and wellness-related behaviors.

Conditions of modeling: In order for a person to successfully reproduce an observed behavior, they have to: (1) pay attention to the model, (2) be able to remember the parts of the behavior, (3) be capable of reproducing the behavior, and (4) want to enact that behavior. We also tend to be more willing to use models who are more like us and who we perceive as having high status or special expertise. This is why wellness messaging tends to be flashy, fast, simple and includes statements of unique expertise or a ton of followers.

Behavioral capability: Remember that none of this is possible unless we have the sheer capacity to act in the ways we want and need to; in other words, we must have the knowledge, skills, and competencies we need to enact a behavior successfully. There are things we simply physically or mentally cannot do at the present time (although we may be able to in the future or under different circumstances). It doesn't matter how much a small child wants to take out the garbage to please their parent, if they are too short or not strong enough to lift the bag, it is beyond their ability to perform this action independently at this time. Our "want to" sometimes exceeds our "can," just as sometimes our abilities exceed our motivation to act.

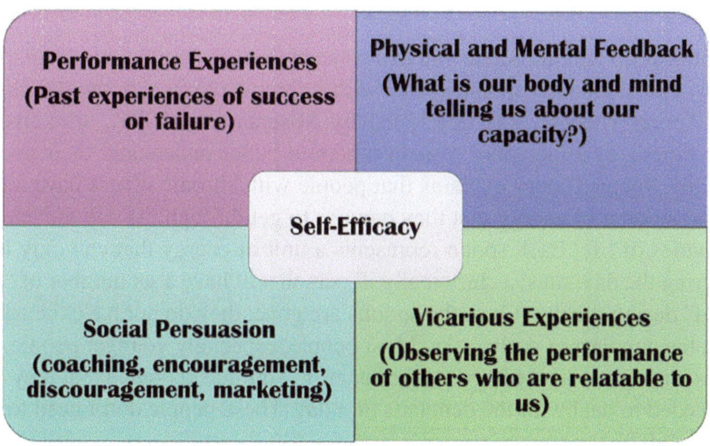

Fig. 5.3 Components of self-efficacy

SCT in general is useful in understanding acquisition of wellness-related behaviors and behavior change, especially how social media influencers and other people might have influence on our behavior. When we perceive our social media favorites to be compelling, knowledgeable, and popular, we will tend to model their behavior and follow their example. There is no inherent problem with modeling health-related behaviors, but we should acknowledge that both beneficial and harmful behaviors can be learned this way.

The concept of self-efficacy has been demonstrated to have a particularly strong connection with a person's ability to make positive changes or, conversely, with the inability to do so. People high in self-efficacy believe they have more control over their wellness, put significant effort into achieving their wellness goals, and are resilient—when failure and set-backs happen, as they do when we pursue our goals, people high in self-efficacy bounce back. Improving self-efficacy is a legitimate target of wellness interventions, and self-efficacy can be developed by:

Experiences of mastery: We build on our past accomplishments. Being successful at small goals leads to confidence that we can be successful in larger goals.

Setting appropriate goals: Setting goals that are achievable and realistic help to successfully achieve them, increasing our mastery and our confidence.

Availability of good models: Surrounding ourselves with people who display the behaviors, drive, and ambition that we want to emulate is how we position our environment to facilitate our goals.

Seek encouragement: We should be our own cheerleader by speaking to ourselves kindly and positively but also seek those who will celebrate our successes and cheer us on toward our goals.

Engage our Coping: Manage emotions by nurturing coping skills, such as exercise, meditation, therapy, being in nature, and self-care.

Wellness Tip: Spoon Theory

This wellness tip will introduce you to a concept that you might find useful, particularly if you or someone you know lives with a chronic physical or mental illness (or both). "Spoon Theory" was developed by Miserandino (2003), who lives with chronic illness, as a metaphor to help others to better understand their needs and limitations. Spoon Theory explains that people with chronic illness have a defined and finite amount of energy that they can use to get through the day and engage in the activities of life. Each spoon represents a unit of energy that can only be used once during the day; thus, a chronically ill person will have a set number of "spoons to spend" during the day. Once the spoons are gone, they do not have the energy to do even the simplest of daily tasks. Most people, especially younger people, have a limitless amount or a very large pool of energy ("infinite spoons") that they can tap when needed to deal with the demands of a day. These people don't need to "count spoons" at all.

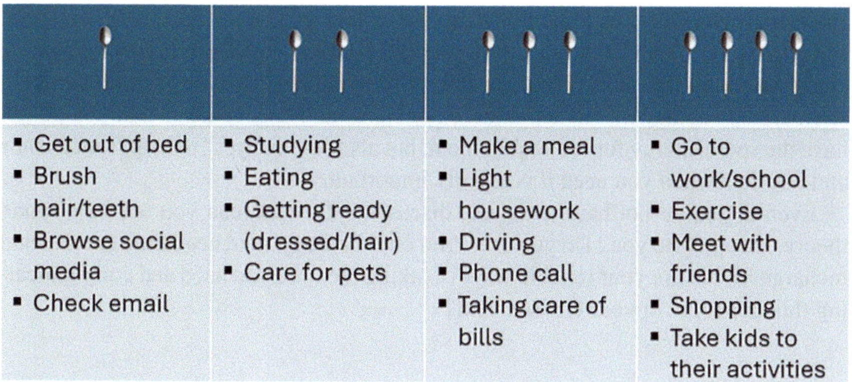

Fig. 5.4 Value of "Spoons"

People with chronic illness struggle to explain to people (or even to justify to themselves) that they just don't have the physical, emotional, or mental energy stores to be able to "keep up" with others or even to get through a regular day (let alone a hard or stressful day). The spoon metaphor is used as a visual representation of what it is like to have real limitations and how these limitations force people with chronic illness to plan out their days very carefully and to decline to participate in certain enjoyable or necessary activities in order to not "run out of spoons" by the day's end.

Figure 5.4 depicts how much each typical daily activity "costs" in spoons. On their best day, someone with a chronic illness could have 12 spoons to spend, but on their worst day they could only have two to spend. How would you spend these spoons? What if you *had* to get something done—like grocery shopping or taking your pet to the vet—but you were low on spoons because you had a test that day? Remember also that even fun/enjoyable activities have an energy cost. For example, just going out to lunch with a good friend involves getting ready, traveling there, conversing through lunch, and getting home, representing the expenditure of many spoons. How do you think these spoons would be recharged? If you are going to work with people (or be a better friend/relative), you should challenge your assumptions about the amount of energy or vitality that people have to deal with life's requirements. Remember, having the energy to get through the day is not only or always about grit, determination, or "willpower." Sometimes people run out of spoons, and that's ok.

Wash Your Spoons

How do you "wash your spoons" to recharge and reset your number of spoons? Sleep should be regenerative and restorative, so we usually get a "new set of spoons" every morning. However, many people struggle with sleep, so they start out each day with few spoons due to tiredness and lethargy. Pain (both physical and emotional) can cause us to be less active, less able to care for ourselves, and more self-protective. Both of these issues require a close working relationship with a compassionate physician, who can help you to increase your spoons. Practicing self-care by saying "no" to activities, excursions, and engagements that you do not have the spare energy for is a requirement, but also saying "yes" to help from friends and families when you need it is equally important.

Even if you do not have a chronic disease or disorder, can you see how spoon theory can apply to you? Do you ever "run out of energy" and need time to relax and recharge? What are your reliable ways of taking the time you need and communicating this to people in your environment?

References

Armitage, C. J., & Conner, M. (2001). Efficacy of the theory of planned behaviour: A meta-analytic review. *The British Journal of Social Psychology, 40*(4), 471–499. https://doi.org/10.1348/014466601164939

Centers for Disease Control and Prevention. (2014). *Disability and health healthy living*. Retrieved from www.cdc.gov/ncbddd/disabilityandhealth/healthyliving.html

Miserandino, C. (2003). *The spoon theory. But you don't look sick*. Archived from the original on 17 November 2019. Retrieved 5 July 2024.

Moss, H. (2005). *Ableism is the wellness issue we're not addressing*. Well and Good. Retrieved from www.wellandgood.com/ableism-issue-in-wellness/

Office of the Surgeon General (US); Office on Disability (US). (2005). *The surgeon general's call to action to improve the health and wellness of persons with disabilities*. Health and Wellness for Persons with Disabilities Today. Retrieved from https://www.ncbi.nlm.nih.gov/books/NBK44662/

Pribadi, E. T., & Devy, S. R. (2020). Application of the health belief model on the intention to stop smoking behavior among young adult women. *Journal of Public Health Research, 9*(2), 1817. https://doi.org/10.4081/jphr.2020.1817

Sheeran, P., Maki, A., Montanaro, E., Avishai-Yitshak, A., Bryan, A., Klein, W. M. P., Miles, E., & Rothman, A. J. (2016). The impact of changing attitudes, norms, and self-efficacy on health-related intentions and behavior: A meta-analysis. *Health Psychology, 35*(11), 1178–1188. https://doi.org/10.1037/hea0000387

Webb, T. L., & Sheeran, P. (2006). Does changing behavioral intentions engender behavior change? A meta-analysis of the experimental evidence. *Psychological Bulletin, 132*(2), 249–268. https://doi.org/10.1037/0033-2909.132.2.249

Chapter 6
Stress and Wellness

What Is Stress?

Stress can be described as an experience of emotional, mental, or physical tension that results from any event, context, behavior, or thought that is perceived as a challenge, problem, or demand. Stress is often perceived as uncontrollable and sometimes as overwhelming. In addition to our stressful experience of mental, emotional, and bodily distress, stress is also defined by how we perceive and interpret these. Stressors are the triggers and causes of our perception of stress. Stressors can be events, people, bodily sensations, information, emotions, and many, many other things! In other words, stress is comprised of our experiences and perceptions, and stressors are the triggers.

The relationship between wellness and stress is complicated, because wellness is not the complete absence of stress—this is impossible. Rather, in the presence of stress, a wellness approach is about reducing our automatic and habitual reactivity to stress by developing reliable ways of responding to it. Stress is an inevitable and unavoidable part of life. Many people erroneously think that it is the social world—specifically other people—that causes us stress. While the social world and people can be a source of stress, it is only one source of many. Even if we lived in a cave away from all people, we would still experience stress—finding food if we're hungry, sourcing clean water, and feeling at risk from the cold or predators would all still be sources of stress. Even gravity is a stress on our body, skin, and joints, and we can't avoid gravity.

S. M. Henney, J. D. Hackett, *Mind-Body Wellness*,
https://doi.org/10.1007/978-3-031-91611-3_6

Types of Stress

There are four primary types of stress—acute stress, episodic stress, chronic stress, and post-traumatic stress. Acute stress is very common and is experienced as immediate and impactful distress in the current moment, and it resolves relatively quickly. As the autonomic nervous system becomes activated, stressed people can experience a racing heart, sweating, lightheadedness, a reduction in decision-making capacity, and feelings of panic. Hormones like adrenaline and cortisol rise, and our bodies are prepped to engage in a fight, flight, or freeze response. What causes acute stress varies—it could be a test, a presentation in front of the class, a car accident or speeding ticket, missing or being late to an appointment, or any of the many things that happen to us during the day. It doesn't really matter if the event is objectively stressful, it only matters that we perceive it to be so.

Episodic stress occurs periodically over time, and it can come in waves or consecutive incidents. These can be regularly occurring and even predictable or seemingly random. The symptoms of episodic stress can resemble those of acute stress, sometimes being less intense and sometimes more, especially if anticipatory anxiety (the anxiety we get when we worry a lot about a future event) is present. We can actually get used to experiencing these waves of stress, as people experience them as part of the pattern of their lives. It can be hard to motivate people to change patterns of episodic stress, because they believe that these stress episodes are "the way life is."

Chronic stress occurs when a person experiences the negative effects of stress consistently over time. Stressors that cause chronic stress can be from all wellness dimensions, such as physical (chronic pain, heart disease), emotional (anxiety, unresolved loss), spiritual (questioning faith), environmental (poor working or living conditions), and so forth. Many of the events of life that we think about as discreet experiences, like marriage, birth, death, moving, changing jobs, and so on can be ongoing stressors, as we strive to adapt to our new normal.

Chronic stress can be very damaging to us as humans in any of the wellness dimensions. As chronic stress progresses, it becomes more associated with physical health and mental health problems over time. In fact, it is one of the most well-researched areas in which we can see the mind/body connection play out. For example, there is substantial evidence that cardiovascular disease is related to chronic mental health conditions, like depression and anxiety, as well as to measures of subjective well-being, such as quality of life (e.g., Cohen et al., 2015). We will discuss more of the research related to chronic stress and wellness later in this chapter.

Post-traumatic stress is often left off the list of types of stress, as it overlaps into the three other categories of stress. However, it is a clinically useful typology, and understanding it can help us to identify, treat, and cope with the effects of trauma. Post-traumatic stress occurs after a person has experienced an overwhelming, uncontrollable, and terrifying event that they are unable to process or resolve in the course of regular life. It proceeds from acute stress in the near-term to episodic or chronic stress reactions over time. It is characterized by a range of symptoms, such as severe anxiety, flashbacks, intrusive thoughts or images, negative mood, insomnia, and irritability, among others. Post-traumatic stress can make the tasks of living—work, relationships, household management, and self-care—difficult or impossible to manage.

Post-traumatic stress can lead to the diagnosis of post-traumatic stress disorder (PTSD), which is typically related to a significant traumatic event, or complex post-traumatic stress Disorder (C-PTSD), which has similar symptoms to PTSD, but more severe and intense, and is the result of repeated and prolonged trauma. PTSD and C-PTSD can be deadly, as they put those who suffer at higher risk of suicide than for other anxiety disorders, even when taking into account coexisting psychological disorders (Sareen et al., 2007). For those suffering from post-traumatic stress, it is essential to engage with a mental health professional with expertise in the treatment of post-traumatic stress to reduce the risk of serious mental health consequences.

Type Vs. Category of Stress

In addition to the types of stress discussed above, stress can also be broken down into different categories. Examples of the categories of stress include:

- Physical/biological
- Nutrition/diet
- Cognitive/intellectual
- Emotional
- Spiritual
- Occupational
- Financial
- Environment/living
- Daily life/daily hassles

It's important to not only know the type of stress but also the category it falls into so that interventions can be targeted and effective. While it is true that some chronic stressors can have an overarching effect on wellness, it is often the case that stress can have differing effects in different categories. For example, a person can be experiencing severe physical stress in terms of illness or disability, but can also find that their spiritual wellness is thriving more than ever. Another person can be going through the emotional stress of loss and grieving but also finds that focusing on positive changes in diet and exercise helps them to cope.

Stress Vs. Anxiety

One may wonder if anxiety and stress are the same. The answer is no, but there is a lot of legitimate overlap. It is true that anxiety is a mental health issue that has many of the same signs as stress reactions, such as racing heart, tension, feelings of dread, and nervousness, but what are the differences? There are some definitions that conclude that anxiety is caused by "internal factors" and stress is caused by "external factors," but this is far too simplistic. Anxiety is worry, fear, and upset that persists even when the trigger goes away or when the trigger is just thought about or imagined. In other words, there does not need to be a real or present stressor for anxiety to occur. On the other hand, as we have learned, stress reactions require a stressor, one that we perceive as negative, distressing, and challenging to our coping mechanisms. Another way to look at this is that anxiety is one possible reaction to stress, but it is not the stressor itself.

Catastrophizing

Catastrophizing occurs when a person always jumps directly to believing that the worst-case outcome will definitely occur, even if other options exist or other outcomes could happen. This is a great example of something that happens "inside the head" and yet is felt throughout the body. Catastrophizers not only focus on the worst outcome, but they also really invest in it and convince themselves of it. For example, a person who is experiencing a relationship break-up might say to themselves, "I'm broken, and no one will ever love me again," or someone who makes a mistake at work might say, "I am a screw-up, and I am going to fail because I always fail." While we do, in fact, sometimes experience poor outcomes, it is seldom as bad as a catastrophizer believes it will be and, sometimes, the catastrophizing itself makes things much, much worse. Catastrophizing thus becomes a stressor in and of itself, with the "doomsday thinking" swirling around in the person's head and being experienced as stress in the body.

Catastrophizing is fundamentally a distorted thought process, but there is some evidence that the body is involved as well. For example, a person feels pain somewhere in their body and perceives it as overwhelming, uncontrollable, and intensely negative. They begin catastrophizing about the pain, including excessive worry, fear, avoidance of activities related to the pain/injury, and intrusive, negative, and repetitive thoughts about the pain/injury. This catastrophizing thought pattern is related to negative pain outcomes like failure of treatment to reduce pain, pain-related disability, and mental health issues (Flink et al., 2013). It is also part of an ongoing feedback loop wherein the body makes the mind pay attention to the pain, and by paying attention to the pain in a catastrophizing way, the pain becomes unmanageable and the source of even more mental distress. In other words, as the person becomes more vigilant and worried about their pain, the pain becomes untreatable by medical means.

Eustress

Can stress ever be positive? Yes! The word "eustress" is used to describe mild to moderate stress that is perceived as beneficial or positive by the person who is going through it. It seems there is an optimal amount of stress that may actually increase our productivity, direct our attention, improve performance, and even enhance enjoyment of life. Examples include enjoying a scary movie, a thrilling roller coaster, or a risky activity like bungee jumping or skydiving. Experiencing eustress from an activity depends on our perception or interpretation of it, which occurs through a process of appraisal. Appraisal means that we evaluate whether the stressor is important for us to react to, and then if the stressor has or will harm or help us and if we have the resources to cope with it (Lazarus & Folkman, 1984). Thus, the same activity, say a zip line, can induce distress in one person and eustress in another. It is even possible that the same event, for example, a deadline on an important project, can have aspects of both eustress (such as increased productivity and focus) and distress (worry and fear of failure).

The Yerkes–Dodson law highlights the empirical relationship between stress and performance (Yerkes & Dodson, 1908). Stress can sometimes improve our performance and, at other times, negatively impact performance. At a basic level, our performance can improve as either physical or mental arousal increases as well…to an extent. When arousal becomes too much, our performance can suffer. Think about the times you've had a test you were nervous about, or you had to give a speech in a public speaking course. These moments may be so anxiety-inducing that it distracts us and interferes with our focus and, as a result, we can't remember needed information, or we stumble over our words. Task complexity and difficulty can impact the relationship between stress and performance. When we are performing an easy task, more anxiety can help us. With difficult or complex tasks, less anxiety is better for us. Additionally, the more familiar we are with a task, the more arousal may benefit us. Think about the musician who walks out on stage and performs incredibly in front of a screaming crowd! For those just learning an instrument they may seem like an impossible feat. For those who have practiced and practiced and practiced though, they may feed off the arousal and excitement and perform so well *because* of their nerves.

The Stress Reactivity Cycle

Stress begins with something that impacts us, and our external environment and internal systems produce a wide variety of stimuli that we perceive through our senses and process via our brain. It is our perception of an event as stressful that causes a response in a brain region called the amygdala, which processes the event as stressful and alerts the hypothalamus to respond. The hypothalamus tells the adrenal glands to release adrenaline, which increases our heart rate, opens our respiration, and sharpens our focus. At the same time, the HPA (hypothalamus–pituitary–adrenal) axis is activated, one result of which is the release of cortisol, which has been called the "stress hormone" because of its release in the stress cycle and because of its pervasive effect on the body. Cortisol is so important to our body's processes that almost all parts of the body have cortisol receptors. Cortisol helps the body manage the deployment of fats, carbohydrates, and protein, suppresses inflammation, regulates blood pressure, and adjusts blood glucose levels. However, cortisol should be a short-term physical solution to an acute stress event. When stress is chronic and cortisol is elevated over time, the result is sub-optimal functioning in several key areas.

What is the difference between reacting to stress and responding to stress? We react automatically rather than respond systematically. The automatic reactivity to stress can cause acute hyper arousal, which can happen often and regularly. When in the midst of acute hyper arousal associated with stress, we can feel a variety of things both mentally and physically, some of which may feel like panic reactions or anxiety or various kinds of bodily distress. This can include racing heartbeat, muscle tightness or weakness, sweating, feeling of impending doom or anxiety, and many more. When hyper arousal as a reaction to stress becomes chronic, we may begin to see its relationship to certain disease processes. This can include high blood pressure, some forms of irritable bowel, insomnia, early waking, back pain, headaches, and more.

Our mental health can also be reactive to the stress hormones, as well as to the cognitive appraisal of the stress itself, resulting in anxiety, depression, insomnia, and so many other symptoms. In turn, these mental health symptoms can become stressors themselves. The ultimate result of the stress cycle, if unresolved, is typically chronic stress. Our evaluation of our own wellness decreases and feelings of distress increase. This leads to feelings of tiredness or exhaustion, general malaise, depression, or adoption of the sick role or even of self-medicating.

Siegel (1999) uses the term "window of tolerance" to describe our typical mental and physiological responses to events around us, including adversity. This window, or optimal arousal zone, is where we function well as our emotions ebb and flow. We are able to effectively deal with daily stress and challenges. At times though, we may experience traumatic events that move us outside of our window and impact our ability to function well. When we are pushed outside of our window, we lose the ability to effectively manage stressors and suffer from overwhelming emotions and intrusive thoughts.

Why We React to Stress Like We Do

There are many different ways that people *could* react to stress, so why does any one person *actually* react the way they do? First, there are genetic effects. Certainly, genetic differences can account for variations in how primed our fight, flight, or freeze response is, in other words, how quickly or slowly we react with fight, flight, or freeze. Temperament, a basic and early disposition toward certain moods and behaviors, likely points us early toward certain patterns of stress reactivity. Our temperament helps determine whether we enjoy being regularly immersed in social activity, if we enjoy skydiving or ziplining, if we are "homebodies," and if we seek change or stability. Each of these is related to whether, how, and with what intensity we react to stress (Akil & Nestler, 2023).

Our life history is also related to our stress response. For example, trauma and abuse history are related to our reactivity to stress. Loss of a parent early in life is related to development of depression later in life, and both parental loss and depression sensitize us and make us vulnerable to stressors throughout life (e.g., Simbi et al., 2020; Slavich et al., 2011). A history of abuse increases likelihood of mental illness symptoms and vulnerability to exacerbation of mental health problems during stressful times. This, in turn, can leave one susceptible to problems in relationships, work, and school and even to re-traumatization. Even the job we choose is related to the psychological, physical, and environmental stress we experience. First responders like police, firefighters, and paramedics and also military personnel collect traumatic experiences of sometimes incomprehensible intensity. This can not only leave them struggling with mental illness symptoms but also leaves them vulnerable to severe exacerbations of symptoms from stressful life events or even day-to-day stressors. However, we don't have to be in the military to have work-related trauma; workers across many job types accumulate traumatic experiences from the workplace, such as abusive bosses or coworkers, workplace accidents, racism, sexism, coworker or client suicide, and coworker or client violence.

Stress from Racism

Racism is a part of our political and public institutions (like housing authorities, voting practices, criminal justice system, and public services), public processes, workplaces, educational institutions, healthcare systems, and economic systems, among others. Every person at one point or another interacts with all of these systems over the course of their lives, and they experience overt or covert discrimination, disparate treatment, microaggressions, and unjust or biased policies and practices. These interactions with the realities of racism in everyday life are associated with a stress reaction called *race-based traumatic stress (RBTS)*. RBTS is experienced when a person's encounters with discrimination, bias, stereotypes, microaggressions, and hate crimes cause them to have physical, mental, and emotional distress and/or injury. The uncontrollable and pervasive nature of negative race-based encounters increases the likelihood of traumatic injury. Like other post-traumatic stress, race-based traumatic stress can result in depression, anxiety, anger, isolation, avoidance, sleep disturbance, and other symptoms. RBTS can be the result of systemic racism, personal experiences, vicarious observations, and/or intergenerational transmission.

Multiple minority stress is the stress experienced by our intersectional identities as members of two or more minority groups, such as being black and LGBT, or disabled, LGBT, and Asian. These multiple and intersecting identities can leave people open to increased social marginalization, stigma, discrimination, and microaggressions. These overlapping stressors compound each other, creating more intense experiences of and reactions to them. Discourse around one identity can also obfuscate another. For example, even physicians and mental health professionals who are trained in culturally competent practice can struggle to adeptly treat a person with multiple minority identities.

The environment can also be a way that our stress responsiveness can increase or be primed. For example, living through a natural disaster or a disaster like a house fire can leave us not only with symptoms of PTSD but also with increased vulnerability to stress over time. When we live in unsafe environments, we are more likely to be a victim of crime and also of repeated offenses. This leaves us primed to react via hypervigilance, insomnia, anxiety, depression, and substance use to the stressors in our environment. Similar reactions to stressors have been found for people living in extreme poverty and for people who are unhoused. Toxic environments, such as those characterized by noise pollution, light pollution, absence of green spaces, and environmental toxins can cause chronic stress and affect our ability to cope with stressful situations.

Our Brain and Body Under Stress

As we discussed in Chap. 1, the brain is one bridge between the mind and the body—it is part of the body and the genesis of the mind and consciousness. Neuroplasticity is the capacity of our nervous system to reorganize and change in response to experience. It is a normal process by which our exposure to environmental conditions such as stress can change our ability to process and cope with those conditions, which can have profound effects on our subsequent behavior, thoughts, and emotions. There are three main ways that stress can affect the brain: (1) Structure, (2) Physical Processes, and (3) Functional Processes.

Structure

Chronic stress can cause changes in the physical structure of the brain, which means that our actual brain architecture changes in response to chronic stress. Chronic stress causes too much "white matter" (the myelin-covered axons) in the brain versus "grey matter" (cell bodies), and also makes the pathway between the amygdala and the hippocampus hardwired and thus more prone to arousal (Chetty et al., 2014). A consistent finding in neuropsychiatry is that the volume of the hippocampus can be reduced by as much as 10% in patients with chronic major depression (Sapolsky, 2000). Additionally, chronic stress can influence the development of Type 2 Diabetes but also have long-term consequences for our cognitive health. Not only is persistent hyperglycemia (high blood sugar) related to stress, but also chronic stress is related to elevated cortisol, which can lead to insulin resistance. Insulin resistance can damage structures in the brain related to cognition, leading to cognitive decline and even dementia states (McEwen, 2017).

Just as an enriched and varied environment can cause beneficial cellular complexity in the brain (Van Praag et al., 2000), stress-filled environments can decrease the number of stem cells that turn into neurons, reducing neuronal density and can kill new brain cells, specifically in the hippocampus (Yassemi & Karalis., 2015).

New brain cells can form in the hippocampus throughout life, and these cells support our memories, some emotions, and our ability to learn new things, yet chronic stress can interrupt this process. Finally, intense, overwhelming, and traumatic stress, such as that associated with PTSD, is related to reduced gray matter in the prefrontal cortex, a region of the brain linked to self-control and emotions (Gold et al., 2016).

Physical Processes

The brain is uniquely able to be both adaptive to and vulnerable to stress. The changes in physical processes associated with stress must be seen in the context of the "dose" of stress, both length and intensity. There is a common saying that "the dose makes the poison," and this is generally true when we think about stress. For example, short-term exposure to certain stress hormones can be helpful and even protective, resulting in what is called allostasis, or the body's and mind's active process of adaptation and returning to homeostasis (balance). However, long-term, intense exposure to stress can be damaging to varying extents to body and mind.

In previous chapters, we reviewed several ways that stress affects the brain and body together, including allostatic load and stress responses. Here, we will give more information on the stress hormones and stress-related inflammation that impact both brain and body. There are several chemicals in the brain, such as neurotransmitters like serotonin, which affect our mood and even the way we think. Chronic stress can alter the processes associated with these chemicals, over time resulting in depressed mood and/or changes in thinking and, particularly, memory (McEwen, 2013).

Inflammation is increasingly being implicated in the development of diseases and disorders of the brain and body. Psychological stress, perceived and modulated by the brain, has been related to poor regulation of the inflammatory process by the immune system because the cellular response to glucocorticoids becomes dysregulated (Cohen et al., 2012). For example, prolonged psychological stress is even implicated in vulnerability to catching colds and subsequent severity and length of illness (Cohen et al., 1991). Autoimmune diseases (like multiple sclerosis and Crohn's disease) are particularly reactive to acute stress, which may activate immune responses like inflammation (McEwen, 2017). There is even some evidence that stress may influence the progression of cancer via the inflammatory response to cancer cells and to cancer treatments (to be clear, however, there is no evidence that stress directly causes cancer) (Eckerling et al., 2021).

Functional Processes

Functional processes are those that demonstrate an ability to perform key life tasks reliably, from daily life tasks like eating, mobility, and bathing to developmental tasks like learning and memory. The structural and physical changes that are related to chronic stress can ultimately result in real-world alterations in functioning. Although stress can have a short-term positive effect in some areas of functioning, such as attention, cognitive processing speed, and recall, at times it can result in a decline in functioning. For example, proliferation of white matter in the brain and reduction in neural volume in key areas of the brain, such as the hippocampus, can make people more vulnerable to mental illness (Abraham et al., 2022), problems with episodic and short-term memory (Kim et al., 2015), and functional symptoms of PTSD (Kim et al., 2015).

Sometimes the result of the impact of stress on brain structure and/or processes is an alteration in functioning. On a casual level, recall back to the time of the novel coronavirus lockdown, when stress was high and typical outlets for stress were restricted. It was easy to observe various anxiety-driven hoarding behaviors, such as amassing large quantities of toilet paper and gasoline. Science has also supported changes in functioning resulting from stress. For example, the rewiring of the neural pathways following chronic stress in the basal forebrain is related to development of addictive behaviors and even compulsive behaviors (Taylor et al., 2014). This helps to explain how stress can facilitate the transition from casual drug use to habitual use—the habit becomes "hardwired" into our brains over time as a result of chronic stress. A final, yet common, example is found with the relationship between stress and disordered executive functioning. Disordered executive functioning impairs our ability to pay attention, manage emotions, organize behaviors, and cope with change. Chronic disordered executive functioning can be seen with diagnoses like ADHD or autism spectrum disorder and can be exacerbated by stress, but short-term disordered executive functioning can also result from stress in people without mental health diagnoses. A likely suspect in how stress relates to impairment of executive functioning is the Hippocampus–Pituitary–Amygdala (HPA) axis and associated release of cortisol (Spencer & Deak, 2017; Tyng et al., 2017).

Health Risks of Chronic Stress

There are many risks to our psychological and physiological health because of chronic stress. Because we are committed to a wellness approach to health, we will list some of the most common stress-related health risks here. Rather than an exhaustive discussion of these risks, in the next few chapters, we will focus on paths of wellness that can help us to mitigate and avoid some of these most common risks:

- Heart disease
- High blood pressure

- Sleep disturbances, such as insomnia and hypersomnia
- Fatigue
- Gastrointestinal distress
- Headaches and migraines
- Weight gain
- Memory and attention problems
- Anxiety and worry
- Depressed mood
- Emotional lability
- Lack of motivation and goal-oriented behavior
- Substance use and abuse

Wow, that's a lot—and this is only a few of the known health consequences of stress. Stress can profoundly impact our ability to live long and fulfilling lives. It benefits us to find ways to proactively stave off stress responses if we can and mitigate our reactivity to stress that we cannot avoid.

- Managing and coping with stress: Managing stress is not simply a matter of avoiding stressors—if it was that easy, no one would be stressed for long. Of course, the reality is that there are many stressors that we simply cannot avoid (work, school, relationships). A stress-reduction plan should not only target the stressor and our reaction to it but also should prepare our minds and bodies to cope with stress in health-promoting ways. Monitoring our bodies, emotions, and thoughts for response to stress and directly intervening with proven techniques is imperative to healthful living. Here are just a few evidence-based techniques to try when inevitable stress happens to us:
  - Identify stress triggers: In order to intervene with our stress, we must first be able to identify what is stressing us out. What worries us, angers us, and makes us upset? This means that we must pay attention to our stress reactions and monitor them closely. For example, it is beneficial to distinguish between internal triggers (like memories or feelings of embarrassment) and external triggers (certain people, places, or situations). In order to improve our capacity to identify triggers, it may be useful to keep a stress journal or use a stress-tracking app.
  - Sleep: Getting sufficient high-quality sleep is a foundation of good health. Poor sleep and not getting enough sleep affects our energy level, brain functioning (such as memory and decision-making), and our gut, heart, and nervous system. Also, remember that alcohol and caffeine consumption directly affect both the quantity and quality of sleep.
  - Relax: Relaxation techniques really do work, but only if people practice them and become competent in their use. For example, progressive relaxation will help to reduce muscle tension and pain. Meditation and yoga can help with cardiovascular symptoms as well as mental clarity and peace. We will learn more about these techniques in upcoming chapters.

- Nurture the self uniquely: Self-care can help prevent reactivity to stress, help us to deal with stress in the moment, and diminish the long-term ramifications of stress. Many, if not most, people are not in the habit of nurturing themselves and may not even be familiar with how to do so. Nurturing the self is not only about providing the basics of living; it is also about providing the enriching and self-affirming experiences that help us develop optimally. We need an enriching environment, some balance of alone and together time, and both support and challenge in order to reach our potential. For some people, music is a proven stress reducer. For others, a quick nap is rejuvenating and increases feelings of wellness. For still others, the social life is where they are most happy and revitalized.

- Eat with health in mind: Food is fuel, but eating well can be complicated. Food is practical, social, emotional, cultural, and many other things. Make a healthful approach to food a priority—this starts in the grocery store or at the menu. There are dietary approaches that have solid science behind them, such as the Mediterranean and DASH (Dietary Approaches to Stop Hypertension) methods. Notice that we are not talking here about "dieting," which is typically focused on calorie or food restriction with the purpose of losing weight. Instead, an approach to food that focuses on wholesome food choices and healthful food preparation is both advantageous and sustainable over time.
- Get moving: Both the physical body and the brain react positively to appropriate exercise. The best thing about exercise is that it is related to lower blood pressure, better average heart rate, and improved emotional state *even when we are not exercising* (Piercy et al., 2018). Exercise is the gift that keeps on giving—both mentally and physically. The good news is that most every movement one can think of can count as exercise, not just sports, going to the gym, or other structured activities, but also walking, yoga, gardening, or even vacuuming. One of the best ways to get our bodies moving is to literally plan it into our day in a manner that is reasonable for us. If "going to the gym" adds stress to our day, we can start out with small changes such as parking a little farther from the door at work or at the grocery store to increase our steps or taking the stairs instead of the elevator.
- Engage with others: A thriving social world and supportive relationships are fundamental to coping with the effects of stress. Even major events—birth, death, loss of job, moving—are made easier through sharing our thoughts and feelings with others. No one makes it through life by themselves, and loneliness makes burdens heavier and more detrimental to our mental health. Relationships that we build and nurture in the good times will help us to withstand life's stresses in the hard times. Also, remember the value of looking outside of ourselves to give of our time and talents to others. The research is clear—volunteering increases our sense of meaning and also perceptions of our mental and physical health (Henney & Hackett, 2019).

Wellness Tip: Laughter

Did you know that laughter really can be the best medicine?

Laughter is how we visibly manifest our feelings of amusement, merriment, and joy (although laughter can sometimes communicate scorn, derision, or nervousness, that's not the laughter we are talking about here). Laughter can be a response to both internal (we can visualize or imagine something funny) or external (we can experience funny things through any sense) cues. Laughter is also social—we tend to like people who "share our sense of humor," and laughing together creates camaraderie and connection.

Gelotology is the study of laughter and how it is related to our mental and physical well-being. The physical benefits of laughter are well known. Laughter activates the autonomic nervous system, with potential cardiovascular benefits (e.g., Fujiwara & Okamura, 2018). Laughter can suppress cortisol and activate the immune system (Kramer & Leitao, 2023), reduce perception of pain (Weisenberg et al., 1998), and induce muscular relaxation and release (Overeem et al., 2004). Preliminary evidence even suggests that laughter can cause changes in brain activity, including release of endogenous opioids (Manninen et al., 2017), which are related to euphoria, pain relief, and positive mood. From a mental and emotional perspective, laughter can reduce distress in social interactions (Monin et al., 2021) and enhance self-reported happiness (Vlahovic et al., 2012). Peterson et al. (2006) argue that humor is an intrinsic strength (which they call a "character strength") in people who deploy it, and it contributes both to physical recovery and a return to subjective well-being.

Since laughter positively affects both body and mind, it is a very attractive therapeutic tool. For such a rich and life-affirming behavior, laughter is inherently simple in its practice—it is free, easy to do, and doesn't require expertise or a specific setting. Nonetheless, these benefits have not stopped the effort to design structured programs designed to use humor as an intervention, such as "humor workshops" and "humor therapy." It is also common to pair laughter with existing wellness techniques, such as "laughter yoga," "laughter meditation," and "laughter wellness." Many of these interventions occur in a group setting, but there is also evidence that online or virtual methods can help increase happiness and, possibly, help to moderate experiences of depression (e.g., Wellenzohn et al., 2016).

It's important to know that you can experience the benefits of laughter without a program or structured intervention. Start this week by paying attention to your laughter—take note of when you laugh, how often you laugh, and how long you laugh. What makes you smile and giggle? What makes you laugh out loud? Who are you with when you laugh? What are you doing? Do you see any trends and patterns? Can you capitalize on opportunities to laugh more? Pinpoint your "laughing strengths," and start laughing for your health!

References

Abraham, M., Mundorf, A., Brodmann, K., & Freund, N. (2022). Unraveling the mystery of white matter in depression: A translational perspective on recent advances. *Brain and Behavior: A Cognitive Neuroscience Perspective, 12*(7), e2629. https://doi.org/10.1002/brb3.2629

Akil, H., & Nestler, E. J. (2023). The neurobiology of stress: Vulnerability, resilience, and major depression. *Proceedings of the National Academy of Sciences of the United States of America, 120*(49), e2312662120. https://doi.org/10.1073/pnas.2312662120

Chetty, S., Friedman, A. R., Taravosh-Lahn, K., Kirby, E. D., Mirescu, C., Guo, F., Krupik, D., Nicholas, A., Geraghty, A. C., Krishnamurthy, A., Tsai, M.-K., Covarrubias, D., Wong, A. T., Francis, D. D., Sapolsky, R. M., Palmer, T. D., Pleasure, D., & Kaufer, D. (2014). Stress and glucocorticoids promote oligodendrogenesis in the adult hippocampus. *Molecular Psychiatry, 19*(12), 1275–1283. https://doi.org/10.1038/mp.2013.190

Cohen, B. E., Edmondson, D., & Kronish, I. M. (2015). State of the art review: Depression, stress, anxiety, and cardiovascular disease. *American Journal of Hypertension, 28*(11), 1295–1302. https://doi.org/10.1093/ajh/hpv047

Cohen, S., Janicki-Deverts, D., Doyle, W. J., Miller, G. E., Frank, E., Rabin, B. S., & Turner, R. B. (2012). Chronic stress, glucocorticoid receptor resistance, inflammation, and disease risk. *Proceedings of the National Academy of Sciences of the United States of America, 109*(16), 5995–5999. https://doi.org/10.1073/pnas.1118355109

Cohen, S., Tyrrell, D. A., & Smith, A. P. (1991). Psychological stress and susceptibility to the common cold. *The New England Journal of Medicine, 325*(9), 606–612. https://doi.org/10.1056/NEJM199108293250903

Eckerling, A., Ricon-Becker, I., & Sorski, L. (2021). Stress and cancer: Mechanisms, significance and future directions. *Nature Reviews. Cancer, 21*(12), 767–785. https://doi.org/10.1038/s41568-021-00395-5

Flink, I. L., Boersma, K., & Linton, S. J. (2013). Pain catastrophizing as repetitive negative thinking: A development of the conceptualization. *Cognitive Behaviour Therapy, 42*(3), 215–223. https://doi.org/10.1080/16506073.2013.769621

Fujiwara, Y., & Okamura, H. (2018). Hearing laughter improves the recovery process of the autonomic nervous system after a stress-loading task: A randomized controlled trial. *BioPsychoSocial Medicine, 12*, 22. https://doi.org/10.1186/s13030-018-0141-0

Gold, A. L., Sheridan, M. A., Peverill, M., Busso, D. S., Lambert, H. K., Alves, S., Pine, D. S., & McLaughlin, K. A. (2016). Childhood abuse and reduced cortical thickness in brain regions involved in emotional processing. *Journal of Child Psychology and Psychiatry, and Allied Disciplines, 57*, 1154–1164. https://doi.org/10.1111/jcpp.12630

Henney, S. M., & Hackett, J. D. (2019). *The development of community engagement from infancy to adulthood.* Routledge.

Kim, E. J., Pellman, B., & Kim, J. J. (2015). Stress effects on the hippocampus: A critical review. *Learning & Memory, 22*(9), 411–416. https://doi.org/10.1101/lm.037291.114

Yassemi, K., & Karalis, K. P. (2015). Neural stem cells respond to stress hormones: Distinguishing beneficial from detrimental stress. *Frontiers in Physiology, 6*, 77. https://doi.org/10.3389/fphys.2015.00077

Kramer, C. K., & Leitao, C. B. (2023). Laughter as medicine: A systematic review and meta-analysis of interventional studies evaluating the impact of spontaneous laughter on cortisol levels. *PLoS One, 18*(5), e0286260. https://doi.org/10.1371/journal.pone.0286260

Lazarus, R. S., & Folkman, S. (1984). *Stress, appraisal, and coping*. Springer.

Manninen, S., Tuominen, L., Dunbar, R. I., Karjalainen, T., Hirvonen, J., Arponen, E., Hari, R., Jääskeläinen, I. P., Sams, M., & Nummenmaa, L. (2017). Social laughter triggers endogenous opioid release in humans. *The Journal of Neuroscience: The Official Journal of the Society for Neuroscience, 37*(25), 6125–6131. https://doi.org/10.1523/JNEUROSCI.0688-16.2017

McEwen, B. S. (2013). The brain on stress: Toward an integrative approach to brain, body, and behavior. *Perspectives on Psychological Science: A Journal of the Association for Psychological Science, 8*(6), 673–675. https://doi.org/10.1177/1745691613506907

McEwen, B. S. (2017). Neurobiological and systemic effects of chronic stress. *Chronic Stress, 1*, 2470547017692328. https://doi.org/10.1177/2470547017692328

Monin, J. K., Feeney, B. C., Tomlinson, J., Levy, B., Clark, M. S., Duker, A., & Gruber, J. (2021). Laughter and short-term blood pressure reactivity in middle-aged and older adult spousal support interactions. *Health Psychology, 40*(11), 764–773. https://doi.org/10.1037/hea0001136

Overeem, S., Taal, W., Ocal Gezici, E., Lammers, G. J., & Van Dijk, J. G. (2004). Is motor inhibition during laughter due to emotional or respiratory influences? *Psychophysiology, 41*(2), 254–258. https://doi.org/10.1111/j.1469-8986.2003.00145.x

Peterson, C., Park, N., & Seligman, M. E. P. (2006). Greater strengths of character and recovery from illness. *The Journal of Positive Psychology, 1*(1), 17–26. https://doi.org/10.1080/17439760500372739

Piercy, K. L., Troiano, R. P., Ballard, R. M., Carlson, S. A., Fulton, J. E., Galuska, D. A., George, S. M., & Olson, R. D. (2018). The physical activity guidelines for Americans. *JAMA, 320*(19), 2020–2028. https://doi.org/10.1001/jama.2018.14854

Sapolsky, R. M. (2000). The possibility of neurotoxicity in the hippocampus in major depression: A primer on neuron death. *Biological Psychiatry, 48*, 755–765. https://doi.org/10.1016/s0006-3223(00)00971-9

Sareen, J., Cox, B. J., Stein, M. B., Afifi, T. O., Fleet, C., & Asmundson, G. J. G. (2007). Physical and mental comorbidity, disability, and suicidal behavior associated with posttraumatic stress disorder in a large community sample. *Psychosomatic Medicine, 69*, 242–248. https://doi.org/10.1097/PSY.0b013e31803146d8

Siegel, D. J. (1999). *The developing mind: Toward a neurobiology of interpersonal experience*. Guilford Press.

Simbi, C. M. C., Zhang, Y., & Wang, Z. (2020). Early parental loss in childhood and depression in adults: A systematic review and meta-analysis of case-controlled studies. *Journal of Affective Disorders, 260*, 272–280. https://doi.org/10.1016/j.jad.2019.07.087

Slavich, G. M., Monroe, S. M., & Gotlib, I. H. (2011). Early parental loss and depression history: Associations with recent life stress in major depressive disorder. *Journal of Psychiatric Research, 45*(9), 1146–1152. https://doi.org/10.1016/j.jpsychires.2011.03.004

Spencer, R. L., & Deak, T. (2017). A users guide to HPA axis research. *Physiology & Behavior, 178*, 43–65. https://doi.org/10.1016/j.physbeh.2016.11.014

Taylor, S. B., Anglin, J. M., Paode, P. R., Riggert, A. G., Olive, M. F., & Conrad, C. D. (2014). Chronic stress may facilitate the recruitment of habit- and addiction-related neurocircuitries through neuronal restructuring of the striatum. *Neuroscience, 280*, 231–242. https://doi.org/10.1016/j.neuroscience.2014.09.029

Tyng, C. M., Amin, H. U., Saad, M. N. M., & Malik, A. S. (2017). The influences of emotion on learning and memory. *Frontiers in Psychology, 8*, 1454. https://doi.org/10.3389/fpsyg.2017.01454

Van Praag, H., Kempermann, G., & Gage, F. H. (2000). Neural consequences of environmental enrichment. *Nature Reviews. Neuroscience, 1*(3), 191–198. https://doi.org/10.1038/35044558

Vlahovic, T. A., Roberts, S., & Dunbar, R. (2012). Effects of duration and laughter on subjective happiness within different modes of communication. *Journal of Computer-Mediated Communication, 17*(4), 436–450. https://doi.org/10.1111/j.1083-6101.2012.01584.x

Weisenberg, M., Raz, T., & Hener, T. (1998). The influence of film-induced mood on pain perception. *Pain, 76*(3), 365–375. https://doi.org/10.1016/S0304-3959(98)00069-4

Wellenzohn, S., Proyer, R. T., & Ruch, W. (2016). Humor-based online positive psychology interventions: A randomized placebo-controlled long-term trial. *The Journal of Positive Psychology, 11*(6), 584–594. https://doi.org/10.1080/17439760.2015.1137624

Yerkes, R. M., & Dodson, J. D. (1908). The relation of strength of stimulus to rapidity of habit-formation. *Journal of Comparative Neurology and Psychology, 18*, 459–482. https://doi.org/10.1002/cne.920180503

Chapter 7
Key Topics in Mind-Body Wellness, Part 1

The body hears everything the mind says
-Anonymous

Our brain and physical body are uniquely constructed to be responsive to our environment—the food and nutrition environment, the presence of health-promoting resources, the presence of health-harming toxins, and physical and mental stressors. Our brain has a characteristic called neuroplasticity, which allows it to grow and adapt as we are exposed to new experiences and stimuli and even in response to stress. In other words, our brain can change in both structures via new neural connections and in function throughout our lives. The path toward wellness undoubtedly involves exposing ourselves to new experiences, environments, knowledge, and people in order to provide our brains with ample opportunities to flourish and mature.

Traditionally, there has been a disproportionate focus on the role of physical health in wellness. This focus has been in contradiction with the direction in which the wellness field is moving, toward mind/body wellness and a whole-person approach to well-being. In this chapter, we will delve into several topics—nutrition, diet, and exercise—that have traditionally been associated with physical wellness, but we will take a different approach to them. These traditional physical topics will be presented from a scientific, anti-pseudoscience perspective, and will include a whole-person approach rather than a narrow focus on physical health.

S. M. Henney, J. D. Hackett, *Mind-Body Wellness*,
https://doi.org/10.1007/978-3-031-91611-3_7

Nutrition

Nutrients

Nutrients are the building blocks of a healthy body and mind. Nutrients fuel our growth and enable us to maintain day-to-day health and repair bodily systems when necessary. There are six fundamental nutrients for optimal human functioning: proteins, carbohydrates, fats, vitamins, minerals, and water. In addition to water, nutrients come in two general forms, macronutrients and micronutrients.

Macronutrients

Macronutrients (also called macros) are proteins, carbohydrates, and fats, which our bodies need in relatively high amounts on a regular basis. Macronutrients fuel our bodily processes, such as growth, repair, and reproduction, and we rely on them for both the energy for and the essential components of these processes. As an example of the importance of macronutrients, the adult brain weighs about 3 pounds, but its energy needs far exceed its relatively small size, as it consumes about 20% of the body's energy usage. An adult needs about 1600 to 2200 calories a day to maintain functioning, depending on age and activity level, which means that it takes between 320 and 440 calories just to think every day.

Proteins have many functions in the body, which include structure, function, and regulation of body processes. Structurally, proteins are the building blocks of cells, muscles, bones, and the immune system. Proteins also regulate the expressions of our genes and generate biochemical reactions through the action of enzymes in the digestive, circulatory, reproductive, and nervous systems. It is not too extreme to say that enzymes run and control our bodies, and they cannot be manufactured without protein sources. Carbohydrates provide energy and fuel for the body, as they are broken down into simple sugars (glucose) in the digestive system. Glucose is used for energy or stored in the liver and muscles or converted to fat. Carbohydrates have a bad reputation in popular culture, particularly relative to weight and metabolism, but high-fiber carbohydrates have an important role in maintaining a healthy body (Blaak et al., 2021). Like carbohydrates, dietary fat provides energy for the body to function. Additionally, dietary fats help to build cell membranes, insulate neurons, absorb vitamins A, D, E, and K, and manufacture and metabolize hormones.

Protein Bars, Drinks, and Powders
People desire added protein in their diet for a variety of reasons. Sometimes people need an easy and portable snack or to replace a meal. Vegans and vegetarians might need extra protein if they are strength/endurance athletes or in certain cases when they are ill or are pregnant or lactating. However, not all protein supplements are created equal:

- Some products can have lots of added sugar, sodium, and fat. Carefully analyze the nutrition label and choose products with the least added sugar (particularly high fructose corn syrup), sodium, and fat.
- Some products have too much protein relative to other macronutrients. Aim for protein supplements with 10–25 g of protein, with fiber to increase the sensation of fullness.
- Overdoing protein can cause constipation. Make sure to drink a lot of water and increase fiber as protein is being increased.
- Many protein products qualify as ultra processed, meaning they have refined proteins as well as additives like emulsifiers. Try to choose products with whole ingredients, such as fruits, whole grains, nuts, and seeds.

A popular way of monitoring nutritional goals is counting macros, which means tracking how much of each macro—protein, carbs, and fats—is being consumed. In many ways, counting macros is the same idea as counting calories; the key difference is that counting macros accounts for where calories come from. Typically, a diet consisting of 20–30% protein, 40–50% carbohydrates, and 20–30% fat is considered reasonable. However, a person's ideal macro ratio is individual to their goals, and the amount of each macro should complement their lifestyle, health status, and activity level (Cai et al., 2022).

Micronutrients

Micronutrients (also called micros) are the vitamins and minerals that support the body's processes and are essential for optimal functioning, disease prevention, and day-to-day wellness. Vitamins are organic—they are made by plants and animals—whereas minerals are inorganic and originate in the earth or water. Some of the most common micronutrients in the body are the minerals sodium, calcium, potassium (K), iron, and magnesium. Water-soluble vitamins (like B vitamins and C) are not stored in the body and must be consumed regularly, whereas fat-soluble vitamins (like A, D, E, and K) are stored in the body in the presence of dietary fat. A varied diet that features choices from all of the macros and includes fruits and vegetables, lean meats, poultry, and fish, low-fat dairy, and whole grains will provide all of the vitamins and minerals that most people require.

This means that for healthy adults with a varied diet, supplementation is usually not required. There are, however, some notable exceptions. Vegetarian and vegan diets can have some nutrient concerns centering around vitamins and minerals found abundantly in meat and dairy products, including B12, D, and Omega-3 fatty acids (Craig et al., 2021). These potential deficiencies can be overcome by supplementation or dietary changes. Pregnant women can help support a healthy pregnancy and infant with a supplement that specifically includes iron and folate. Finally, older people can have deficiencies based on aging, such as poor absorption or reduced variety of foods, as well as specific deficiencies, such as lower vitamin D because less time is spent outdoors.

Herbal products (also called herbal supplements, botanicals, or phytomedicines) are plant-based products used as capsules, powders, liquids, teas, lotions, gels, or in the bath or shower. The use of herbal remedies and wellness elixirs dates back to early human history, and herbs are still used today in many traditional medicine preparations. They are different from conventional supplements, in that the FDA considers them food, so they are not as well-regulated in terms of testing, purity, and labeling as supplements. Some of the herbs in common use are described in Table 7.1, although this is just a selection of the many herbs that have been used for human health and wellness purposes. Never start taking a new herb without

Table 7.1 Common herbal preparations: possible uses and risks

Herb	Delivery method	Possible uses[a]	Risks
Aloe vera	– Lotion, gel	– Skincare	– Skin irritation
		– Burns, sunburn	– Allergic reaction
	– Juice, latex	– Inflammation	– Drug interactions
		– Diabetes	– Stomach upset
			– Diarrhea
Chamomile	– Tea	– Relaxation	– Drug interactions
		– Anti-stress	
	– Compress	– Inflammation	– Skin irritation
	– Lotion, oil		– Allergic reaction
Echinacea	– Tea	– Infections, particularly colds	– Stomach upset
	– Capsule		– Headache
	– Lotion	– Inflammation	– Allergic reaction
Garlic	– Food	– Reduce cholesterol	– Odor
	– Capsule	– Reduce blood pressure	– Heartburn
			– Bleeding
Ginger	– Tea	– Nausea and vomiting	– Stomach upset
	– Food		– Heartburn
	– Candy/ gummy		
Green tea	– Tea	– Cognition	– Digestive issues
		– Weight management	– Caffeine-related symptoms (racing heart, headache)
		– Heart disease markers	
	– Lotion, oil	– Inflammation	– Skin irritation
		– Aging/wrinkles	
		– Antioxidant	
Turmeric	– Food	– Inflammation	– Stomach upset
	– Capsule	– Reduce joint pain	– Kidney stones
		– Antioxidant	– Reduce the effect of some pain relievers

[a] No herb listed has clear, evidence-based effects substantiated by multiple high-quality studies. All should be used at dosages recommended by a physician, and none should be used by pregnant or lactating women without supervision by a doctor

consulting a physician. Most herbs that have any effect on the human body and mind have side effects that can increase with dose or delivery method, and all have the potential to interact with other herbs and/or medications.

The supplement industry is a money-making machine, with over $200 billion in worldwide sales, but it is poorly regulated and potential quality problems around dosing and purity are of great concern (Cadwallader, 2022). It is important to practice discernment in choosing supplements, paying close attention to supply chain, quality, and brand name. We should be wary of advertisements, social media influencers, and even people we know who "oversell" the benefits of supplements, remembering that any supplement that promises beauty, anti-aging, slim physique, to cure disease(s), or to "protect the brain" needs to be evaluated with a critical lens.

"Primal" and "Ancestral" Vitamins

"Primal" and "Ancestral" vitamins are dietary supplements made from the organs and tissues of grassfed, antibiotic-free, and free-range animals. Organs and fluids like blood, liver, heart, and spleen are freeze-dried and constructed in pill form. The philosophy behind this product is that our ancestors were more vigorous, energetic, and healthy than us, and ancestral vitamins represent a return to nature and wholesome, sustainable living. The problem is that our ancestors did not enjoy a vital, long life—in fact, they lived sicker, more dangerous lives with shorter lifespans than we enjoy today (life expectancy was about 35–40 in the Bronze Age (5000 BC) and only reached 50 by the end of the nineteenth century).

"Primal" and "Ancestral" vitamins are part of the "nature is always healthy" and "live like our ancestors" pseudoscience craze. While the importance of a diet rich in a variety of whole foods is clear, this is not necessarily the diet that most of our ancestors ate. Our ancestors intermittently had very poor diets, and they had many food-related risks, including food-borne illness, vitamin and mineral deficiencies, and high saturated fat levels. The biggest issue, however, is the lack of any substantive evidence that ancestral vitamins have any of the claimed health benefits, such as "detoxification" and improved digestion, immunity, and metabolic functioning. Instead, people who take ancestral vitamins may experience upset stomach, diarrhea, vitamin and iron overload, rashes, and, in rare cases, liver damage and vitamin A or copper toxicity. Pregnant and nursing women should not take ancestral vitamins, and everyone should speak with their healthcare provider before starting new supplements.

For healthy adults, there is no known benefit to "superdosing" any vitamin or mineral. For those with specific deficiencies, health conditions, or diagnoses, the appropriate supplementation is based on if the micronutrient is water or fat-soluble and the person's age, weight, and health condition(s). Vitamin and mineral toxicity is possible with excessive supplement use, particularly for the fat-soluble vitamins since they accumulate in the body. Vitamin A toxicity, for example, can cause nausea, headache, intracranial pressure, and even coma and death. There is a saying that "the poison is in the dose," meaning that anything can become toxic if we ingest enough of it (this is true for everything—even vitamins and even water!). Thus, it is healthy for both body and mind for us to be prudent about supplement use.

Vitamins and Drip Bars

Drip bars are a wellness marketing concept which encourages customers to purchase an intravenous infusion of vitamins, electrolytes, and other nutrients within a boutique or spa-like atmosphere. A popular drip is called a "Myers' cocktail," which was developed by Dr. John Myers more than 50 years ago to help support patients who presented with a variety of symptoms. The Myers cocktail, its derivatives, and other IV products are widely popular but have little science behind them. The "studies" of wellness IV cocktails are largely anecdotal or of dubious quality.

These drips (also called IV vitamin therapy) are advertised to improve health and wellness in a variety of ways, including as an anti-aging treatment, to "boost immunity," reduce stress, eliminate hangovers, or to reduce the effects of food poisoning and jet lag. However, there are also claims that IV vitamin therapy can address health conditions like fibromyalgia, pain, allergies, migraines, asthma, infections, premenstrual syndrome, depression, and anxiety. It is very unlikely that any treatment, even our most advanced therapies, can have such far-reaching effects—Remember that anything that promises to cure everything is most likely pseudoscience.

The best candidates for IV Vitamin Therapy are people who are unable to eat (due to illness or injury), who have a condition that prevents absorption of nutrients or vitamin pills (such as cystic fibrosis or inflammatory bowel disease), who are severely dehydrated from overexertion or illness, or who have specific (confirmed) vitamin deficiencies. Risks of the drip bar concept are largely to the pocketbook—these are expensive procedures marketed by a for-profit business. Furthermore, the industry is not well-regulated, and IV Vitamin Therapy is not without medical risks, such as IV infiltration, drug interactions (such as magnesium with antihypertensives), overdosing on specific ingredients, nerve damage, low blood pressure, and fluid overload (Shane-McWhorter, 2024). Anyone considering IV Vitamin Therapy should consult with their healthcare provider first to discuss risks and benefits.

Diet and Dieting

A Healthful Diet

The word "diet" is used in so many ways that it can be hard to discern what is. A diet is what and how much a person eats; in other words, it is the type and quantity of food we ingest. A good diet is based on a practice of eating healthful foods at the right times in appropriate amounts while avoiding toxins and ultra-processed foods. The U.S. Department of Health and Human Services, Office of Disease Prevention and Health Promotion (2024) publishes dietary guidelines designed to provide direction on "what to eat and drink to meet nutrient needs, promote health, and prevent disease." Herman et al. (2022) designed a simulation that projected what the benefits would be 30 years into the future if Americans followed these dietary guidelines. The study found that following the guidelines could reduce heart disease (the largest mortality source of Americans) by about 10% and save almost $60 billion in healthcare costs (Herman et al., 2022). The benefits to our society and to us as individuals of a better approach to food are palpable. Wellness across all domains rests on appropriately fueling one's body and providing the foundation for growth, repair, and reproduction. A healthful diet has several hallmarks:

Variety: A healthful diet includes a range of foods, including fresh and whole foods.

Macronutrients: Carbohydrates, proteins, and fats are included in proportions that support energy, growth, and maintenance needs.

Micronutrients: Vitamins and minerals, especially those the body doesn't manufacture, are included in the food choices.

Calories: The calories ingested every day are matched to energy needs, age, and activity level.

Reasonable limits on established risk factors: Limit intake of salt, saturated and trans-fats, refined sugar, and alcohol.

Hydration: Drink enough simple water to stay hydrated, based on climate and activity level. Sugar-sweetened or artificially sweetened drinks have little dietary value.

How to Identify a Fad Diet

We do not need to drink pickle juice and eat cauliflower rice to be healthy. Many of the diet fads that we hear about—cleanses, supplements, unique food combinations, food group restrictions—do not make us more well, but they do make us feel like we are actively and purposefully trying to improve our wellness. Too much wellness spending is in the "why not try it" category, rather than the "it has legitimate research supporting it" category. Is this useful to us? Perhaps, as long as the diet fad is not actively dangerous, and it doesn't take the place of a healthier alternative. It's also important to note that just because a diet or foods trend on social media doesn't mean they are fads. Some culturally relevant foods and drinks like Yuzu, kimchi, Yerba mate, and Kombucha tea will trend on social media and can be an interesting and healthful addition to a diet.

Fad diets tend to be extremely restrictive and have rigid rules about acceptable foods, supplements, and additives. In particular, they will eliminate certain foods or food groups, ban specific ingredients, label a certain food or food group as harmful and dangerous, and have a list of acceptable vs unacceptable foods. Remember that what we include in our diet is just as or more important than what we exclude. Fad diets always exaggerate the benefits of the diet, promising weight loss with little effort, to cure diseases or eliminate symptoms, and that this diet will work when nothing else has.

Almost all proponents of fad diets will end up trying to sell us something, often a product that is very expensive or increasingly expensive over time. Additionally, when we start to figure out that the budget-breaking supplements or foods aren't working, more products are added on, increasing our monetary commitment. Fad diets and associate supplements and products rely on the sunk-cost fallacy for continued expenditures, meaning that people are reluctant to give up on something that they have invested heavily in; they would rather continue to double down on their spending even when they know they are not realizing the weight loss or health gains they expected. The fact is that fad diets, products, plans, and supplements often produce weight loss in the short term when motivation is high, but many people (not all) regain the weight regardless of diet type (e.g., Anderson et al., 2001). Remember, if it sounds too good to be true, it probably is.

Most fad diets have risks, most of which are undisclosed when people are discussing the diet. Some of the common risks are dehydration and intestinal difficulties (like constipation or diarrhea), as well as hunger and fatigue. If practiced rigorously for a long time, some fad diets can even negatively impact our organs, metabolism, or other body functions. Fad diets can also have mental health risks, such as guilt, anxiety, and frustration around food choices and setbacks in adherence to the diet. As depicted in Fig. 7.1, this results in people feeling bad about themselves in relation to the diet, which can lead to self-blame, negative body image, and return to the diet cycle with a new fad diet.

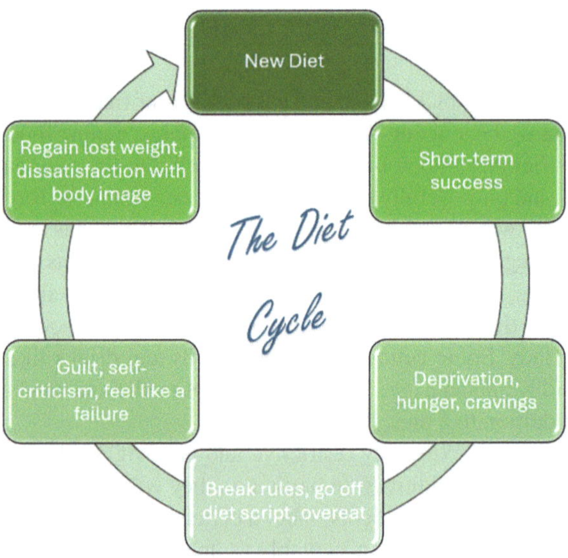

Fig. 7.1 The diet cycle

Dieting and Diet Culture

Dieting refers to a restrictive and often temporary eating plan, typically for the purpose of losing weight or maintaining a thin physique. There is dieting advice everywhere, from the doctor's office to social media, and while some of the advice is well-meaning and some are even evidence-based, most modern dieting advice is provided for the purpose of clicks, likes, marketing, and product sales. The only way to lose weight is to consume fewer calories than are expended or burned (a calorie is a unit of energy provided to the body by food). This is called a calorie deficit. People do not want to believe this is true, as calorie deficits are hard to accomplish and maintain, but it is true at every stage of life. It is difficult to design a calorie-deficit eating plan while still feeling full and fulfilled by food, but it is possible. Food is key to weight loss—avoiding most calorie-dense, sugary, ultra-processed foods and instead choosing foods that have a balanced mix of protein, carbs, and fat, as well as necessary fiber and nutrients. Foods that are "calorie deficit killers" when used in excess (no one is telling us not to cook with a small amount of oil), include:

- Fatty meats, including poultry with skin.
- Oils, particularly vegetable oils like corn oil.
- Refined carbs (white bread, white rice, white pasta, granola, sugary cereals).
- Sugary drinks (regular soda, juice, sports/energy drinks).
- Fried foods (chips, doughnuts, fried chicken).
- Full-fat dairy (milk, some yogurts, ice cream).
- Alcohol.

Even though a calorie deficit is necessary for weight loss, this does not equate to weight loss being a valuable, worthy, or even important goal for any particular individual. Goals around weight loss and body size should be personal and reflect one's own values, wants, and needs. Unfortunately, we live in a society where critical and negative attitudes and beliefs about thin vs fat bodies and the "right" way to eat abound. Diet culture is the embodiment of our cultural fixation on thinness and dieting; it reflects societal expectations about appropriate weight and a social disdain for fat bodies. Diet culture assumes that there is some moral superiority to being thin, that the scale dictates worth, and, above all, that being thin equals being healthy and attractive. Signs that diet culture is at work include restrictive food rules that often include eliminating whole food groups, labeling food as "good" vs "bad" or "clean" or "real," exercise for "gains" and not for joy or uplift, and body shaming. These aspects of diet culture can lead to disordered eating and an unhealthy relationship with both food and one's own body. Diet culture encourages us to be judgmental and ugly to others around weight and food choices.

Mind-Body Approaches to Eating

There is no type of diet that is inherently healthy. Whether people choose to eat meat or not, follow a popular diet plan, or take a bunch of supplements does not indicate that they are eating a high-quality diet. Indeed, it is possible to have a low-quality plant-based diet and a high-quality meat-based diet and, of course, vice-versa (Thomas et al., 2023). What mind-body methods bring to the issue of diet and nutrition is an approach or a mindset about food that is different from traditional diets. We will review some of these techniques here.

Mindful Eating

Mindful eating is an approach to eating that centers on the physiological and psychological experience of eating. The goal is to turn "mindless eating" into a purposeful and mindful act. This approach is meant to not only characterize eating as a pleasant, wholesome, and natural process, but it also encourages awareness of what is right for one's unique body and mind. It encourages a new relationship with food, one that should make us feel well in mind and body. Mindful eating typically has the following components:

Slow down: Practice mindful enjoyment of food and drinks by relaxing into eating. It takes time for our brain and body to realize we are full, and slowing down helps to identify and listen to satiety cues.

Be fully aware: Savor each bite or sip, noticing the taste, texture, and overall flavor through our five taste senses (sweet, sour, salty, bitter, and umami). Digestion starts with chewing, so chew each bite with intent to understand and enjoy.

Notice what our body is saying: We typically feel like we should eat when we are fatigued, have a headache, feel hunger, or have a rumbling stomach, but do we always stop when we feel full and satisfied? These are our body's cues to eat or stop eating.

Practice a compassionate and nonjudgmental approach: We can quiet the outer and inner food noise by connecting with our food and how it nourishes our body instead of the messages, marketing, and self-criticism that surrounds food.

Create an eating space: Mindful eating discourages multitasking while eating, and instead suggests that creating an intentional time and space for eating without distractions (i.e., turn off the TV, step away from work, etc.) improves our ability to pay attention to the experience of eating.

Intuitive Eating

Intuitive eating has many of the same components as mindful eating, but it much more clearly centers self-care, self-compassion, and listening to our body and mind (Tribole & Resch, 2020). The first pillar of intuitive eating is the rejection of diet culture and dieting, which contributes to unhealthy and disordered eating. There are no "right" foods, right time to eat, or right amount of calories to consume, according to this philosophy. Instead, intuitive eating at its core is about eating when we are hungry (whenever that is) and stopping when we are full. Specifically, intuitive eating equips people to reject the negative messages surrounding food and to embrace the body and mind's wisdom about when and how much to eat. However, in order to do this, one must learn to listen to the hunger cues of the body and mind. In intuitive eating, one learns to identify the actual cues of hunger and to notice and dismiss the other cues (advertisement, boredom, sensory cues like smells, and social cues like family dinners or other people eating). Weight loss is not necessarily the goal of intuitive eating (although it can happen), but rather the goal is developing a healthy relationship with food and a positive body image. Indeed, honoring our body regardless of shape, size, ability, or age is a core belief of intuitive eating. Some practices of intuitive eating include:

Hunger awareness: Becoming aware of emotional and physical triggers for hunger and learning to pay attention to the cues that signal a true hunger state. We should not eat if we are not hungry, even if it is "time to eat."

Fullness awareness: It is often difficult to stop eating, especially if there is food left on the plate/in the container. Learning to monitor the body's cues (fullness, decreased appetite, less interest) and the mind's cues (satisfaction, feeling "done") by slowing down and paying attention can help.

Develop nonfood coping mechanisms: Emotions can trigger eating, so learning how to cope with negative emotions through social interactions, going out into nature, or mindfulness is an important part of intuitive eating. Being content and fulfilled is a whole-person endeavor and does not only have to do with food.

Holistic Nutrition (Also Called Holistic Eating)

Holistic nutrition is an approach that considers the whole person—body, mind, lifestyle, and environment—when choosing how, when, and what to eat. Holistic nutrition doesn't only focus on food, because this method emphasizes the interconnectivity of mind and body as the locus of action and includes lifestyle and healthy living coaching in concert with healthy eating. This way of approaching nutrition also emphasizes incorporating stress management, mindfulness, self-care, and a growth mindset into our daily activities. Like the other mind-body techniques, holistic nutrition promotes diets rich in whole foods that are minimally processed, the avoidance of additives and preservatives, and a mindful approach to the body's hunger and satiety cues and typical eating patterns. Some holistic nutritionists focus on the relationship of diet to problematic physical and mental symptoms or to specific disorders, such as autism spectrum disorders, diabetes, and autoimmune disorders. While diet, approached from a whole-person perspective, may be able to help manage certain symptoms, clients must be wary of holistic nutrition advice that follows the "food-as-medicine" perspective, which oversells the possible benefits of dietary interventions and often excludes conventional medicine altogether. However, if we desire a planful way to approach food that takes into account our self-concept, our lifestyle, and our environment, then holistic nutrition may be an avenue to explore.

Health at Every Size (HAES)

HAES is an approach that opposes a traditional focus on weight and weight loss and instead focuses on healthy living and body positivity (Association for Size Diversity and Health, 2024). In essence, this approach is about discovering health, not losing weight, and aims to combat the stigma, self-judgment, and exclusion that occurs for people in larger bodies. In addition to advocating for size inclusivity and respect for all bodies generally in society and in healthcare in particular, HAES emphasizes building healthy eating and movement habits instead of a hyperfocus on weight. The HAES perspective asks us to examine whether our purpose is to encourage and support healthful behaviors or to punish fatness? Although this approach requires more study, it does have potential to alter the way we think about weight and health and the way we approach healthy living interventions and programming for people of all sizes (Penney & Kirk, 2015).

Plant-Based Diets

The most well-known plant-based diets are vegan and vegetarian diets. A vegan diet features no animal products of any kind, whereas a traditional lacto-ovo-vegetarian diet excludes meats, fish, and seafood, but typically allows dairy and eggs. Vegan and vegetarian diets are often perceived as mindful diets. Veganism, in particular, reflects a philosophy of thoughtful, intentional food choices and compassion for animals in all aspects of lifestyle (not just food). Plant-based diets are actually the most common diets worldwide and are more sustainable, requiring less land, water, and energy resources than meat-forward diets (Pimentel & Pimentel, 2003). In addition to a sustainability-focused lifestyle, plant-based diets seem to have notable health benefits, including lowered cholesterol (Wang et al., 2015), reduced risk of cardiovascular disease (Kim et al., 2019), decreased inflammatory markers and body weight (Thomas et al., 2023), and preventing and treating Type 2 diabetes (McMacken & Shah, 2017). It is interesting to consider that some studies have found that plant-based diets are related to depression in adults, but this is a complicated finding with some contradictory evidence, indicating that further research is needed (Jain et al., 2022). It is worth noting that, like all specialized diets, vegan and vegetarian diets are not inherently healthy, and vegan and vegetarian diet quality can vary extensively. These diets require careful, purposeful planning if one is going to cover the micros and macros necessary for a thriving body and mind.

The Myth of Detox and Cleanses

The human body has two sources of toxins, those originating in the body like urea and lactic acid (called endotoxins), and those whose source is outside of the body like chemicals, pesticides, and pollutants (called exotoxins). If a person believes their body is being overwhelmed by toxins, they might be tempted to buy products or supplements and engage in cleanses or detox diets. Such products and programs promise a wide range of benefits, from fighting fatigue, migraines, pain, digestive troubles, and inflammation to guaranteeing effortless weight loss.

The good news is that the body has a built-in detoxification system—The liver is specially designed to detoxify the body, and it is good at it! Other organs also assist in detoxification, such as the skin (the largest organ), lungs, and kidneys. This doesn't mean that we can eat, drink, and breathe in any toxin with no effect; too much of any toxin can overwhelm our natural detoxification processes. However, this would typically be a medical emergency or be associated with a known treatment of proven effectiveness. Furthermore, the first step to addressing an extreme toxic exposure is not to get a cleanse, it is to remove the toxin from the person's environment immediately.

The detoxes and cleanses are not without risk. Some call for fasting (including water or juice fasting), reduction to one food or type of food, herbs, teas, or supplements, and others call for sweating, intensive exercise, and even laxatives and enemas. In addition to the high cost of some of these products, the physical risks of these measures can include dehydration, digestive issues, electrolyte imbalances, metabolic acidosis, and disruption of intestinal flora. There is little evidence that cleanses and detoxes can lead to long-term weight loss, although brief water-weight loss can occur.

We can help our organs, particularly our liver, effectively clear both endogenous and exogenous toxins by taking these steps:

- Stay well hydrated, as dehydration stresses the liver and other organs, making it difficult to clear toxins.
- Limit fatty and fried foods which, when eaten in excess, can lead to fatty liver.
- Wear sunscreen, don't smoke, and be prudent about alcohol intake. Alcohol itself is a toxin that people who partake voluntarily add to their body, and overuse is legitimately bad for all body systems.
- Eat a balanced diet and exercise regularly as part of a healthy lifestyle.

Food Quality

"Avoid processed food" is advice that almost everyone has heard, and "I don't eat processed food" is a type of virtue signaling around food that is also common. The problem with these statements is that *all* agriculturally based food that is purchased in a store is processed, some more so than others, via washing, cleaning, cutting, heating, and even packaging. What we really desire is minimally processed foods, which doesn't substantially change the nutritional value of the food item, such as washing carrots or steel-cutting oats. Normally processed foods may have a higher level of processing or added ingredients, but still retain most of their nutritional value, such as pasteurizing raw milk or canning vegetables. On the other hand, we should look carefully at our consumption of ultra-processed foods, which are foods that have been substantially altered to include or are wholly made from starches, fats, and sugars derived from other foods (like high fructose corn syrup or carrageenan) and tend to include preservatives, artificial flavor and/or color, and lots of salt. More than 70% of packaged food and drink sold in the US qualifies as ultra-processed (Baldridge et al., 2019). Many of us have gotten so used to the taste and texture of ultra-processed chips, chicken nuggets, lunch meat, soft drinks, sweetened juice, canned soups, and hot dogs and sausages that less-processed alternatives don't taste as good to us and can have an unpalatable "mouth feel".

Ultra-processed food consumption can raise the risk of a variety of negative health outcomes, such as high blood pressure, heart disease, Type 2 diabetes, and even certain types of cancer (Lane et al., 2024). For example, in a large study of food consumption and health status, Wang et al. (2022) found a 29% higher risk of colorectal cancer among men who consumed the highest amount of ultra-processed foods. Limiting intake of ultra-processed foods is a valid and science-based approach to healthier nutrition. One way to do this is to become educated on how to read food labels. American Heart Association (2023) suggests:

1. Understand what the serving size is for the product.
2. Find both calories per serving and per container and consider how these fit into total daily intake.
3. Check trans fats, saturated fats, sugars, and sodium. Avoid trans fats if possible and limit the others.
4. Look for the daily value (%DV) calculation of beneficial nutrients and use the "5–20 rule" to evaluate it. The product is low in a nutrient if the %DV is 5% or less, and it is high in a nutrient if the %DV is 20% or more (based on a 2000-calorie diet).

When looking at the ingredients list, check the order first, as ingredients will be listed by weight in descending order. Then look for allergens, added sugar (can be called many things, like dextrose, fructose, brown rice syrup, and high-fructose corn syrup), and other additives. Remember, however, that just because something is a chemical (or has a chemical-sounding name) does not mean it is inherently toxic or harmful. For example, words like Pyridoxine (vitamin B6), Acetic Acid (Vinegar), Ascorbyl palmitate (fat-soluble vitamin C), and steviol glycosides (sweetener from the stevia plant) sound "bad for you," but are actually good (or at least neutral). A good rule of thumb is to choose products with the shortest possible list of ingredients. For example, bread could be just flour, water, salt, and yeast, and pasta just flour and water (or flour, water, and eggs), but bread and pasta found on the grocery shelves typically have added emulsifiers (to prevent separation of ingredients) and preservatives (to keep items fresh longer). Thus, when shopping it is useful to compare different brands for the product and choose the one that most closely meets both dietary and financial needs.

Organic Foods

The increase in demand for organic foods is tied to the rise in consumer health consciousness and the desire to avoid normally- and ultra-processed foods. According to the Pew Research Center (2016), typical consumers believe that organic produce is more healthful than conventionally grown produce, and the overwhelming majority of those who purchase organic foods do so for health reasons. However, the actual health benefits of organic-labeled foods are not entirely clear. There are some directly observable differences from conventionally farmed foods, such as a reduction in heavy metals and pesticide residues, and higher concentrations of antioxidants (e.g., Barański et al., 2014), though this is not consistent across all organic-labeled foods.

Organic and natural are not the same thing, despite what consumers may believe, and there are different levels of organic food labeling. For example, the "USDA Organic" label means that the food must contain 95% organic content, whereas the "made with organic" label only needs 70% organic content. Also, there are many myths and misunderstandings related to organic products and farming processes (e.g., Paarlberg, 2021). Organic farmers also use pesticides, albeit ones "labeled" as natural, that can include copper sulfate which accumulates in the soil. Compost, which is a primary fertilizer and soil conditioner on organic farms, has a massive carbon footprint. There are concerns related to the expense of organic food, as well as the more intensive methods required to efficiently farm clean, edible food at the scale required to meet market demands. Organic farming is highly inefficient in terms of labor and land, requiring more land and producing less yield. Indeed, most organic foods available in grocery stores are produced by large industrial farms, not local or small farms as most people believe.

In terms of the health outcomes associated with organic foods, it is possible that the primary drivers of improved health markers in adults consuming greater amounts of organic foods are the lifestyle choices associated with increased health consciousness and not necessarily from the organic food itself. Organic foods can be a part of living a healthy lifestyle, but the actual nutritional value of the products and the ways we produce them might not meet the expectations of those who perceive them as being far more healthy and good for the environment. The message is to be an informed consumer and to clearly understand the benefits and limitations of eating organic foods.

Hydration

Good hydration is a basic foundation of physical health in every sense of the term. Proper hydration is necessary for optimal functioning of all parts of our body, including our brain. Dehydration can cause intense thirst, dry mouth, headache, dizziness, confusion, muscle cramps, dark urine, and fatigue. These are not only unpleasant symptoms, but they can also be dangerous. Many people have heard that we should drink eight, eight-ounce glasses of water a day (the "8 × 8" advice), but this is simply a rule of thumb. There is no one amount of water one should drink, as the optimal amount is based on temperature, exertion, and medical status. If the ambient temperature is high, the person is physically active, and/or has a fever or is on diuretic medications, they should definitely hydrate at a higher volume. On the other hand, healthy people going about their everyday lives can hydrate less than a gallon a day and be fully fit (Valtin, 2002). Also, it is a myth that intake of caffeinated beverages causes dehydration, as at a moderate intake level, caffeinated beverages do not negatively affect hydration (Grandjean et al., 2000).

Hydration fads

IV hydration spas are booming businesses, driven largely by social media and influencers. IV hydration is a lifesaving measure for severely dehydrated people or those too ill to drink by mouth. Outside of these conditions, however, there is no indication that IV hydration has any health benefits. Save this money and just drink a glass of water.

Water additives come in a variety of forms, from simple sugary sweeteners to fruit-based additives to electrolytes or to those claiming to work like IVs. While these may make the water taste better, and thus make one more likely to drink, the cost is high and the added wellness benefits are few. One possible benefit is to electrolyte-enhanced water after a heavy workout or when taking diuretics; the replenishment of salt, potassium, and (typically) sugar can assist people to recover quickly from a heavy workout. However, water "enhanced" with fruit or electrolytes does not hydrate a person any better than plain old H20. For example, although watermelon is chock full of water, adding it to water doesn't make the drink more effective—it's all just water in the end. Similarly, "oxygen enhanced" water doesn't actually improve oxygen intake—one breath of air covers this (Piantadosi, 2006).

Raw water, or unfiltered and untreated water, sounds healthy and even preferable to treated water. With waterborne illness being the number one cause of diarrheal death and sickness worldwide, raw water is not quite the healthy choice that it sounds like.

A final word about hydration… Misinformation about hydration and tap water, as well as pervasive and targeted marketing, have led us to a large demand for single-use plastic water bottles, which contribute to our disastrous plastic waste problem. A better alternative is reusable water containers, which have in turn become a big business to the tune of hundreds of millions of dollars a year.

Exercise and Fitness

Physical activity, the expenditure of physical energy through movement, is a general way to describe human movement. Somewhat more specific is exercise, which is goal-oriented physical activity that features planned and repetitive physical movement. Don't get caught up in traditional or rigid ideas of what exercise is. Traditional notions of exercise include running, swimming, biking, and lifting weights, but walking, dancing, roller skating, gardening, yoga, and even hula or pickleball are also fun and worthwhile forms of exercise. The goal of exercise can be fun and pleasure, but people often exercise with a goal of physical fitness, which is the ability of our physical self to perform the activities of life (work, play, home, social) while experiencing feelings of vigor, health, and well-being. Exercise can be further broken down into types:

Endurance exercise (also called aerobic exercise): These exercises increase heart rate and rate of breathing and typically focus on large muscle groups. They feature longer durations of physical effort under a lower load. In addition to cardiovascular and respiratory benefits, endurance exercises help build stamina, which is the mental and physical ability to sustain prolonged effort. The role of endurance exercise in building and maintaining health over the lifespan cannot be overstated. For example, in a review of studies concerning cardiovascular disease (CVD) and aging, Seals et al. (2019) state, "Regular aerobic exercise is the most evidence-based strategy for reducing CVD risk with aging in both men and women."

Strength training (also called resistance training or weight training): These exercises focus on making muscles work against resistance. They feature exercises of short duration under a higher load. Strength training is great for the body, with research suggesting cardiovascular, muscular, and weight management improvements (e.g., Tyler & Thanos, 2023), but it is also good for the mind, with benefits including enhanced cognitive functioning, decreased reports of pain, and reduction in symptoms of anxiety and depression (e.g., O'Connor et al., 2010). Strength training can be particularly advantageous when combined with other forms of exercise.

Flexibility: This refers to a person's ability to move a joint or joints through the range of movement without pain, allowing for free, smooth, and efficient movement. The extent and limitations of flexibility vary widely between people. However, there are many benefits to reasonable flexibility, including lowered risk of injury, relief of pain (such as lower-back pain), and improved athletic performance (such as swimming strokes and swinging a golf club). There are also risks to flexibility exercises, especially when taken to an extreme, including hypermobile joints that don't provide the stability needed for normal functioning, elevated injury risk, and lowered strength as ligaments become too loose.

Balance: This type of training typically targets the muscles that keep us upright and maintain our posture, specifically the core muscles and legs. The goal of balance training is stability and, of course, better balance. Exercises like single-leg balancing, sidestepping, leg swings, and yoga can help improve and maintain balance. As we age, it becomes particularly important to avoid falls, maintain a healthy posture, and preserve flexibility and mobility, as these will help us to preserve our independence.

Mind-body exercises: This is a range of techniques that purposefully incorporate both physical and mental aspects of fitness, including intentional movement, mental focus, and, often, conscious control of breathing. Examples of mind-body exercises include yoga, qigong, tai chi, and Pilates. We will learn more about these techniques in Chap. 9.

Benefits of Regular Exercise

It is well-established that engaging in regular physical activity has beneficial effects on both body and mind. It has been said that "sitting is the new smoking," highlighting the risks of a sedentary lifestyle. Being sedentary is clearly associated with risk of death and disability from all causes, but particularly from cardiovascular disease, respiratory disease, and (in some studies) cancer (Chang et al., 2024; Proper et al., 2011). The type of activity is less important than getting moving, and even modest increases in physical activity can reduce all-cause mortality. Kirk et al. (2009) found that strength training of only 11 minutes three times a week increased metabolic rate by an average of 7.4%—an additional 125 calories/day! However, larger increases in activity (not necessarily intensity) can be associated with greater benefits. For example, in a study of more than 4800 adults, Saint-Maurice et al. (2020) found that those who took 8000 steps a day had a 51% decrease in all-cause risk of death over those who took 4000 steps a day. Finally, exercise is vital for any weight management plan, but it must be combined with healthy eating and calorie control for both weight maintenance and weight loss. Exercise alone in the presence of an unhealthy diet will not typically be effective for managing weight (if that is one's goal).

Exercise is good for the brain as well. Aerobic exercise can have a positive effect on cognitive performance (Chang et al., 2012), attention and executive functioning (Smith et al., 2010), and memory (Loprinzi et al., 2023). As we age, exercise can help us stave off cognitive decline and progression toward dementia (e.g., Omura et al., 2020). There is evidence that exercise, particularly more intense exercise, can help reduce the symptoms of anxiety and depression (e.g., Martinsen, 2005; Noetel et al., 2024), but it is unclear if this effect differs from that of psychotherapy and medication.

Hormone Balancing
The fad of hormone balancing is all the rage on social media, but the general concept has been around for a lot longer than TikTok has. Hormone balancing relies on the idea that the reason people feel sluggish, have head or body aches, and can't lose weight is because the timing and quantity of their hormones are in a state of imbalance. Hormones act as chemical messengers in the body, and they have effects in almost every area of human functioning. Abnormalities in hormonal systems are revealed in real medical testing and diagnoses, which can require treatment with medication or lifestyle changes. However, the very nature of the global effect of hormones on the body makes them an easy target for pseudoscience. The vagueness of the definition of "imbalance," the rejection of typical testing procedures and standard ranges, and the idea that "fixing" a hormone imbalance will "fix everything" are all pseudoscience red flags. There is a substantial difference in efficacy and risk profile between what a doctor prescribes as the result of medical testing and the "products" peddled by wellness influencers and nonmedical practitioners. A good example is supplemental testosterone for low testosterone levels, as determined by medical testing. When a low testosterone level is confirmed via testing, the lifestyle and functional health benefits may outweigh the risks, but when supplemental testosterone is added to someone in the normal range, the potential risks of heart disease, prostate cancer, and blood clots become more concerning.

MacKendrick and Troxel (2022) examined 25 books authored by medical doctors about hormone imbalance. They found that, "Hormone balance is a fantasy that is less about restoring a so-called 'natural' baseline of hormone function, and more about engineering the molecular body through demanding and expensive lifestyle and consumer projects" (p. 7). There is a pointed lack of evidence that hormone balancing, as peddled by influencers and nontraditional practitioners, has any legitimate medical effect. Further, almost all books, websites, and influencers in the hormone-balancing space are selling products, programs, and diet plans that are expensive, untested, and unregulated.

Functional Fitness

Functional fitness is the physical capacity to engage in activities that support and sustain the activities of everyday life. Functional fitness exercises look like or mirror the physical actions we perform as we go about our typical day from cleaning to mowing to grocery shopping—even to getting out of chairs or carrying children. Examples of functional fitness activities include strength training (to be able to carry heavy bags of groceries), pushing and pulling exercises (to be able to reach to put away dishes or get things down from shelves), squatting (to be able to pick up children), and incline walking (to be able to walk up stairs or walk from our car to our office). Other functional fitness activities will include flexibility, squatting, lunging, rotating, and core strength. The priority is on natural movements that encourage our muscles to work in harmony to make our daily tasks easier and with less risk of injury. As we age, loss of strength, flexibility, and mobility is related to physical and cognitive decline, but functional exercise can help avoid injury and maintain our strength, balance, memory, and thinking capacity (e.g., Liu et al., 2014).

Fitting in Exercise

Our lives are hectic and full. It can be overwhelming to try to fit one more thing into a week filled with family, work, school, commuting, shopping, cooking, cleaning, and paying bills, let alone taking care of ourselves and our health. Fitting in exercise is not as simple as, "if it is important to you, you will find a way," as this kind of message is both patronizing and dismissive of real-life problems. The most important parts of fitting in exercise are making a plan as to when and how we will exercise, and then giving ourselves permission not to be perfect. For very busy people, life *will* intervene, and treating ourselves with grace when that happens will help us to stay motivated. Some other tips for fitting in exercise include:

Don't rely only on willpower. Instead, make a reasonable plan with a good chance of working, and then tweak it as needed along the way. Identify the best time to work out and then schedule it, just like scheduling a meeting or picking up a child from school.

We should know the reasons we work out. It's important to embrace why we work out, as this will provide initial and ongoing motivation to continue.

A workout buddy will help keep us accountable and on track.

Be efficient when exercising, as taking longer to do less will make an already busy life seem unbearable.

Take classes, as these have the advantage of a set start time and a defined length.

Parents should find a gym with childcare.

Keep workout clothes and shoes in the car. Stopping at home before working out after work will often kill the motivation to go back out to the gym.

Figuring out how and where we like to exercise keeps us engaged. There is absolutely no need to torture ourselves with exercises we do not like. If people like the outdoors, then they should exercise there, but if they don't, then they should invest in a gym membership—there are a wide variety of activities available either indoors or out.

Change a routine that is not working. Change can be good for us!

Tech can help. Take advantage of the many apps, programs, and products that can help to plan, monitor, and track a fitness journey.

Wellness Tip: Trauma and the Body

Trauma is your reaction to any experience, or the memory of any experience, that you perceive as distressing, disturbing, painful, or upsetting. This means that any event can be traumatic, even events that other people perceive as neutral or positive. Two-thirds or more of university students report a history of trauma, with almost one in ten having symptoms commensurate with post-traumatic stress disorder (e.g., Read et al., 2011; Smyth et al., 2008). There are many factors that influence our perception of trauma, including our trauma history, personality factors, perception of control over the situation (vs perceived helplessness), and existing mental health concerns (such as depression, anxiety, drug and alcohol use, etc.).

It's important to note that trauma is not the experience itself, but your reaction to it, which in turn relies on your perception of it. Here are some things to know about trauma reactions:

- Common
- A reaction to an event or series of events
- Rely on your perceptions of events
- Can be mild, moderate, or extreme and acute, short-term, or chronic
- Can overwhelm your ability to cope

Experiences of trauma can change you. For example, trauma early in life can alter the brain's processing of perceptual cues and the brain connections concerned with emotional regulation (Herzberg & Gunnar, 2020). This means that trauma can alter both brain structure and brain function. Other functions of your body and mind are also affected by trauma, including your immune, digestive, and cardiovascular systems, as well as your hormonal responses, sleep, and stress reactivity processes. Post-traumatic stress, for example, is related to a variety of physical illnesses, such as cardiovascular disease and asthma, as well as to autoimmune disorders like inflammatory bowel disease and also to metabolic syndrome and diabetes (Katrinli et al., 2022). Inflammatory processes in the body and the brain have been identified as one important link between post-traumatic stress and physical disease and disorder.

It is important to seek and receive treatment as soon as possible after the trauma, in order to mitigate long-term effects on the mind and body. People who experience trauma require a support system to offer both immediate support and ongoing comfort and aid. Enlisting the assistance of mental health professionals helps reduce the severity, frequency, and functional impact of trauma reactions. Mental health professionals include medical doctors for prescription medication (such as antianxiety, antidepressant, and MDMA-assisted therapy) and therapists using techniques such as cognitive behavioral therapy, exposure therapy, Eye Movement Desensitization and Reprocessing Therapy (EMDR), narrative therapy, virtual reality therapy, and mind-body cognitive therapy. Complimentary mind-body techniques such as yoga, paced breathing, tai chi, and exercise provide relief for acute symptoms. Now is the time to take care of yourself by working with professionals to heal your trauma—by doing so, you are protecting your future mind and body wellness!

References

American Heart Association. (2023). *Understanding food nutrition labels.* Retrieved from https://www.heart.org/en/healthy-living/healthy-eating/eat-smart/nutrition-basics/understanding-food-nutrition-labels

Anderson, J. W., Konz, E. C., Frederich, R. C., & Wood, C. L. (2001). Long-term weight-loss maintenance: A meta-analysis of US studies. *The American Journal of Clinical Nutrition, 74*(5), 579–584. https://doi.org/10.1093/ajcn/74.5.579

Association for Size Diversity and Health. (2024). *Health at every size principles.* Retrieved from https://asdah.org/haes/

Baldridge, A. S., Huffman, M. D., Taylor, F., Xavier, D., Bright, B., Van Horn, L. V., Neal, B., & Dunford, E. (2019). The healthfulness of the US packaged food and beverage supply: A cross-sectional study. *Nutrients, 11*(8), 1704. https://doi.org/10.3390/nu11081704

Barański, M., Srednicka-Tober, D., Volakakis, N., Seal, C., Sanderson, R., Stewart, G. B., Benbrook, C., Biavati, B., Markellou, E., Giotis, C., Gromadzka-Ostrowska, J., Rembiałkowska, E., Skwarło-Sońta, K., Tahvonen, R., Janovská, D., Niggli, U., Nicot, P., & Leifert, C. (2014). Higher antioxidant and lower cadmium concentrations and lower incidence of pesticide residues in organically grown crops: A systematic literature review and meta-analyses. *The British Journal of Nutrition, 112*(5), 794–811. https://doi.org/10.1017/S0007114514001366

Blaak, E. E., Riccardi, G., & Cho, L. (2021). Carbohydrates: Separating fact from fiction. *Atherosclerosis, 328*, 114–123. https://doi.org/10.1016/j.atherosclerosis.2021.03.025

Cadwallader, A. B. (2022). Which features of dietary supplement industry, product trends, and regulation deserve physicians' attention? *AMA Journal of Ethics, 24*(5), E410–E418. https://doi.org/10.1001/amajethics.2022.410

Cai, J., Chen, Z., Wu, W., Lin, Q., & Liang, Y. (2022). High animal protein diet and gut microbiota in human health. *Critical Reviews in Food Science and Nutrition, 62*(22), 6225–6237. https://doi.org/10.1080/10408398.2021.1898336

Chang, Q., Zhu, Y., Liu, Z., Cheng, J., Liang, H., Lin, F., Li, D., Peng, J., Pan, P., & Zhang, Y. (2024). Replacement of sedentary behavior with various physical activities and the risk of all-cause and cause-specific mortality. *BMC Medicine, 22*(1), 385–314. https://doi.org/10.1186/s12916-024-03599-2

Chang, Y. K., Labban, J. D., Gapin, J. I., & Etnier, J. L. (2012). The effects of acute exercise on cognitive performance: A meta-analysis. *Brain Research, 1453*, 87–101. https://doi.org/10.1016/j.brainres.2012.02.068

Craig, W. J., Mangels, A. R., Fresán, U., Marsh, K., Miles, F. L., Saunders, A. V., Haddad, E. H., Heskey, C. E., Johnston, P., Larson-Meyer, E., & Orlich, M. (2021). The safe and effective use of plant-based diets with guidelines for health professionals. *Nutrients, 13*(11), 4144. https://doi.org/10.3390/nu13114144

Grandjean, A. C., Reimers, K. J., Bannick, K. E., & Haven, M. C. (2000). The effect of caffeinated, non-caffeinated, caloric and non-caloric beverages on hydration. *Journal of the American College of Nutrition, 19*(5), 591–600. https://doi.org/10.1080/07315724.2000.10718956

Herman, P. M., Chen, A. Y.-A., & Sturm, R. (2022). Improving diet quality in US adults: A 30-year health and economic impact microsimulation. *American Journal of Preventive Medicine, 63*(2), 178–185. https://doi.org/10.1016/j.amepre.2022.01.022

Herzberg, M. P., & Gunnar, M. R. (2020). Early life stress and brain function: Activity and connectivity associated with processing emotion and reward. *NeuroImage, 209*, 116493. https://doi.org/10.1016/j.neuroimage.2019.116493

Jain, R., Larsuphrom, P., Degremont, A., Latunde-Dada, G. O., & Philippou, E. (2022). Association between vegetarian and vegan diets and depression: A systematic review. *Nutrition Bulletin, 47*(1), 27–49. https://doi.org/10.1111/nbu.12540

Katrinli, S., Oliveira, N. C. S., Felger, J. C., Michopoulos, V., & Smith, A. K. (2022). The role of the immune system in posttraumatic stress disorder. *Translational Psychiatry, 12*(1), 313–313. https://doi.org/10.1038/s41398-022-02094-7

Kim, H., Caulfield, L. E., Garcia-Larsen, V., Steffen, L. M., Coresh, J., & Rebholz, C. M. (2019). Plant-based diets are associated with a lower risk of incident cardiovascular disease, cardiovascular disease mortality, and all-cause mortality in a general population of middle-aged adults. *Journal of the American Heart Association, 8*(16), e012865. https://doi.org/10.1161/JAHA.119.012865

Kirk, E. P., Donnelly, J. E., Smith, B. K., Honas, J., Lecheminant, J. D., Bailey, B. W., Jacobsen, D. J., & Washburn, R. A. (2009). Minimal resistance training improves daily energy expenditure and fat oxidation. *Medicine and Science in Sports and Exercise, 41*(5), 1122–1129. https://doi.org/10.1249/MSS.0b013e318193c64e

Lane, M. M., Gamage, E., Du, S., Ashtree, D. N., McGuinness, A. J., Gauci, S., Baker, P., Lawrence, M., Rebholz, C. M., Srour, B., Touvier, M., Jacka, F. N., O'Neil, A., Segasby, T., & Marx, W. (2024). Ultra-processed food exposure and adverse health outcomes: Umbrella review of epidemiological meta-analyses. *BMJ Clinical Research, 384*, e077310. https://doi.org/10.1136/bmj-2023-077310

Liu, C., Shiroy, D. M., Jones, L. Y., & Clark, D. O. (2014). Systematic review of functional training on muscle strength, physical functioning, and activities of daily living in older adults. *European Review of Aging and Physical Activity, 11*(2), 95–106. https://doi.org/10.1007/s11556-014-0144-1

Loprinzi, P. D., Roig, M., Tomporowski, P. D., Javadi, A.-H., & Kelemen, W. L. (2023). Effects of acute exercise on memory: Considerations of exercise intensity, post-exercise recovery period and aerobic endurance. *Memory & Cognition, 51*(4), 1011–1026. https://doi.org/10.3758/s13421-022-01373-4

MacKendrick, N. A., & Troxel, H. (2022). Like a finely-oiled machine: Self-help and the elusive goal of hormone balance. *Social Science & Medicine, 309*, 115242. https://doi.org/10.1016/j.socscimed.2022.115242

Martinsen, E. W. (2005). Exercise and depression. *International Journal of Sport and Exercise Psychology, 3*(4), 469–483. https://doi.org/10.1080/1612197X.2005.10807319

McMacken, M., & Shah, S. (2017). A plant-based diet for the prevention and treatment of type 2 diabetes. *Journal of Geriatric Cardiology, 14*(5), 342–354. https://doi.org/10.11909/j.issn.1671-5411.2017.05.009

Noetel, M., Sanders, T., Gallardo-Gómez, D., Taylor, P., Del Pozo Cruz, B., van den Hoek, D., Smith, J. J., Mahoney, J., Spathis, J., Moresi, M., Pagano, R., Pagano, L., Vasconcellos, R., Arnott, H., Varley, B., Parker, P., Biddle, S., & Lonsdale, C. (2024). Effect of exercise for depression: Systematic review and network meta-analysis of randomised controlled trials. *BMJ Clinical Research, 384*, e075847. https://doi.org/10.1136/bmj-2023-075847

O'Connor, P. J., Herring, M. P., & Caravalho, A. (2010). Mental health benefits of strength training in adults. *American Journal of Lifestyle Medicine, 4*(5), 377–396. https://doi.org/10.1177/1559827610368771

Omura, J. D., Brown, D. R., McGuire, L. C., Taylor, C. A., Fulton, J. E., & Carlson, S. A. (2020). Cross-sectional association between physical activity level and subjective cognitive decline among US adults aged ≥45 years, 2015. *Preventive Medicine, 141*, 106279. https://doi.org/10.1016/j.ypmed.2020.106279

Paarlberg, R. (2021). *Resetting the table: Straight talk about the food we grow and eat.* Knopf.

Penney, T. L., & Kirk, S. F. (2015). The health at every size paradigm and obesity: Missing empirical evidence may help push the reframing obesity debate forward. *American Journal of Public Health, 105*(5), e38–e42. https://doi.org/10.2105/AJPH.2015.302552

Pew Research Center. (2016). *The new food fights: U.S. Public Divides Over Food Science.* Retrieved from https://www.pewresearch.org/internet/wp-content/uploads/sites/9/2016/11/PS_2016.12.01_Food-Science_FINAL.pdf

Piantadosi, C. A. (2006). "Oxygenated" water and athletic performance. *British Journal of Sports Medicine, 40*(9), 740–741. https://doi.org/10.1136/bjsm.2006.028936

Pimentel, D., & Pimentel, M. (2003). Sustainability of meat-based and plant-based diets and the environment. *The American Journal of Clinical Nutrition, 78*(3 Suppl), 660S–663S. https://doi.org/10.1093/ajcn/78.3.660S

Proper, K. I., Singh, A. S., van Mechelen, W., & Chinapaw, M. J. M. (2011). Sedentary behaviors and health outcomes among adults: A systematic review of prospective studies. *American Journal of Preventive Medicine, 40*(2), 174–182. https://doi.org/10.1016/j.amepre.2010.10.015

Read, J. P., Ouimette, P., White, J., Colder, C., & Farrow, S. (2011). Rates of DSM-IV-TR trauma exposure and posttraumatic stress disorder among newly matriculated college students. *Psychological Trauma Theory Research Practice and Policy, 3*(2), 148–156. https://doi.org/10.1037/a0021260

Rohrmann, S., Cassidy, A., & Kühn, T. (2023). Association of healthful plant-based diet adherence with risk of mortality and major chronic diseases among adults in the UK. *JAMA Network Open, 6*(3), e234714. https://doi.org/10.1001/jamanetworkopen.2023.4714

Saint-Maurice, P. F., Troiano, R. P., Bassett, D. R., Graubard, B. I., Carlson, S. A., Shiroma, E. J., Fulton, J. E., & Matthews, C. E. (2020). Association of daily step count and step intensity with mortality among US adults. *JAMA: The Journal of the American Medical Association, 323*(12), 1151–1160. https://doi.org/10.1001/jama.2020.1382

Seals, D. R., Nagy, E. E., & Moreau, K. L. (2019). Aerobic exercise training and vascular function with ageing in healthy men and women. *The Journal of Physiology, 597*(19), 4901–4914. https://doi.org/10.1113/JP277764

Shane-McWhorter, L. (2024). *Intravenous vitamin therapy (Myers' cocktail).* Merk Manual. Retrieved from https://www.merckmanuals.com/home/special-subjects/dietary-supplements-and-vitamins/intravenous-vitamin-therapy-myers-cocktail#Side-Effects_v61151925

Smith, P. J., Blumenthal, J. A., Hoffman, B. M., Cooper, H., Strauman, T. A., Welsh-Bohmer, K., Browndyke, J. N., & Sherwood, A. (2010). Aerobic exercise and neurocognitive performance: A meta-analytic review of randomized controlled trials. *Psychosomatic Medicine, 72*(3), 239–252. https://doi.org/10.1097/PSY.0b013e3181d14633

Smyth, J. M., Hockemeyer, J. R., Heron, K. E., Wonderlich, S. A., & Pennebaker, J. W. (2008). Prevalence, type, disclosure, and severity of adverse life events in college students. *Journal of American College Health, 57*(1), 69–76.

Thomas, M. S., Calle, M., & Fernandez, M. L. (2023). Healthy plant-based diets improve dyslipidemias, insulin resistance, and inflammation in metabolic syndrome. A narrative review. *Advances in Nutrition, 14*(1), 44–54. https://doi.org/10.1016/j.advnut.2022.10.002

Tribole, E., & Resch, E. (2020). *Intuitive eating: A revolutionary anti-diet approach* (4th ed.). St. Martin's Publishing Group.

Tyler, J., & Thanos, P. (2023). Raising the bar for public health: Resistance training and health benefits. *International Journal of Strength and Conditioning, 3*(1), 195. https://doi.org/10.47206/ijsc.v3i1.195

U.S. Department of Health and Human Services, Office of Disease Prevention and Health Promotion. (2024). *Dietary guidelines for Americans*. Retrieved from https://health.gov/our-work/nutrition-physical-activity/dietary-guidelines

Valtin, H. (2002). "Drink at least eight glasses of water a day". Really? Is there scientific evidence for "8 x 8"? American journal of physiology regulatory, integrative and comparative. *Physiology, 283*(5), 993. https://doi.org/10.1152/ajpregu.00365.2002

Wang, F., Zheng, J., Yang, B., Jiang, J., Fu, Y., & Li, D. (2015). Effects of vegetarian diets on blood lipids: A systematic review and meta-analysis of randomized controlled trials. *Journal of the American Heart Association, 4*(10), e002408. https://doi.org/10.1161/JAHA.115.002408

Wang, L., Du, M., Wang, K., Khandpur, N., Rossato, S. L., Drouin-Chartier, J. P., Steele, E. M., Giovannucci, E., Song, M., & Zhang, F. F. (2022). Association of ultra-processed food consumption with colorectal cancer risk among men and women: Results from three prospective US cohort studies. *BMJ Clinical Research, 378*, e068921. https://doi.org/10.1136/bmj-2021-068921

Chapter 8
Key Topics in Mind-Body Wellness, Part 2

This chapter will begin with a topic that most people find is foundational to their experience of mind-body wellness—sleep—and will continue from there with an overview of additional topics related to mental wellness and caring for our mental well-being. We cover sleep first because no book on mind-body wellness would be complete without attention to sleep. Sleep affects almost every process of our body and brain, and if we are not sleeping well, the effects impact our lives almost immediately. Lack of sleep can cause problems with attention, focus, decision-making, depression, and irritability, and chronic sleep deficit is associated with greater risk of heart disease, obesity, and diabetes (Colten & Altevogt, 2006). A person does not have to meet the clinical guidelines for a sleep disorder to struggle with sleep and to experience the effects of poor sleep.

Sleep

Good sleep is one of our most important daily wellness activities. We spend a lot of our life sleeping or trying to sleep, and many spend too much time sleepy, groggy, and in sleep debt. The optimal amount of sleep for thriving physically and mentally depends on age and health. Healthy adults need at least 7 hours of sleep, while infants, children, and teens will need more (National Sleep Foundation, 2020), yet a majority of college students (and more than a third of adults overall) report problems with sleep and associated daytime tiredness (Hershner & Chervin, 2014). There are few things as tortuous to our psyches, as detrimental to our mood, or as disabling to our physical wellness as being chronically sleep deprived.

In addition to daytime sleepiness, people experience a range of both physical and mental consequences of low sleep and sleep debt. In the physical realm, these problems include an increased risk of high blood pressure, weight gain, diabetes, and low sex drive. People who are sleepy also have a higher incidence of accidents of all

S. M. Henney, J. D. Hackett, *Mind-Body Wellness*,
https://doi.org/10.1007/978-3-031-91611-3_8

types, including household accidents, workplace accidents, and motor vehicle accidents. In fact, drowsy driving accounts for upwards of 90,000 auto accidents and 800 deaths per year (National Highway Traffic Safety Administration, n.d.). On the mental and emotional side, sleepiness can affect our mood, increasing our risk for depression (in the long term) and sadness or feeling blue (in the shorter term), but also making us more susceptible to anxiety, irritability, and anger. Sleepy people are less motivated in both big ways (getting to work, meeting deadlines, etc.) and smaller ways (preparing a healthy meal, consistent hygiene, etc.) and often have problems concentrating, thinking clearly, and making good decisions. These and other consequences of poor sleep can have devastating effects on our interpersonal relationships, our work life, and our school success, which makes attaining and maintaining consistently high-quality sleep of sufficient quantity crucial to personal wellness across multiple dimensions.

Finally, just as insomnia is a legitimate and debilitating mental and physical health issue that can be addressed with lifestyle and medical intervention, oversleeping can lead to negative outcomes as well if not addressed. Oversleeping, or hypersomnia, can be defined as sleeping more than nine hours at one time or in one 24-hours period, and has been associated with headaches, depression, and cardiovascular disease, among other outcomes (e.g., Ohayon et al., 2013). Engaging the senses with bright lights and a warm room, drinking cold water or taking a cold shower, having our loudest alarm being farthest from the bed, making social appointments, and getting sunlight first thing in the morning can help with patterns of oversleeping.

Sleep Hygiene

Sleep hygiene means engaging in the behaviors, habits, and environments that promote sleep, which both help us to fall asleep and stay asleep. Getting the right amount of sleep is a balance between doing things that promote sleep and avoiding other things that are barriers to sleep (see Table 8.1). First, if we are struggling with sleep, sleep can't be fixed until we pinpoint exactly what's wrong. Identifying patterns and barriers to good sleep will point us to the solution. One way to do this is to monitor sleep for seven nights using a sleep log, sleep journal, or a sleep tracking app (there are many to choose from). Next, look at the results and identify patterns, benefits, and barriers to sleep. What is working right? What feels good and helps facilitate sleep? Is it possible to pinpoint behaviors or conditions that are negatively affecting sleep? We should analyze what is in our control and what is not. Sometimes our neighbors are loud or we cannot afford to keep the air conditioning as low as we would like it to be, and we may not be able to control these things. However, there are many things that are within our control about sleep, especially bedtime routines and sleep schedules. Whenever possible (hopefully on a consistent basis), we should prioritize going to sleep and waking up at the same time. Finally, we should see a doctor if there is an ongoing struggle to address poor sleep on our own.

Table 8.1 Getting those ZZZs

Promoting Good Sleep	Barriers to Good Sleep
•Go to bed and get up at the same time every day •Bed is only for sleep and "romance" •Fully dark room at night, lots of morning sunlight •Cool sleeping area •De-stress with relaxing music, yoga, or meditation •Warm or hot shower or bath •Exercise (but not right before bed)	•Stop or limit caffeine, alcohol, nicotine three hours before bed •Stop or limit screen time 30 min to one hour before bed (reduce blue light) •Avoid long daytime naps •Don't go to bed hungry *or* full •No liquids one hour before bed

Sleep Aids

About a third of adults between the ages of 18 and 64 say that they don't get enough sleep, and college students in particular are in chronic sleep deficit, reporting both low sleep quantity and quality (Centers for Disease Control and Prevention, 2024). Not only do we have too much to do and not enough time to get everything done, but it is also common to struggle with "turning off" our bodies and minds so that we can sleep. Stress can cause us to be sleepless, with worry, rumination, and exposure to stressful events being related to increased risk of insomnia (e.g., Drake et al., 2014; Kalmbach et al., 2018). It is no wonder that people seek out ways to help themselves both fall asleep and stay asleep. Remember that what we do during the day—getting up at the same time, exercise, morning sunlight—sets us up for good sleep at night. In addition to the mind/body techniques like meditation, yoga, and progressive muscle relaxation covered in Chap. 9, here are some things to try (note that people should not take any teas, supplements, or ingest any sleep aid without consulting their doctor, particularly if they are pregnant or trying to become pregnant):

- Sound: White noise (even, flat sound), violet noise (higher frequency, masks tinnitus), nature sounds, music, and many other sound-based sleep aids work almost like a lullaby to signal the mind to shut off and the body to relax. Sleep apps and internet tools featuring sound-based sleep aids are plentiful and free or low-cost.
- Herbal teas: Chamomile, valerian root, and lavender are among the herbal sleep aids that have been studied for their soporific effects. Chamomile flowers, for example, have a flavonoid called apigenin, which appears to increase drowsiness (note that excessive use of apigenin, including in supplement form, can have unwanted side effects, so consult a doctor before use).
- Supplements:

  - *Melatonin*: The pineal gland in the brain produces melatonin to help regulate sleep and circadian rhythms. Our 24-hours circadian rhythms, when functioning properly, help us to wake up and sleep at the right times, which in turn influence how alert or tired we feel. Travel, exposure to light at night, illness, stress, overwork, and aging can cause changes in melatonin production, leading to sleep problems. Melatonin supplements are extremely popular because they work for most people, are cheap and readily available, and have a low side-effect profile.
  - *Magnesium*: This is typically taken in the form of magnesium glycinate, a mineral that helps the body to regulate neural activity, muscle function, and blood pressure, as well as the development of bones. Like melatonin, magnesium supplementation is readily available and appears to have low side-effects when taken as directed (watch out for digestive upset), but more high-quality research is needed (e.g., Arab et al., 2023).
  - *Plants and herbs*: Valerian root, lavender, CBD, and ginseng are just a few of the plants and herbs that are in common use as supplements for sleep. Such supplements are readily available at the store, and they are popular because they have the reputation for being "natural sleep remedies." However, it's important to note that even plant-based and herbal supplements can be dangerous. For example, kava had a period of popularity on social media for its purported ability to produce calm, relaxation, and sleepiness. However, kava has also been associated with severe liver damage, indicating that consumers should be very careful about the type and amount they ingest. Remember, just because someone says "try this" on social media doesn't mean it's safe, and every "natural" thing is not without risks and side effects (sometimes severe ones).

- Prescription sleep aids: About 6% of American adults take sleep medication every night, while 12% take it some or most days (Reuben et al., 2023). For some people, these are last-option ways to address chronic insomnia. Prescription sleep aids can work, but they do have a high side-effect and risk profile. Often, prescription sleep aids are associated with difficulty waking, daytime drowsiness, impaired concentration and memory, and even drowsy driving and increased risk of household accidents. Some people develop tolerance to these medications, meaning they must take more over time to have the same effect. Others have withdrawal symptoms, such as rebound insomnia, which makes it hard to stop. It is essential to work closely with a physician when taking prescription sleep aids and to always read the medication's warning label.

Sleep Fads

Like most types of wellness behaviors, sleep is not immune to fads and pseudoscience. Some sleep fads are popular and possibly ultimately harmless, but untested, while others are extremely concerning and possibly dangerous. An example of the latter is "mouth taping," which encourages breathing through the nose by placing a piece of tape over the mouth, thereby supposedly reducing snoring, bad breath, and sleep apnea. However, this practice can be dangerous for people with narrow/ obstructed nasal passages or large tonsils. Other, less dangerous, sleep fads include:

Sleep drinks and sleep mocktails, such as lettuce water, tart cherry juice, and the sleepy girl mocktail.

Bed rotting/hurkle-durkling, which involves spending long periods of time in bed without sleeping, often to read, scroll, or watch TV (this is not advised for people with a history of deep vein thrombosis or depression).

Sleep games, such as Pokémon Sleep™, that reward people in the game for the quality of their sleep.

What all of these have in common is a lot of social media talk and little evidence of effectiveness. Like every human behavior, they have risks, but these can be mitigated if the techniques are used appropriately.

Understanding Mental Wellness

Mental wellness is more than the absence of mental illness, it is a set of internal attributes that includes a positive outlook, a tendency toward growth and self-improvement, acceptance of the self, a consistent, reliable approach to fulfilling social relationships, and realistic and clear thinking. Mental wellness is dynamic and changes with our environment and circumstances; it allows us to be flexible and proficient in dealing with life's challenges. We might rightly ask how this is different from mental health, and in truth it is a difficult and perhaps unnecessary distinction. Even the World Health Organization (WHO) incorporates mental well-being into their definition of mental health as, "a state of mental wellbeing that enables people to cope with the stresses of life, realize their abilities, learn well and work well, and contribute to their community" (World Health Organization, 2022).

However, mental wellness is not a "state" to be achieved—it is always changing, dynamic, and occurring within our current life context. Writing about achieving and maintaining mental health, Youssef-Morgan (2024) states, "Importantly, optimal functioning is not the absence of negative emotions, experiences, or events. Optimal functioning does not come about through the elimination of negativity, challenges, difficulties, conflict, or suffering. Rather, optimal functioning involves a balance between positivity and negativity to achieve optimal outcomes that evolve over time, such as growth, development, and positive change."

Consider Fig. 8.1, for example, which shows ways that mental health and mental wellness can be viewed in relation to each other. The ideal situation is when a person consistently feels subjectively well and experiences no or mild symptoms of mental illness. The most challenging situation occurs when a person has severe symptoms of mental illness and also cannot identify subjective feelings of well-being in their life. However, most people are somewhere between these extremes and travel

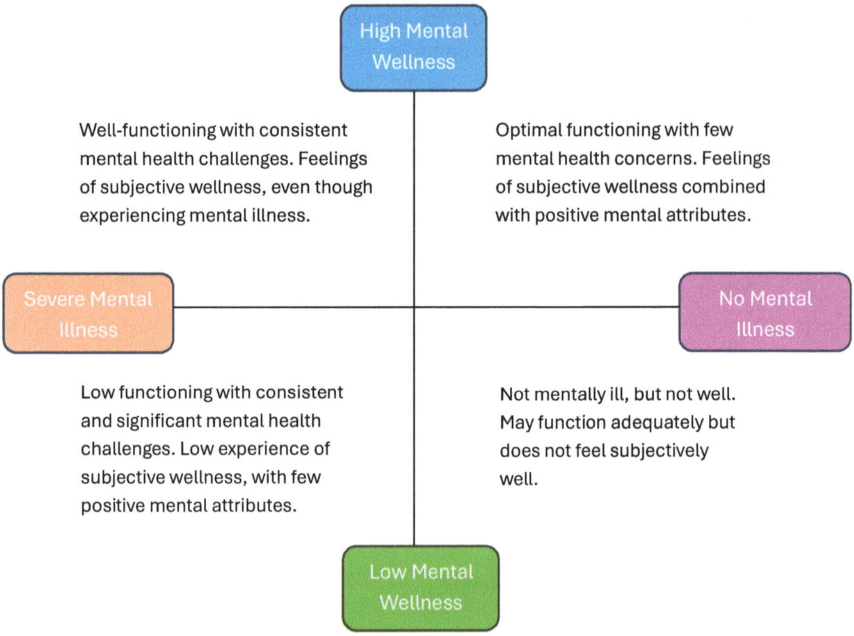

Fig. 8.1 The relationship between mental wellness and mental health

between feeling well along with some mental health challenges and feeling subjectively unwell even with few mental health symptoms. Why is this? It probably has a lot to do with context, changing life circumstances, and, particularly, changes in the stage of life we are in. Our needs of every kind—mental, physical, spiritual, relational—change as we age, and one stage of life can bring hardships that challenge our coping, whereas another can bring more self-understanding and peace.

The Benefits of Mental Wellness

Helping professionals have traditionally focused on treatment of mental illness, with more narrow attention on reducing behavioral, emotional, and cognitive problems. However, just reducing troubling symptoms like anxiety, sadness, or distress doesn't improve mental wellness by itself (Seligman, 2011). The good news is that the focus is shifting from only addressing symptoms to developing and supporting assets of wellness, such as a positive approach to life, strong social skills, building resilience and coping, and exploration of meaning and purpose in life. By not only focusing on problems, we can look at how the whole person functions in their environment and provide support to shape positive personal resources that can help people cope and function better, even in the presence of mental health symptoms. The key personal resources and assets include:

- Belonging and sense of place.
- Understanding of life's meaning and purpose.
- Resilience and coping.
- Supportive and fulfilling relationships.
- Satisfaction with work and play.
- Freedom to be who we are and to express our potential.
- Feelings of joy, contentment, and fulfillment.
- Positive mental outlook.

Understanding Mental Illness

One of the common questions people ask about mental illness is whether mental illness is a physical disease or a product of a disordered environment (i.e., are people "born mentally ill" or "made mentally ill" by the environment)? The answer, for most people, is "both"—there are genetic, biological, and physical contributions to mental illness, but all mental illness occurs within an environmental context that can make expression of mental illness symptoms more or less likely and more or less severe. Thus, like mental wellness, the presence of mental illness is not a rigid yes or no proposition, as there are varying presentations, intensities, and durations of symptoms of mental illness. Furthermore, the symptoms of severe mental illness can be extremely disruptive to one's life, but reducing the severity and intensity of symptoms can move a person to a healthier level of functioning. In other words, people with symptoms of mental illness typically move up and down a continuum of severity, depending on context, stressors, and treatment effectiveness (see Fig. 8.2).

Mentally healthy people tend to experience positive emotions, fulfilling relationships, resilience in the face of challenging circumstances, make good decisions about their health and well-being, and practice necessary self-care. On the other hand, people struggling with severe mental illness can have negative emotional worlds, exhibit problems with making and keeping relationships, spiral into more severe symptoms in the face of stress, often make poor decisions (sometimes leading to physical danger or substance abuse), and have notable lapses in self-care. However, people are able to travel along the continuum of mental health and mental illness. With effective treatment, symptoms of severe mental illness can become more manageable, and some level of functional living can be developed. On the other hand, severe or persistent stressors or trauma can cause someone who is functioning with better mental health to move into moderate or more severe symptoms.

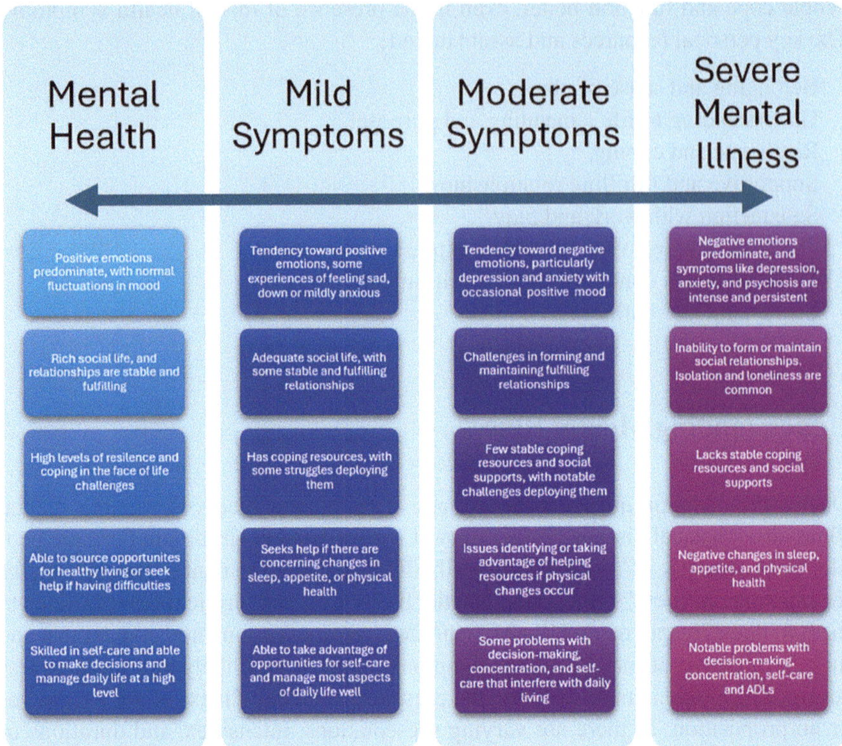

Fig. 8.2 The mental health—mental illness continuum

Mental Health Treatments

There are many different types of therapy, but the therapies with the most high-quality and abundant research are the traditional modalities that have been used and studied for many years. This section will provide an overview of these traditional forms of therapy, as they are pertinent to learning about mental wellness. Each of these types of therapy (except biological/medical therapies) can be accomplished in individual therapy, group therapy, dyadic or couples therapy, and family therapy.

Behavior therapy: This group of therapies is concerned almost entirely with the factors that produce and maintain observable behavior. Behavior therapy uses techniques like aversion therapy (substance abuse disorders), systematic desensitization (phobias), and applied behavior analysis (autism spectrum disorder) with the goal of changing specific unwanted behaviors. True behavior therapy can provide substantial relief relatively quickly, as long as the target behavior is well-defined and the treatment accurately addresses it.

Cognitive-behavior therapy: A shorter-term therapy that targets both behavior and thoughts that are difficult for the client. During a therapy session and outside of therapy via homework, CBT therapists support clients to identify and develop new ways of dealing with thoughts and behaviors that are causing them hardship in life. By replacing these problematic thoughts and behaviors with more functional thoughts and behaviors, the patient's life is more productive and fulfilling.

Humanistic therapy: A longer-term talk therapy that focuses on personal growth, self-understanding, and achievement of our authentic, whole self. Clients achieve change through introspection, being truthful about one's behaviors and motivations, and development of self-awareness. This is the traditional therapy that is most comparable with contemporary mind-body therapies, as most types of humanistic therapy focus on the whole person (rather than just thoughts, feelings, or behaviors).

Psychodynamic psychotherapy: This is a long-term type of talk therapy in which the goal is for the client to become increasingly aware of the connection between their conscious thoughts, emotions, behaviors, and their unconscious thoughts, feelings, and urges.

Biological/medical therapies: The most common biological mental health treatment is medication. Psychiatric medications address the chemical pathways that influence our thoughts, feelings, and behaviors. For example, SSRI medications like sertraline (Zoloft®), paroxetine (Paxil®), and escitalopram (Lexapro®) are popular psychiatric medications that are used for the treatment of depression and anxiety. These are different from nonprescription psychoactive drugs, which include alcohol, nicotine, and caffeine, and illegal psychoactive drugs, like amphetamines, LSD, and heroin. However, drugs are not the only biological therapies. There are also brain stimulation therapies that are used to treat chronic, severe depression, like electroconvulsive therapy (ECT) and transcranial magnetic stimulation (TMS) that have shown success for hard-to-treat cases (Berlim et al., 2013). Of course, as has been discussed in this text, diet and exercise changes can also assist in addressing mental health and are key parts of any plan to improve and maintain mental wellness.

Are Psychiatric Medications Good or Bad?

Every teacher in the area of psychological health and wellness has been asked to provide a perspective on whether psychiatric medications "work" or are "good" or "worth it" to treat mental health problems. A competent and fact-based answer is…it depends. Like all medications, psychiatric medications have drawbacks and side effects, some of which can be quite distressing to people taking them. On the other hand, when appropriately used and monitored, these medications can be life-saving and life-affirming treatments that can very much improve the person's quality of life.

In the case of mild to moderate mental illness, it is typically best to start with therapy and see if that provides relief. If there are suicidal thoughts or other severe symptoms, if troubling symptoms persist, or if the person deteriorates in functioning, then evaluation for psychiatric medications is warranted and should happen relatively quickly. The balance of the research in this area has shown that the combination of therapy and medication is appropriate for many patients and gives more relief—and, importantly, long-term change—than either one alone. Note that it takes weeks, sometimes up to 6–8 weeks, for some psychiatric medications to work, and therapy is an important part of the treatment picture during this time.

Remember that, to be useful, medication doesn't have to be the only answer, but it can be part of the whole answer. The sum of all this is that we are whole beings, both biological in nature and also with an emergent mind and consciousness through which we interact with our world. Let's not think in duality—mind (therapy) vs body (medication)—but instead with mind *and* body as part of solutions to human suffering and as part of every path toward human wholeness.

How to Enhance Mental Wellness

Everything we do or don't do and every choice we make or don't make influences our mental wellness. We do not have to take pricey "brain boosting" supplements, attend a wellness retreat, or even engage in a specific type or length of mental health therapy to be mentally well. What we do need is to be aware of just how important our lifestyle choices and behaviors are to our mental well-being. Walsh (2011) argues persuasively that, "...mental health professionals have underestimated the importance of unhealthy lifestyle factors in contributing to multiple psychopathologies, as well as the importance of healthy lifestyles for treating multiple psychopathologies, for fostering psychological and social well-being, and for preserving and optimizing cognitive capacities and neural functions" (p. 579). In other words, those who evaluate and treat us for mental health concerns do not fully realize and/or account for the importance of lifestyle choices in creating and maintaining both mental illness and mental wellness. Figure 8.3 presents a variety of ways to enhance mental wellness. Suggestions on how to implement some of these strategies include:

Take care of physical health: This might include a reasonable diet, regular exercise, appropriate and necessary medication, hydration, avoiding smoking, and a moderate approach to alcohol. As we have learned, good sleep habits create a positive outlook, more energy, cognitive function, social relationships, and emotional regulation. It should be clear by this point that we really cannot talk about mental health without looking at ourselves as biological beings.

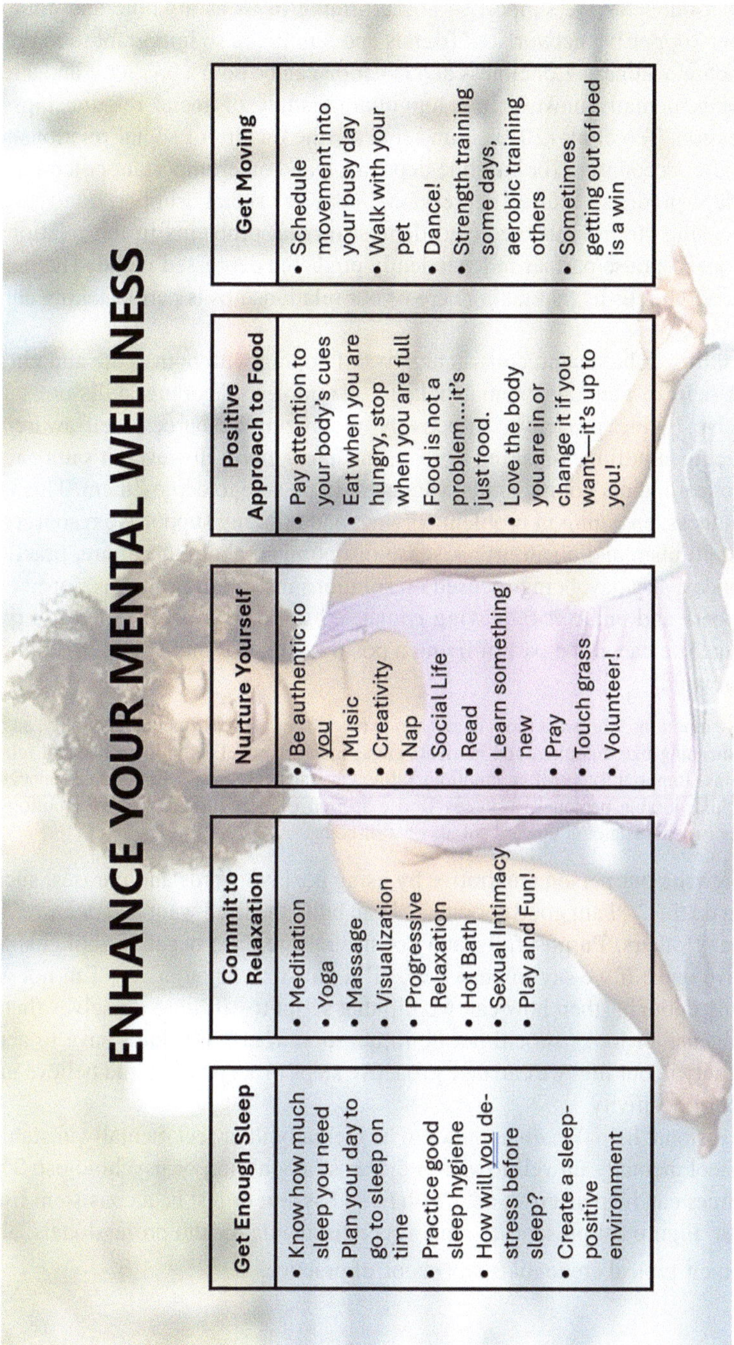

Fig. 8.3 Ways to enhance mental wellness

Good relationships help us feel good: We should pay attention to which relationships in our lives are supportive and affirming of us as a whole and complete person. Supportive networks of friends and family are so important to maintaining mental wellness. Loneliness and isolation can be both a predictor and a result of being mentally unwell. In a longitudinal study of social relationships and depression, Teo et al. (2013) found that, "...the quality of social relationships–even after accounting for baseline depression and other important potential confounders–predicts future depression." Lower social support and higher relationship strain both predicted depression and problems in the relationship with one's spouse/partner independently predicted depressed mood. The bulk of the research tells us that taking care of our relationships is part of taking care of ourselves.

Coping skills: Reliable and consistent ways of coping with both acute and chronic stress help to maintain mental balance. Examples of coping skills are taking initiative, being proactive, effectively mobilizing resources, self-awareness, practicing mindfulness, taking a break, and many more. However, it's not enough just to learn about coping skills, we've got to be able to deploy them. This takes planfulness, engaging in problem solving, and utilizing supportive resources.

Nurture optimism and positivity: A sense of optimism about the future, practicing gratitude every day, being focused on solutions instead of problems, forgiveness (of others and ourselves), staying connected to positive people, and a thriving spiritual life can all be part of living a positive life. Garland et al. (2010, p. 860) state it well,

> Positive emotions…broaden thought and action repertoires, increase mental flexibility, augment meaning-based coping, and motivate engagement in novel activities and social relationships. Importantly, positive emotions, although transient, have lasting consequences; they build durable personal resources whose accrual triggers further positive emotions, leading to self-sustaining upward spirals of well-being.

We can rewrite our personal narrative by using positive words and phrases, such as "I can do this," "I am good enough," "I can build the life I want and deserve," and so many others. Purposefully and consistently replace negative thoughts with positive ones. If we say to ourselves, "I'm not smart enough" or "I'm not good looking enough," then how can we flip that script to affirm to ourselves that our intelligence or looks should not be in question at all? We don't have to accept negativity in our life; we can take proactive steps to act positive and believe in the power of positivity.

Get professional help. We do not have to be mentally ill or feel mentally unstable or even feel mentally unwell to visit a therapist, counselor, or psychologist. These resources can help us grow, deal with life's hassles, or just be a consistent listening ear. Figure 8.4 presents the main types of mental health professionals, along with their typical credentials and scope of practice.

Counselor Broadest term for mental health professional.

- Can have many different degrees, such as a bachelor's degree, a licensed clinical dependency counselor, a minister, a social worker, just to name a few, or sometimes no degree at all.
- Can add richly to life within their own specialty area, such as religious figures who offer pre-marital counseling or teachers who offer career counseling.
- Be careful about counselors with no degree and no license, especially if you are experiencing moderate to severe mental health challenges.

Therapist Term for several different approaches and educational backgrounds.

- Provide treatment to individuals, couples, families, and groups.
- Can be licensed or unlicensed (depending on jurisdiction), and they have degrees such as an MSW, MA, or other advanced degree.
- Cannot prescribe medication unless they are also licensed as a medical professional, like an MD or DO, physician assistant, nurse practitioner, or similar.

Psychologist Typically PhDs, MD/PhDs, or PsyDs

- High level of training in mental health and mental illness.
- Can prescribe medication, depending on jurisdiction.
- More likely to treat patients with severe mental illness.
- More likely to have done or be doing research in the course or treatment of mental illness and the maintenance of mental health.

Fig. 8.4 Types of mental health professionals

Reducing Health and Wellness Disparities through Culturally Competent Practice

People of color often suffer from barriers to accessing and fully utilizing high-quality and culturally relevant physical and mental healthcare. Culturally competent care can be defined as, "the ability of providers and organizations to effectively deliver health care services that meet the social, cultural, and linguistic needs of patients" (Georgetown University Health Policy Institute, n.d.). Culturally and linguistically appropriate services (CLAS) approach each patient as an individual, with individual preferences, needs, and experiences (Department of Health and Human Services Office of Minority Health, n.d.). The standards of CLAS means delivering care that is "equitable, effective, understandable, and respectful." Culturally competent healthcare benefits us (both nationally and individually) by improving health outcomes, increasing utilization of preventive services, lowering costs for management of chronic conditions, and increasing healthcare quality, patient safety, and patient satisfaction.

Cultural competence is a process, not an achievement. It is obtained over time and with effort through self-evaluation, reflection, and acknowledgment of the potential for bias and bias-based behavior. Nonetheless, even people who are culturally educated and aware have biases. Cultural humility is recognizing that understanding and knowledge of others is limited by one's own privilege, experiences, and personal characteristics.

For those interested in going into a career in any aspect of mental healthcare, physical healthcare, or the health-related social services, it is their responsibility to engage in culturally competent practice. It is incumbent on each of us who are or will be working with people to pay attention to the cultural aspects of our practice and to change our behaviors and approaches when they do not match the high standards of ethical practice with people of different races and ethnicities. Providing the exact same treatment to every client (equal care) may seem like the ethical thing to do, but the ethical practice is to provide the client with the treatment they need, considering their individual history, condition, and way of life (equitable care). This includes, of course, accurately identifying and acting on their cultural, ethnic, linguistic, and identity needs

Happiness

The concept of happiness is deeply embedded in popular culture. We are supposed to live happily ever after with our spouse, have a happy birthday and a happy new year, be happy-go-lucky, and let's not forget "don't worry, be happy." But what does it really mean to be happy? Happiness is a sticky subject—people want to be happy, but it turns out that happiness is hard to define and even harder to measure. This is because common definitions like "positive subjective well-being" or "feelings of pleasure and contentment" are mostly indistinguishable from satisfaction, general positivity, or positive emotion. Some definitions of happiness include the experience of joy or delight, but this seems to imply very strong emotion, whereas people may experience happiness as lighter and less intense. Defining happiness with such intensity may also, unfortunately, make it seem unattainable or unrealistic to some. How we look at happiness may have something to do with our culture. Cultures that emphasize individualism may characterize happiness more in terms of individual emotions, such as joy, excitement, and pleasure. On the other hand, more collectivist cultures may define happiness more in terms of harmony, contentment, and amity.

Seligman (2002) describes three pathways to happiness. The first is to maximize the opportunity for positive emotions and minimize the experience of negative emotions, which he calls The Pleasant Life. We can achieve this by doing the things we enjoy, such as eating foods we like, having fun with friends, or walking the dog. The second is to engage fully and deeply with the activities and pursuits that both nurture and cultivate our skills, competencies, and personal strengths, which is The

Good Life. This involves losing ourselves in the process of using our abilities to the fullest, resulting in an intense and positive personal experience of fulfillment. The final path we walk toward happiness involves committing our time, talents, and service to a cause greater than ourselves, which is The Meaningful Life. This engages our sense of purpose and, ultimately, by uplifting others and contributing positively to society, we uplift ourselves. Perhaps the most important part of Seligman's theory is that it implies we can build, grow, and nurture happiness through purposeful activity. Thus, we should not only see happiness as something we "have" or even something that is simply "pleasure seeking." Furthermore, happiness is not to be found in a supplement, a paid program, or a workshop. Instead, it is an investment in a profound pursuit of positivity, meaning, and connection that, when taken together, form our personal recipe for happiness.

Mind-body techniques like gratitude journaling and mindfulness can improve happiness levels by increasing awareness of positive experiences and reducing stress. Diener, Lucas, and Scollon (2006) observe that people tend to underestimate their positive emotions and overemphasize emotional intensity when recalling emotional moments. Learning to pay attention to positive emotion and muting the intensity of negative emotion can help us to fully experience happiness in the moment. Diener, Tamir, and Scollon (2006) discuss the concept of hedonic adaptation (also called the hedonic treadmill), which is the idea that no matter what we do or how many emotionally intense experiences we have, we have an average level of happiness that we tend to balance towards. We are working hard at happiness, but we are really running in place to achieve the same level of happiness. It actually does not matter if our experiences are strongly happy or sad, we have a baseline level of happiness where we spend the majority of our emotional life. For example, we may be joyful and emotionally "high" in the period around a new relationship or our wedding or we may be sorrowful or depressed in the time around the death of a loved one or loss of a job, but we will tend over time to return to our typical level of happiness.

Psychological Capital

What are the mental assets that can help us live more satisfying lives? One construct is called psychological capital (PsyCap), which is defined by four psychological states: hope, self-efficacy, optimism, and resilience (Youssef-Morgan & Luthans, 2013). Hope encompasses our ability to envision a positive and meaningful future as well as our willingness to work to achieve it. Hope is inspiring and motivating, and it is key to moving forward toward our goals. Self-efficacy is our belief in our ability to do the things we want and need to do to live a good life. Self-efficacy can be our confidence in a specific activity, like our ability to train successfully for a 5 K, or in relation to a bigger or more wide-ranging goal, like our belief in our ability to parent a child. Lack of self-efficacy can stop or block us from trying, whereas high self-efficacy means we think we can, so we try. Optimism is a positive outlook and the belief that good things will happen in the future. It is a mindset of positivity and belief that, even if bad things happen, there is the possibility of better days ahead. Optimism is different from hope, because optimism is a mental attitude or approach, whereas hope is action oriented. Finally, we can see resilience when people experience hardship and are able to function and maintain mental health through the difficulties. Resilient people can adapt to and overcome many types of adversity, as they have developed a consistent set of assets and skills that they proficiently deploy as the need arises.

PsyCap has been used extensively in the study of organizational behavior and workplace wellness, with high PsyCap being related to work performance, satisfaction, and engagement, and low PsyCap associated with burnout, absenteeism, and high stress (e.g., Avey et al., 2011). Considering the amount of time we spend at work over our lives and our investment of mental and physical resources there, PsyCap must be considered as part of our personal potential for wellness. Indeed, PsyCap is associated with qualities that are associated with success in roles outside of a traditional workplace, such as leadership, activism, creativity, and organization. Youssef-Morgan (2024) describes PsyCap as, "characterized by an internalized sense of agency, control, and intentionality that promotes a positive outlook, the choice of challenging goals, and the investment of energy and resources in their pursuit despite obstacles," which one can easily see would make the confluence of hope, self-efficacy, optimism, and resilience an asset for people beyond work.

Living with Intention

Living with intention means that we mindfully align our behaviors, decisions, and goals with our values and vision, rather than letting other people's actions and opinions, environmental pressures, or our own impulsiveness determine our path. Life comes at us fast, and it is full and busy—It is easy to lose track of what is meaningful in service of putting out fires.

Living with intention involves frequent self-reflection, including through scheduled self-check-ins, meditation, journaling, prayer, wellness coaching, or counseling. These activities help us to be in the present moment, to clarify what matters most, and to separate the "big deals" from the "little deals." living with intention also involves creating daily routines that incorporate intentional behaviors, including dedicating time to meaningful relationships, engaging in activities that spark joy, and pursuing personal growth. It also helps to set boundaries with technology and to manage time effectively. Intentionality helps us to prioritize the activities, attitudes, approaches, and relationships that make us live within our core beliefs and to be true to ourselves.

Psychological Richness

Closely aligned with the concept of psychological capital is the idea of psychological richness as a wellness asset. This concept states that true flourishing is defined by a rich wash of both positive and negative emotions and experiences across our lives, and that we can only grow, change, and bloom into fullness when we experience the full depth and complexity of human experience. This defies the traditional view that the good life is defined by positivity, happiness, or pleasant experiences. Oishi and Westgate (2022) state, "psychologically rich lives are uniquely associated with curiosity, openness to experience, and willingness to defy systems. Complexity and difficulty fuel psychologically rich experiences, and informant and self-reports converge in suggesting that psychological richness grows over time in response to perspective-changing life experiences."

Thus, psychological richness develops when we not only focus on the positive aspects of the good life, but also when we have the courage and willingness to try new things, seek out new experiences and people, to engage with diversity, and to face the obstacles and hurdles of life with courage. Experiences that develop psychological richness include:

Overcoming challenges: Working through important life events, like loss of a loved one, a significant accident, or a natural disaster can help us to grow, develop resilience, and be grateful for what and who we are. The process of overcoming difficulties changes our perspective, enhances adaptability, and molds our depth of character.

Openness to diverse experiences: This involves actively searching out new experiences and engaging with cultures, perspectives, and lifestyles other than our own. These experiences can be positive and affirming, but also challenging, confusing, and unsettling. Both positive and negative experiences are equally valuable and teach us about ourselves, foster empathy, engender open-mindedness.

Intellectual exploration: Also called intellectual curiosity, this is a willingness to engage with complex issues and topics, such as ethics or politics, which encourages critical thinking, promotes a mindful view of the world, and opens one to meaningful dialogue with others.

Embracing complexity: Relationships, workplace politics, creative activities, and even day-to-day life are filled with mixed messages, a wide variety of opinions, and endless options. It is important to accept or at least to be able to work with ambiguity and to be able to maintain a strong sense of self and purpose within a complex system.

Giving of the self: Community involvement, volunteerism, donation of personal resources, and acts of kindness enrich others' lives, but also contribute strongly to our sense of living our values, being a member of the global community, and integrating the well-being of others into our worldview. It is not always easy to fit volunteerism into our schedule, to include giving in our budget, or even to identify what types of giving align with our values, but it is part of a rich and vibrant life to commit to improving the world outside of ourselves.

Psychological Flexibility

The ability to adapt to changing circumstances and to respond to life's challenges with versatility is a mental asset called psychological flexibility. Key components of psychological flexibility, as described in the Hexaflex model (Hayes et al., 2011), are: (1) awareness of one's own thoughts, feelings, and perceptions, (2) being present in the here and now, (3) acceptance of one's inner world, both positive and negative, (4) ability to separate from one's thoughts and feelings so as not to be overtaken or ruled by them (cognitive defusion), (5) knowing what matters and has meaning (values), and (6) commitment to actions that reflect one's values. Acceptance and commitment therapy (ACT) is a specialized type of therapy that utilizes these six elements to assist clients to build the psychological asset of flexibility.

People high in psychological flexibility can choose to respond to changing situations and challenging people in ways that maintain their wellness and align with their values, including in the workplace and in relationships. For example, psychological flexibility has been identified as being related to good ratings of job performance (Bond & Flaxman, 2006), improvement in mental health (Fledderus et al., 2010), and students' feelings of self-efficacy in the college environment (Jeffords et al., 2020). In a large study of the relationship between psychological flexibility and individual and relational well-being, Twiselton et al. (2020) found that a person's psychological flexibility was related to better relationship quality, via higher positive emotionality and lower negative emotionality. Finally, the Covid-19 lockdown provided a real-life test of psychological flexibility for many people, and the research generally reveals the importance of context when considering psychological flexibility—primarily, within the context of a large-scale environmental stressor, as psychological flexibility goes up, mental health and wellness also improve (Pakenham et al., 2023).

Self-Esteem and Wellness

The notion of self-esteem is truly a crossover concept, with clear implications for the relationship between mind and body. Our self-esteem is the subjective evaluation of our goodness and how well we are performing in the areas of our life we feel are important (Yang et al., 2016). In other words, self-esteem reflects how we see and evaluate ourselves. Low self-esteem is often accompanied by feelings of unhappiness. How we feel about ourselves directly impacts feelings of contentment and life satisfaction. Feeling down makes it difficult to truly enjoy life. Moreover, low self-esteem is associated with anxiety, especially in social situations. Concerns about how others view us can lead to avoiding social situations or experiencing anxiety when we are interacting with others. Because of its relationship to mental health problems, low self-esteem is a diagnostic criterion for several mental health issues (American Psychiatric Association, 2013). Self-esteem directly impacts our sense of worthiness in that low self-esteem can generate a sense of being unworthy.

Feeling this way causes us to avoid others and not pursue challenging tasks that would bring about a sense of accomplishment.

Low self-esteem is often reflected in our perception of self-efficacy, or our view on how well we can perform a specific task. With high self-efficacy, we are more likely to perceive success in our endeavors. In contrast, low self-efficacy means we do not think we will be successful. High self-esteem and feeling confident improve our performance in key areas. For instance, academically we perform much better when we feel good about ourselves and approach our studies with confidence. At a general level, this positively impacts our physical and psychological health, as well as social acceptance (Jordan et al., 2017).

While there is some cross-cultural variability, greater self-esteem is associated with more life satisfaction, happiness, and experiencing fewer negative moods (Baumeister et al., 2003). Lower self-esteem leads to poorer physical health and a reduced ability to recover from illness (Stinson et al., 2008). When we experience lower self-esteem our motivation to engage in health-promoting behaviors, such as exercise and attending medical appointments, is diminished. Ironically, physical activity can directly increase self-esteem and can be a great way to address feeling down (Zamani Sani et al., 2016).

Earned esteem occurs when, over time, a person builds a vision of themselves based on actions and behaviors, rather than feelings or emotional evaluations. In other words, earned esteem comes from achieving goals and overcoming difficult tasks. It is one thing to set goals for ourselves, but when we achieve them, we feel a sense of accomplishment and mastery. The confidence we build as a result of these successes encourages us to continue to grow and set even more goals.

Wellness Tip: Positive Self-Talk

Feeling "less than?" Stressed? Overwhelmed? Think about how you talk about yourself to yourself. Most people have an internal dialogue, and for almost everyone, this includes situational self-talk and evaluative self-talk. Situational self-talk is typically context-related, and it may happen regularly when you are interacting with some people or in some situations, but not ever/often in others. Evaluative self-talk happens when we judge ourselves, sometimes harshly and irrationally and other times kindly and realistically.

Situational self-talk can be motivating, encouraging, and we sometimes experience this in the form of "pep talks" or "psyching ourselves up." Evaluative self-talk can be hopeful, pragmatic, and authentic. Table 8.2 presents examples that can help to identify differences in positive self-talk.

Situational self-talk can also be negative, such as when we consistently affirm the negative qualities of a place (like our workplace) or people (neighbors, in-laws, etc.) to ourselves. Evaluative negative self-talk is common and occurs when we say derogatory, hurtful, and even irrational things to ourselves over a real or perceived flaw or failure. As we beat ourselves up over something, our inner critic can be

Table 8.2 Positive situational self-talk vs. evaluative self-talk

Scenario	Situational self-talk	Evaluative self-talk
Public presentation	Stepping up to the podium and saying to yourself, "I am prepared for this. I will do great"	Finishing the presentation and saying to yourself, "Even though I was nervous inside at first, I really did a great job being poised and professional"
Work meet-and-greet	Walking into the room to interact with future colleagues, "I can do this. I've done this before. I'm going to be ok"	During the meet-and-greet, "I am making eye contact and smiling at people. This is helping me connect, and I feel good!"

Table 8.3 Negative situational self-talk vs. evaluative self-talk

Scenario	Situational self-talk	Evaluative self-talk
Doing poorly on a test	"I hate this school and this teacher. They want me to fail"	"I'm dumb. I shouldn't even be in college"[a]
Being ghosted at the end of a relationship	"Relationships are horrible. I am miserable. I give up. I'm never doing this again"	"I'm not even worth saying goodbye to. No one will ever want me forever"

[a] This is also called "imposter syndrome," which has a large negative self-talk component. You doubt yourself and have a significant fear of being exposed as a fraud or as incompetent

detrimental to our mental and physical health. Table 8.3 includes examples of different types of negative self-talk.

The good news is that positive self-talk can be learned, and negative self-talk can be unlearned or reduced. This can be done through cognitive therapy, through mindfulness, through specific and targeted self-talk exercises, and by other means. Try to use the "three Cs of self-talk" to grow your positive self-talk abilities:

- *Catch the thought*: Be aware and mindful of your thoughts and when positive versus negative self-talk occurs.
- *Check the thought*: When negative self-talk occurs, pause and interrupt it by acknowledging it and considering alternatives.
- *Change the thought*: Switch modes to positive self-talk. At first, you will need to have some go-to phrases to help yourself orient to positivity, such as, "I can do this," "I am ok," or "I will find a way."

Also remember that practice makes perfect. You can do something simple today to help yourself: Practice talking to yourself in a kind, supportive, and uplifting way. The way you talk to yourself can empower you or defeat you...uplift your best qualities to yourself and have a practice of positive self-talk. Remember that you deserve to value yourself and love yourself, so talk to yourself as if you are worthy and loveable. Start today with saying one positive thing about yourself each time you sit or stand:

- "I'm ok…this is just temporary."
- "I love who I am."
- "I am not always perfect, but I am always trying."
- "I am enough."

References

American Psychiatric Association. (2013). *Diagnostic and statistical manual of mental disorders* (5th ed.). American Psychiatric Association. https://doi.org/10.1176/appi.books.9780890425596

Arab, A., Rafie, N., Amani, R., & Shirani, F. (2023). The role of magnesium in sleep health: A systematic review of available literature. *Biological Trace Element Research, 201*(1), 121–128. https://doi.org/10.1007/s12011-022-03162-1

Avey, J. B., Reichard, R. J., Luthans, F., & Mhatre, K. H. (2011). Meta-analysis of the impact of positive psychological capital on employee attitudes, behaviors, and performance. *Human Resource Development Quarterly, 22*(2), 127–152. https://doi.org/10.1002/hrdq.20070

Baumeister, R. F., Campbell, J. D., Krueger, J. I., & Vohs, K. D. (2003). Does high self-esteem cause better performance, interpersonal success, happiness, or healthier lifestyles? *Psychological Science in the Public Interest: A Journal of the American Psychological Society, 4*(1), 1–44. https://doi.org/10.1111/1529-1006.01431

Berlim, M. T., Van den Eynde, F., & Daskalakis, Z. J. (2013). Efficacy and acceptability of high frequency repetitive transcranial magnetic stimulation (rTMS) versus electroconvulsive therapy (ECT) for major depression: A systematic review and meta-analysis of randomized trials. *Depression and Anxiety, 30*(7), 614–623. https://doi.org/10.1002/da.22060

Bond, F. W., & Flaxman, P. E. (2006). The ability of psychological flexibility and job control to predict learning, job performance, and mental health. *Journal of Organizational Behavior Management, 26*(1-2), 113–130. https://doi.org/10.1300/J075v26n01_05

Centers for Disease Control and Prevention. (2024). *FastStats: Sleep in adults.* Retrieved from https://www.cdc.gov/sleep/data-research/facts-stats/adults-sleep-facts-and-stats.html

Colten, H. R., & Altevogt, B. M. (2006). *Sleep disorders and sleep deprivation: An unmet public health problem.* National Academies Press.

Department of Health and Human Services Office of Minority Health. (n.d.). *Culturally and linguistically appropriate services (CLAS): What, why and how.* Retrieved from https://thinkculturalhealth.hhs.gov/assets/pdfs/class-infographic-what-why-how.pdf

Diener, E., Lucas, R. E., & Scollon, C. N. (2006). Beyond the hedonic treadmill: Revising the adaptation theory of Well-being. *American Psychologist, 61*(4), 305–314. https://doi.org/10.1037/0003-066X.61.4.305

Diener, E., Tamir, M., & Scollon, C. N. (2006). Happiness, life satisfaction, and fulfillment: The social psychology of subjective Well-being. In P. A. M. Van Lange (Ed.), *Bridging social psychology: Benefits of transdisciplinary approaches* (pp. 319–324). Lawrence Erlbaum Associates Publishers.

Drake, C. L., Pillai, V., & Roth, T. (2014). Stress and sleep reactivity: A prospective investigation of the stress-diathesis model of insomnia. *Sleep, 37*(8), 1295–1304. https://doi.org/10.5665/sleep.3916

Fledderus, M., Bohlmeijer, E. T., Smit, F., & Westerhof, G. J. (2010). Mental health promotion as a new goal in public mental health care: A randomized controlled trial of an intervention enhancing psychological flexibility. *American Journal of Public Health, 100*(12), 2372–2372. https://doi.org/10.2105/ajph.2010.196196

Garland, E. L., Fredrickson, B., Kring, A. M., Johnson, D. P., Meyer, P. S., & Penn, D. L. (2010). Upward spirals of positive emotions counter downward spirals of negativity: Insights from the broaden-and-build theory and affective neuroscience on the treatment of emotion dysfunctions and deficits in psychopathology. *Clinical Psychology Review, 30*(7), 849–864. https://doi.org/10.1016/j.cpr.2010.03.002

Georgetown University Health Policy Institute. (n.d.). *Cultural competence in health care: Is it important for people with chronic conditions?* Retrieved from https://hpi.georgetown.edu/cultural/

Hayes, S. C., Strosahl, K. D., & Wilson, K. G. (2011). *Acceptance and commitment therapy: The process and practice of mindful change.* Guildford Press.

Hershner, S. D., & Chervin, R. D. (2014). Causes and consequences of sleepiness among college students. *Nature and Science of Sleep, 6*, 73–84. https://doi.org/10.2147/NSS.S62907

Jeffords, J. R., Bayly, B. L., Bumpus, M. F., & Hill, L. G. (2020). Investigating the relationship between university students' psychological flexibility and college self-efficacy. *Journal of College Student Retention: Research, Theory & Practice, 22*(2), 351–372. https://doi.org/10.1177/1521025117751071

Jordan, C. H., Zeigler-Hill, V., & Cameron, J. J. (2017). Self-esteem. In V. Zeigler-Hill & T. Shackelford (Eds.), *Encyclopedia of personality and individual differences*. Springer.

Kalmbach, D. A., Anderson, J. R., & Drake, C. L. (2018). The impact of stress on sleep: Pathogenic sleep reactivity as a vulnerability to insomnia and circadian disorders. *Journal of Sleep Research, 27*(6), e12710. https://doi.org/10.1111/jsr.12710

National Highway Traffic Safety Administration. (n.d.). *Drowsy driving*. Retrieved from https://www.nhtsa.gov/risky-driving/drowsy-driving

National Sleep Foundation. (2020). *How much sleep do you really need?* Retrieved from https://www.thensf.org/how-many-hours-of-sleep-do-you-really-need/

Ohayon, M. M., Reynolds, C. F., & Dauvilliers, Y. (2013). Excessive sleep duration and quality of life. *Annals of Neurology, 73*(6), 785–794. https://doi.org/10.1002/ana.23818

Oishi, S., & Westgate, E. C. (2022). A psychologically rich life: Beyond happiness and meaning. *Psychological Review, 129*(4), 790–811. https://doi.org/10.1037/rev0000317

Pakenham, K. I., Landi, G., Cattivelli, R., Grandi, S., & Tossani, E. (2023). Identification of psychological flexibility and inflexibility profiles during the COVID-19 pandemic. *Journal of Clinical Psychology, 79*(10), 2225–2250. https://doi.org/10.1002/jclp.23536

Reuben, C., Elgaddal, N., & Black, L. (2023). *Sleep medication use in adults aged 18 and over: United States, 2020. NCHS Data Brief, no 462*. National Center for Health Statistics. https://doi.org/10.15620/cdc:123013

Seligman, M. E. P. (2002). *Authentic happiness: Using the new positive psychology to realize your potential for lasting fulfillment*. Simon and Schuster.

Seligman, M. E. P. (2011). *Flourish: A visionary new understanding of happiness and Well-being*. Free Press.

Stinson, D. A., Logel, C., Zanna, M. P., Holmes, J. G., Cameron, J. J., Wood, J. V., & Spencer, S. J. (2008). The cost of lower self-esteem: Testing a self- and social-bonds model of health. *Journal of Personality and Social Psychology, 94*(3), 412–428. https://doi.org/10.1037/0022-3514.94.3.412

Teo, A. R., Choi, H., & Valenstein, M. (2013). Social relationships and depression: Ten-year follow-up from a nationally representative study. *PLoS One, 8*(4), e62396. https://doi.org/10.1371/journal.pone.0062396

Twiselton, K., Stanton, S. C. E., Gillanders, D., & Bottomley, E. (2020). Exploring the links between psychological flexibility, individual Well-being, and relationship quality. *Personal Relationships, 27*(4), 880–906. https://doi.org/10.1111/pere.12344

Walsh, R. (2011). Lifestyle and mental health. *The American Psychologist, 66*(7), 579–592. https://doi.org/10.1037/a0021769

World Health Organization. (2022). *Mental health*. Retrieved from https://www.who.int/news-room/fact-sheets/detail/mental-health-strengthening-our-response

Yang, J., Xu, X., Chen, Y., Shi, Z., & Han, S. (2016). Trait self-esteem and neural activities related to self-evaluation and social feedback. *Scientific Reports, 6*(1), 20274. https://doi.org/10.1038/srep20274

Youssef-Morgan, C. M. (2014). Advancing OB research: An illustration using psychological capital. *Journal of Leadership & Organizational Studies, 21*(2), 130–140. https://doi.org/10.1177/1548051813515512

Youssef-Morgan, C. M. (2024). Psychological capital and mental health: Twenty-five years of progress. *Organizational Dynamics*. https://doi.org/10.1016/j.orgdyn.2024.101081

Youssef-Morgan, C. M., & Luthans, F. (2013). Psychological capital theory: Toward a positive holistic model. In A. B. Bakker (Ed.), *Advances in positive organizational psychology* (pp. 145–166). Emerald Group Publishing. https://doi.org/10.1108/S2046-410X(2013)0000001009

Zamani Sani, S. H., Fathirezaie, Z., Brand, S., Pühse, U., Holsboer-Trachsler, E., Gerber, M., & Talepasand, S. (2016). Physical activity and self-esteem: Testing direct and indirect relationships associated with psychological and physical mechanisms. *Neuropsychiatric Disease and Treatment, 12*, 2617–2625. https://doi.org/10.2147/NDT.S116811

Chapter 9
Supporting Mind-Body Wellness

A Paradigm Shift

Around the beginning of the twenty-first century, an interesting paradigm shift began in the field of psychology. The shift brought a focus on human flourishing. That is, instead of a concentration on what is "wrong" with people or what needs to be "fixed," psychologists began to consider what factors help encourage positive human functioning. What factors influence positive development, allow for people to work on what is important to them and allow us to live up to our full potential. In short, this shift in focus puts an emphasis on promoting aspects of our lives that make us happy, feel fulfilled, and encourage us to work towards our maximum capacity.

Thriving, Meaning, and "Living a Good Life"

What does it mean to thrive? Or, to "live a good life?" Is it having abundant money, so we'll never want for anything? While lottery winners show greater general life satisfaction, despite what we may think of these winners, they are not happier than those of us who have not won the lottery (Lindqvist et al., 2020). The extra money may increase life satisfaction, but it does not necessarily impact one's affective sense of well-being. Surely, financial stability is nice, but it does not mean we are happy with other aspects of our lives. This money will not directly improve our health and/or the quality of our close relationships or make all the other issues we worry and stress over simply disappear. If we ask 100 people "What does it mean to live a good life?", we may receive 100 different answers! It is subjective—while for some it may rest on having a healthy romantic relationship, for others living a good life may hinge on having a successful career.

S. M. Henney, J. D. Hackett, *Mind-Body Wellness*,
https://doi.org/10.1007/978-3-031-91611-3_9

The question of happiness and what it means to live life to the fullest is clearly not a recent area of thought. Aristotle considered the good life and suggested it is an ultimate goal that arises from an understanding of how our values and self-beliefs provide a concrete vision or destination for how to live our life. According to Western Kenyan philosopher, Chaungo Barasa, we should strive for what he calls *humanization*—the perfection of human life (Smith et al., 2002). In this perspective, the path to humanization is through knowledge. As a result, education is highly valued and prioritized. When we humanize, we are fully living our human virtues. Living life to the fullest, achieving our true potential, and living a life that brings satisfaction and contentment are themes emerging in multiple philosophical and psychological perspectives.

While there are many different ways we could think about thriving or living a good life, it is hard to imagine anyone able to thrive and feel they live a good life if their mind and body are disconnected or imbalanced. Research in several key disciplines (e.g., psychology, neuroscience, psychoneuroimmunology) has clearly illustrated how our thoughts and emotions impact our bodies. In essence, the connection between the processes in our minds and our physical bodies allows for the mind to influence our bodies and our bodies to influence our minds.

Mind-body medicine involves techniques to assist the mind's capacity to influence the body's functions and symptoms, while simultaneously recognizing the body's ability to impact our minds (Astin et al., 2003). This perspective is at odds with the reductionist approach that characterizes much of modern western medicine. A reductionist view takes complex problems and breaks them into smaller and simpler basic units. This creates a tendency to seek out a singular explanation for an illness or an observed behavior. Like a car mechanic, we expect our doctor to point us to the cause of what is happening to us. To be clear, many medical advances have happened with this view. A more nuanced and complex perspective may consider dietary habits, sleeping patterns, other physical and mental health issues, stress and stress management, the quality of close relationships, and subjective sense of well-being. Mind-body medicine incorporates a broader view to examine how the interaction between mind, body, and behavior promotes health.

Work in mind-body medicine distinguishes between top-down and bottom-up interventions (Taylor et al., 2010). Top-down interventions begin through the mental processes in our cerebral cortex. In other words, these interventions involve conscious and intentional mental activities. Meditation and mindfulness are great examples of this approach. We engage mentally with a focus on our thoughts and emotions. Their neurological activity in turn influences the endocrine and nervous system, with meaningful changes within our body. In contrast, bottom-up interventions involve the transmission of sensory information from the periphery (like sensory organs or tissues) to higher levels of the nervous system, such as the brain. Activities centered on breathing and physical movements such as yoga, tai chi, and Qigong stimulate the nervous, immune, and endocrine systems, resulting in changes to our psychological states. In practice, the "no duality" perspective encourages us to recognize and engage in behaviors that promote the connection between mind and body. This requires a recognition of what practices or activities we can do that benefit both the mind and body. Examples of these behaviors are found around the world. While some of these practices are supported by empirical research, others have not been empirically reviewed or have aspects without research support.

Mind-Body Practices

Meditation

Meditation practices, an umbrella term that describes a variety of techniques, represent a growing area of interest for researchers and the general public. These practices are not new. In fact, early written records of meditation appeared around 1500 BCE in the Indian Vedas (ancient religious writings considered the oldest scriptures in Hinduism). The Vedas encourage meditation as a way to experience divinity by turning our attention inward through contemplative meditation.

When we meditate, we are training ourselves to increase attention and awareness. It is an attempt to "quiet our mind" and focus on the present moment. Closing our eyes for just a few minutes and concentrating on just breathing can highlight just how much our mind wanders. Thoughts just seem to appear in our minds—we quickly think about the other tasks we have planned during the day, what we want to make for dinner, or worry about whether we'll make it to the gym today. Meditating is our chance to tame the mind and be a bit more present in the moment. Emerging work indicates meditation can restructure our brains and produce widespread changes while activating emotional and cognitive centers (Afonso et al., 2020; Austin, 2013).

Transcendental meditation and mindfulness meditation are two of the more common meditation practices in the United States. Both forms of meditation have the same goal—to still our thoughts and produce greater awareness and clarity. Transcendental meditation involves breaking our usual mental activity by focusing on a specific word or phrase (e.g., Om, Om mani padme hum, I am that I am). Increasing our focus on a specific object allows our mind to become more attentive in the moment. The word or phrase may or may not have a specific meaning, rather the repetition is what is important during the meditative session. Repeating the word helps to settle our minds, breaking the constant intrusion of thoughts and concerns, and generating a deeper awareness within us. The goal is to reach a state of transcendental consciousness, which is characterized by heightened awareness and wakefulness where one experiences greater energy and understanding.

Mindfulness meditation, a 2500-year-old Buddhist practice, involves staying present in the moment by maintaining an alert and aware state and letting thoughts move in and out of our mind. With mindfulness meditation, we focus on our thoughts and sensations as we experience them. When our mind naturally wanders, we can observe our breathing or count our breaths to bring us back into the moment. The belief is that our minds have an innate tendency to revisit and think about the past and to ruminate about a future that will likely never happen. In other words, we spend our present moments often stuck in the past or thinking of the future. The fear is that we may move through life as if we are on autopilot and miss out on the beauty of our lives and the world around us as a result. Research suggests our minds wander almost 50% of our waking time and this wandering predicts unhappiness (Killingsworth & Gilbert, 2010). In contrast, our ability to be mindful predicts a greater sense of well-being in our daily lives. Mindfulness, centering ourselves through deep breathing, allows us to be fully present in the moment. One of the more frequently used definitions of mindfulness comes from Kabat-Zinn (1994; pg. 4), who describes it as awareness that arises through "paying attention in a particular way: on purpose, in the present moment and nonjudgmentally." In this state, we are more aware of our body's sensations, thoughts, and consciousness, and we're more open and accepting (Bishop et al., 2004; Kabat-Zinn, 2003).

Guided meditation is another popular approach. These sessions incorporate an instructor who leads and helps guide the meditative practice. One daunting issue for many people is how to start a meditation practice. These guided sessions take the mystery out of the process. Popular Apps like Headspace, Calm, and Ten Percent Happier offer subscribers access to a library of guided meditations. These apps use prerecorded sessions that are available on demand and make meditation accessible for most people. With many prerecorded sessions, it provides users with the freedom to meditate when it works in their schedules. However, we do not need a subscription to one of these services to start, as there are also guided meditations available for anyone on YouTube. In many of these guided sessions, the content of the meditation is important. The topics may focus on specific mantras related to death and suffering, lovingkindness, or compassion. These guided meditations are a great way to remove the mystery and uncertainty over how to start a meditation practice.

Physical and Mental Health Benefits of Meditation

There are several reasons people choose to meditate: as part of an attempt to work through psychological and/or emotional issues, to reduce stress, and to seek a better understanding of self. Whatever the reasoning might be for starting a meditation practice, research shows meditation positively impacts both our physical and mental health. An increase in the number of randomized control trials involving mindfulness interventions provides us with the ability to examine the effects of these interventions. Mindfulness should improve our emotional regulation skills, increasing our resilience and coping with stress. As a result, stress-related physical health issues should improve. This is, in fact, what we see! Studies found mindfulness interventions reduced pain for those suffering from chronic back pain (Morone et al., 2016), pain severity and interference were reduced amongst chronic pain opioid-abusing patients (Garland et al., 2014), and mindfulness reduced daily level stress, pain-related catastrophizing, disability, and fatigue amongst adults with rheumatoid arthritis (Davis et al., 2015).

An important physiological defense for humans is a healthy and well-functioning immune system. Experiencing prolonged stress can generate physiological changes known as a "stress response," resulting in changes in the adrenal medullary hormone system, the HPA axis, and our sympathetic nervous system. Mindfulness meditation is associated with reductions in proinflammatory processes and with increases in anti-inflammatory and immunity biomarkers (e.g., Jedel et al., 2014; Malarkey et al., 2013; Moynihan et al., 2013). There is additional research suggesting meditation may impact the aging process. The telomere theory of aging suggests telomere length is a clear marker of aging in people. Telomeres are structures found on the ends of chromosomes that help protect DNA. As our cells divide, the length of the telomeres is reduced. Eventually, however, the telomeres are no longer able to protect the cell and cells begin to die. Meditation is associated with increases in enzyme activity that guards against cell aging by regulating telomere length (e.g., Black & Slavich, 2016; Dasanayaka et al., 2021).

Some of the most powerful data showing the effectiveness of mindfulness interventions is in the impact on mental health. Mindfulness interventions reduce the likelihood of depression relapse by 50% amongst individuals who had previously experienced three or more episodes of depression (Ma & Teasdale, 2004). There is additional evidence that those at greater risk of relapse, such as those who've had four or more previous episodes or who experienced childhood trauma, benefit even more from these interventions. For those who are acutely depressed or suffer from an anxiety disorder, mindfulness interventions are an effective way to reduce symptoms (Strauss et al., 2014).

Reviewing this research begs the question, what is the process through which meditation and mindfulness affects us? One process through which meditation positively impacts our health is through cultivating self-compassion (e.g., Carmody et al., 2009; Neff & Germer, 2013). Self-compassion is the recognition, awareness, and sympathy toward our own sufferings and failures. We are often more tolerant of others' failures than we are of our own. Recognizing we are human and, like all other humans, are not perfect generates a greater tolerance of our shortcomings. The impact of mindfulness on reducing our stress response explains the positive health outcomes associated with the practice. At the neurobiological level, mindfulness increases our stress-regulatory pathway. More specifically, our prefrontal regulatory regions can inhibit activity in the stress-processing regions of our body, like the amygdala, and can reduce our physiological stress reactions (e.g., the activation of sympathetic nervous system with increases in heart rate and blood pressure, and rapid breathing) (Creswell & Lindsay, 2014).

Yoga

The word yoga is derived from a Sanskrit word that means "union" or "join with." This implies that one of the core purposes of yoga is harmony of mind and body, but it also encompasses exploration of other connections, such as with the spirit, the social world, nature, or one's emotions. As a spiritual practice, yoga's roots in India stretch back more than 5000 years. In the west, yoga is often viewed as more of an exercise and relaxation technique. For many, regardless of whether the practice is taken on with a spiritual intent or not, it is a way to balance the mind and body. There are well-documented benefits associated with practicing yoga. The movements associated with the practice release neurotransmitters impacting happiness (Büssing et al., 2012), ease stress and feelings of anxiety (Lemay et al., 2019; Saeed et al., 2010), improve sleep (Kumar, 2010), and improve inflammatory biomarkers (Bower et al., 2005; Falkenberg et al., 2018).

Typically, yoga combines physical postures or poses (called asanas) with breathing techniques (called pranayama) and meditation. Yoga postures focus body and mind on one goal, freeing both from other less immediate concerns. There are many types of yoga practice, and here are a few of the most widely practiced:

Ashtanga Yoga: This yoga is practiced with a series of postures that are performed in an exact order and become increasingly difficult as one advances up the six levels of poses. It is described as "dynamic and flowing," with attention to achieving physical flow through movement and balance. This yoga practice builds muscle tone, physical strength, and endurance. Ashtanga yoga is physically intense, but it does not result in tiredness or exhaustion, rather in renewed energy and vitality.

Bikram Yoga (also called Hot Yoga): This type of yoga is composed of a set of 26 poses over a 90-minute class and takes place in a humid, heated room. The purpose of the heat is to facilitate muscle stretching and to encourage free perspiration, and this yoga can increase flexibility, relieve stress, and induce muscle relaxation. Since the poses are in sequence, once the poses are learned it frees the mind to roam or to concentrate on the sensations of the body. It is important to note that the heat increases the risk of dehydration, heat stroke, and other heat-related symptoms, so it is important to check in with ourselves and drink water while practicing Hot Yoga.

Hatha Yoga: This is a common type of yoga in gym environments and online videos. It focuses on mastering specific postures (like mountain, tree, and downward-facing dog), while breathing through and meditating on each pose. Calmness and stillness of body and mind are desired outcomes of the poses. Iyengar Yoga is a subtype of Hatha Yoga that follows a meticulous sequence of poses.

Vinyasa Yoga: This type of yoga focuses on smooth transitions from one pose to another in a series of fluid motions matched with controlled breathing. Vinyasa yoga is one of the more physically demanding types of yoga, and it can be challenging to master. Power Yoga is a subtype of Vinyasa Yoga that is even more fast-paced and focused on building strength.

Yin Yoga: This is a slower type of yoga, focused on holding poses for long periods of time (sometimes, with practice, for 5 minutes or longer). This yoga stretches the joints and connective tissue (like ligaments and fascia) in what has been described as "deep stretching," rather than focusing on the major muscles like other types of yoga. Yin yoga is part of a type of yoga called "restorative yoga," which can help build flexibility, physical and mental balance, and mobility. It can be a useful post-workout meditative practice, as the long poses provide moments of mental clarity and openness.

Table 9.1 Other Eastern approaches to mind-body wellness

Technique	Description
Qigong and Tai Chi	Qigong and Tai Chi are self-healing and energy-cultivation exercises. An ancient Chinese practice, these exercises combine body movements with deep breathing and mental focus. The goal is to balance Qi with our body, which practitioners believe to be the vital energy that flows along certain channels, or meridians, throughout our bodies. The purported benefits of these practices are similar to those of mindfulness meditation. In addition, research suggests the movements associated with Qigong and Tai Chi, paired with controlled breathing, alters the autonomic system and attenuates stress related to the hypothalamus-pituitary-adrenal axis
Acupuncture	Acupuncture, aligned with the philosophy of Qi, is used to balance energy flow within us. Practitioners believe that Qi can be blocked, and imbalance in our energy is the result. Acupuncture involves placing needles along the channels or meridians where Qi flows. Practitioners believe these needles open blocked channels and help to improve health and well-being. The research concerning acupuncture typically has methodological concerns that make interpretation and application difficult. Questions about the role of the placebo effect and the validity of causal claims regarding the efficacy of acupuncture remain
Ayurveda	Ayurveda, a natural approach to medicine, began in India more than 3000 years ago. This perspective views disease as the result of an imbalance or stress within one's consciousness. Treatment revolves around re-establishing harmony between mind and body. Interventions begin with a purification process and are uniquely created for each person to address nutritional needs, yoga, meditation, massage, and social engagement

One of the many benefits of yoga is that most types can be done virtually anywhere—home, a class, outside in nature, or while traveling. Yoga ranges from simple beginner level to extremely complex and advanced. For people who want to begin practicing yoga or maintain an established practice, there are many types of in-person classes available, but there are also guiding videos online, subscription online services, and apps available. If a person is not typically physically active, has any health conditions, or has pain anywhere in the body, they should check with a doctor before starting yoga. Also, make sure to have a yoga mat or a nonslip surface to practice on—safety first to avoid injury!

In addition to yoga, there are many other mind-body techniques that originate or are heavily practiced in Asia and the pacific islands. Some of these approaches are detailed in Table 9.1.

Breathwork

The practice of breathwork centers on conscious, intentional control of breathing. Slow controlled breathing can help calm us down and focus us on the present moment. Breathwork can be used on its own to relax, focus, and empower, but it is also often used in conjunction with or as a core feature of yoga, meditation, progressive relaxation, and other mind-body techniques. When we control our breathing, it moderates the communication sent from our respiratory system and quickly influences brain regions involved in the regulation of behavior, thought, and emotion (Philippot et al., 2002). A meta-analysis reviewing 15 clinical studies focusing on breathwork found breathwork interventions significantly reduce distressing anxiety symptoms for people diagnosed with anxiety disorders (Banushi et al., 2023).

The first step of any breathwork journey is to learn our normal pattern of breathing through mindful attention to our breathing across a variety of situations. Here are some of the most common types of breathwork:

Abdominal Breathing: From a sitting position or laying down, place one hand on the abdomen and one on the chest. Taking deep and long breaths through the nose, focus on expanding the abdomen (picture the belly like a balloon filling with air), hold for a second or two, then pull in the belly button to exhale. Try to have the chest and ribs be neutral (meaning, try not to breathe in or exhale using chest muscles). Abdominal breathing is efficient and effective in improving breathing and inducing calm, as it exercises the diaphragm and engages the full range of breath capacity.

Paced Breathing: The goal of paced breathing is to exert both mental and physical control on breathing, which can help to interrupt anxiety spirals, slow physiological responses to stress (like rapid heart rate or heavy breathing), and induce feelings of calm. There are a variety of ways to pace our breathing, which can be used in conjunction with other breathing techniques (like abdominal breathing) or with meditation and yoga. One variation is to breathe out for twice as long as we breathe in, meaning that if we breathe in for 5 seconds, we will breathe out for 10 seconds. Another variation is 4–7-8 breathing, in which we inhale for four counts, hold for seven counts, and exhale for eight counts. The final type is "box breathing," which entails inhaling for four counts, holding for four counts, and exhaling for four counts.

Alternate Nostril Breathing: For this technique, start by gently pressing the right thumb onto the right nostril to block air flow, and inhale slowly and deeply through the left nostril. Then switch the pressure to the left nostril and exhale through the right. Inhale on the right and continue switching back and forth. The primary benefits of alternate nostril breathing are to strengthen respiration and regulate heart rate through conscious attention.

There are additional breathing techniques, such as Breath of Fire (rapid abdominal breathing) and Holotropic Breathwork (continuous breathing pattern of rapid, deep breaths) that are used therapeutically to address psychological and emotional distress. These techniques, particularly Holotropic Breathwork, have been described as facilitating "altered consciousness" and assisting to "rewire the brain." However, these techniques can cause hyperventilation and alter blood chemistry in ways that can cause fainting and seizures. These techniques should never be practiced alone, without the guidance of a trained practitioner, or without consulting with a physician first. When practicing any type of breathwork, however, we should always pay attention to the cues of our body, and if we start to feel unwell, lightheaded, or dizzy, then *stop immediately*, sit down, and breathe normally.

Progressive Muscle Relaxation (PMR)

As a relaxation technique, PMR can help to control stress, anxiety, and insomnia and can assist with managing pain. The mind-body philosophy behind PMR is that mental calmness also requires physical relaxation. To practice PMR, start by tensing the toes, holding for 5 seconds while paying attention to the sensation of tension, then releasing the hold and relaxing the muscle completely while focusing on the sensation of muscle relaxation. Then tense and release the top of the feet, then the bottom of the feet, then the ankles, progressing all the way up the body. PMR can also be done from the head down (starting with the scalp) or from the hands in, and it can also incorporate breathwork (breathe in while tensing the muscles, breath out as the muscles are released). This technique builds awareness of where tension is held in the body and also empowers practitioners to actively improve well-being by releasing tension and purposefully creating relaxation. A clear advantage of this technique is that it can be done anywhere—watching TV, reading or studying, before sleep, or at our desk.

Massage

Many of us likely view massage as a luxurious spa experience. The benefits, however, extend beyond a simple day of pampering. A massage is the rubbing of our body's soft tissue, including skin, muscles, tendons, and ligaments. The process can be relaxing and was an early tool used by humans to help address pain. In a massage session, our body responds by decreasing our stress response. As a result, cortisol levels decrease, and both serotonin and dopamine increase. These neurotransmitters are closely linked to happiness and a greater sense of well-being. The benefit to the mind from massage's intervention with the body provides another great example of the intricate connection between the two. Research reviewing the effectiveness of massage found massage therapy to be effective in reducing pain after surgery, as well as short-term and long-term pain.

There are several types of massage. Each approach has some variation in technique and different foci on the body.

Traditional Massage (sometimes referred to as Swedish Massage): Typically involves circular movements and kneading with long smooth strokes, used to manipulate muscles, tendons, and ligaments. This approach increases blood and lymph circulation, improves the delivery of oxygen and nutrients to tissue cells, removes toxins, tissue damage, and inflammation, and encourages relaxation. This helps assist our body's self-healing process and aids in pain reduction.

Sports Massage: Many athletes and weekend warriors rely on Sports Massages (often called Performance Massage) to help with repetitive motion injuries. This specialized form of massage is aimed at enhancing athletic performance and promoting post-event recovery. Muscle groups involved in a specific sport are targeted using direct or trigger point pressure, focused squeezing, and rhythmic tapping to treat muscle soreness, fatigue, and help prevent injuries.

Deep Tissue Massage: Utilizes firmer pressure, heavy heel of the hand pressure, and more intense finger pressure on specific tight spots. This approach targets tight muscles and tendons to release the tightness using slow, high-pressure strokes and deep finger pressure. This type of massage is great for sore muscle, muscle tightness, and chronic muscle pain.

Lymphatic Drainage Massage: A gentler massage technique that helps move lymphatic fluid through the lymphatic system and into the bloodstream. Precise rhythmic strokes are used to help pump lymphatic fluid, open and close small capillaries, and enhance reabsorption of lymph back into the lymphatic vessels. This massage technique helps remove toxins and tissue fluid retention, reduces pain, and promotes a sense of relaxation.

Visualization and Guided Imagery

Visualization is our ability to use our mind's eye. If someone asks you how many windows your house or apartment has, you will likely mentally walk around or through your place and count the number of windows. Incredibly, when we are doing this, the part of our brain that is engaged is the same area activated when we are actually viewing the scene (Pearson et al., 2015). Visualization or mental imagery is strongly associated with emotions. The process activates emotions in the same way that real-life experiences do for us (e.g., Holmes & Mathews, 2010). Preliminary work has found positive imagery to enhance positive emotions (Nelis et al., 2012) and decrease depression (Torkan et al., 2014). Guided imagery is a type of visualization that can be used in psychotherapy to create images and scenes of healing, calm, and wellness. Guided imagery can also be used to walk through the solution to a problem or to visualize success in a scenario that is meaningful to us, such as asking our boss for a raise, winning a sports championship, or quitting smoking.

Aromatherapy

Aromatherapy is the practice of using essential oils to enhance well-being. The oils are typically derived from plants using mechanical means (like squeezing or crushing) or through distillation. Essential oils can be inhaled, usually from a diffuser or via heating, or a diluted form can be applied to the skin via lotions, gels, or massage (always thin essential oils with a carrier oil before applying to skin). Some people use aromatherapy misters or sprays to scent their pillows and bed sheets, believing this leads to good sleep and pleasant dreams. Others use aromatherapy steaming pods in the shower or add essential oils to their bath. Aromatherapy can be used to complement traditional medicine, and people often use pleasant smells to reduce anxiety, induce relaxation, and help to cope with pain. It is important to note that the subjective value of the aroma—whether it is perceived as favorable, stimulating, intense, or arousing—appears to be a key to its reported effects (Herz, 2009). Research on aromatherapy is often of poor quality with small samples, but there is some evidence that subjective well-being and self-reports of mood and reported pain levels may be improved via aromatherapy (e.g., Herz, 2009). Aromatherapy and essential oils are a companion to, not a replacement for, conventional medicine.

Grounding (Also Called Earthing)

Grounding has been around for hundreds, perhaps thousands of years, and has been referred to as an "authentic" mind/body technique. Grounding refers to mindfulness-based techniques that help anchor us in the present moment. This enhances self-soothing and release of care through actions that center around immersion in the natural world and/or focus on a perceptual experience via one of our body's senses. Grounding develops skills that can help distract us from unwanted memories or anxious feelings, as sometimes we all need a break from the things that are distressing us. Figure 9.1 lists several categories and types of grounding techniques. While practicing any of these techniques, the goal is to clear the mind, calm the body, and experience them fully in the moment.

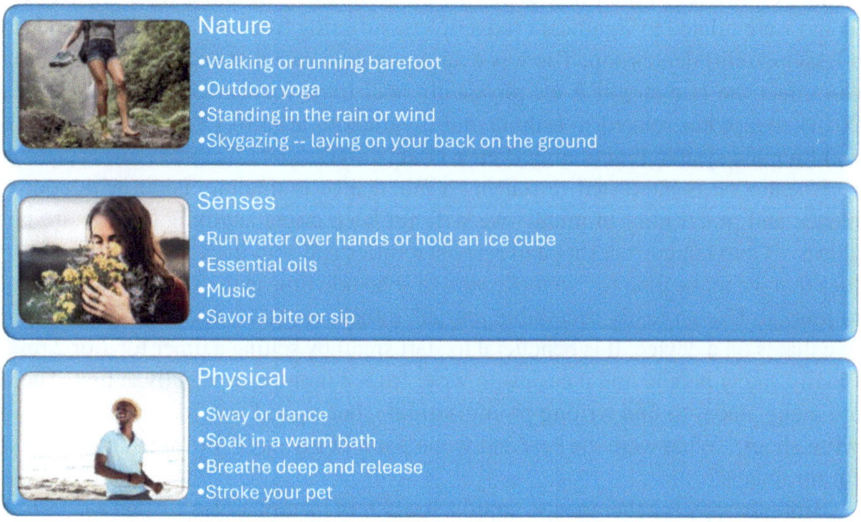
Nature
•Walking or running barefoot
•Outdoor yoga
•Standing in the rain or wind
•Skygazing -- laying on your back on the ground
Senses
•Run water over hands or hold an ice cube
•Essential oils
•Music
•Savor a bite or sip
Physical
•Sway or dance
•Soak in a warm bath
•Breathe deep and release
•Stroke your pet

Fig. 9.1 Grounding techniques

Journaling and Bibliotherapy

Journaling can be a powerful tool for working through thoughts and emotions that are troublesome and/or persistent. Journaling is an expressive endeavor in that it is not only about the act of "getting it down on paper," but it is also about discovering a way to articulate what has been overwhelming, inaccessible, or even vaguely discernable in our inner world. Journaling does not have to be done "in a journal," but rather it can be accomplished through writing or typing or voice recording anywhere—in a formal journal, on a pad of paper by our bed, on our phone, in the sand, or by any means that we can graphically represent our thoughts. Journaling can be a formal "sit down and write a paragraph" process, or it can be more stream of consciousness, wherein words or phrases are written as they come into conscious perception. Gratitude journaling is a specific kind of positive journaling focused on those things that we are grateful for, wish to express thanks for, and appreciate about our lives and the people in them. Journals can even be topical, including topics like dreams, diet or food journey, relationship progress, or any other personally important topic.

Journaling is a low-cost, easily implemented, nonmedical intervention that can be used by itself as a positive wellness tool to increase self-understanding or to work through problems of life. It can also be used in conjunction with other interventions like therapy or medication to help patients cope with mild to moderate mental health symptoms. In a meta-analysis of studies of expressive and gratitude journaling, Sohal et al. (2022) found that even small amounts of journaling (two to four sessions) were related to significant reduction in suffering from anxiety, PTSD, and (to a lesser extent) depression. There is even some evidence that expressive journaling can affect the rate at which we physically heal from wounds (Koschwanez et al., 2013), symptoms related to asthma and rheumatoid arthritis (Smyth et al., 1999), and immune system functioning (Petrie et al., 2004).

If someone is interested in starting a practice of journaling, begin with convenience and practicality in mind—we will not keep doing anything that we are not able to fit into our current scope of responsibilities and activities. We maintain activities that we make time for, so make sure to schedule time at the same time each day to journal. Use an easily accessible journal, either one that can easily be carried or one that is on a device. It is beneficial to start small by setting a timer for 1 or 2 min. Finally, many people find it easiest to write from a prompt, especially at first. There are many places to find writing prompts online, but a good way to start is simply to write about, "What were the best and worst parts of my day?" or "What am I thankful for today?"

Bibliotherapy is a therapeutic approach wherein therapists use written works like stories, poems, fiction, and biographies to facilitate discussion of specific issues in the therapeutic session. The goal is to take a specific issue, say relationships or life dissatisfaction or parenting, and facilitate insight into related emotions and behaviors through reading. Bibliotherapy is often used in association with or as an accompaniment to another therapeutic approach. A meta-analysis of bibliotherapy found that it helps relieve mild to moderate symptoms of depression compared to standard treatment or no treatment (Gualano et al., 2017). Bibliotherapy has the advantage of being able to incorporate authentic cultural and/or gender elements into the therapeutic process, and it can also be useful for people who are undergoing treatments or conditions that limit their mobility (e.g., McCoy & McKay, 2006). Another benefit of bibliotherapy is that it can be used with all ages. It is very common to enlist a book to help children understand complex topics, such as grief and loss, divorce, or puberty (e.g., Arruda-Colli et al., 2017). One can also engage in bibliotherapy without the assistance of a therapist by using self-help books or literature related to existing concerns. However, it is wise to be careful in choosing self-help books to avoid pop psychology and also to avoid traumatizing or retraumatizing oneself with works that do not write about specific issues in terms that can be processed independently.

Biofeedback

The current shift in medicine is moving us from disease management to a greater focus on health promotion and prevention. This shift requires us to be more actively involved in monitoring our well-being. Biofeedback requires the use of our mind-body connection to observe and self-regulate changes within our body. According to the Association for Applied Psychophysiology and Biofeedback (AAPB, n.d.), biofeedback is "...a process that enables an individual to learn how to change physiological activity for the purposes of improving health and performance." These measurements can include physiological activity such as brain waves, heart function, breathing, muscle activity, and skin temperature. Receiving this information allows us to more accurately notice physiological changes. The goal is, over time, for us to continue to notice these changes without the continued use of an instrument.

Technology provides a convenient way to support the use of biofeedback. Products like the Apple Watch monitor physiological changes in heart rate, breath, and can detect irregular heart rhythms. In addition, this technology allows us to track our sleeping patterns, menstrual cycles, and can even let us know when our cardio level is too low. This technology makes monitoring changes associated with biofeedback easier and more definitive. By noticing these physiological changes, we can become more aware of our bodies and learn to control pain to some extent.

Chiropractic

Chiropractic care is concerned with the healing, maintenance, and proper functioning of the musculoskeletal system. Chiropractic treatments are designed to support the healing processes of the body, reduce pain, and enhance health and wellness. Clients particularly seek this type of care when dealing with back and neck pain, headaches, arthritis, reduced range of motion due to pain, and sciatica. Chiropractors use a range of treatments to assist clients to regain and maintain both function and pain reduction or elimination, such as:

Spinal Adjustment: Typically done through a "Diversified Technique" (but many other manipulation techniques are possible), this involves the manual manipulation of the spine.

Extremity Adjustment: Manipulation of joints other than the spine, such as shoulders, hips, wrists/hands, and feet.

Activator Method: Involves the use of a hand-held instrument to direct a quick, low-force thrust to the spine or joints.

Heat or ice therapy: Used to relax the muscles, lower inflammation, and reduce the perception of pain.

Movement-Based Massage (also called Active Release): Facilitates soft tissue release and healing through application of pressure along with movement of the affected area.

Electrical Stimulation: Typically, a transcutaneous electrical nerve stimulation (TENS) unit is used to deliver low-voltage electrical current to an area to block pain or alter the perception of pain.

It is important to note that chiropractors are not medical doctors, but they can be part of the care team when a person feels they need additional intervention around an issue that is resistant to conventional medical treatment, or the person wants to pursue nonmedical approaches. Goertz and colleagues (2018) compared usual care for lower back pain (medication, physical therapy, self-care) with usual care plus chiropractic care in a sample of active-duty military personnel. They found that usual care plus chiropractic was modestly more effective over the short term in lowering self-reported pain and level of disability and decreasing medication use.

Overall, the research on chiropractic care is mixed at best, and in general the techniques show little to modest benefit over conventional care for headache or back and neck pain. For example, Bronfort et al. (2012) divided patients with neck pain into three groups receiving medication, spinal adjustment, or home exercise with advice (HEA). Both the spinal adjustment and HEA groups reported better pain management than the medication group, but there were similar outcomes for pain with spinal adjustment or HEA. At least some of the benefits of chiropractic are subjective in that patients are highly satisfied with chiropractic care and believe it makes them feel better (e.g., Herman et al., 2018; Jensen et al., 2023), but more large-scale, well-designed studies are needed to clarify the benefits of chiropractic for specific disorders and specific populations.

Nature

There are many advantages to living in modern times. It is, however, in stark contrast to how we evolved as a species where we spent the majority of our lives outside. Vitamin D production is triggered when we are exposed to sunlight. Vitamin D is often referred to as the sunshine vitamin! When we experience Vitamin D deficiency our bodies struggle to absorb calcium and phosphorus, and we increase our risk for bone pain, bone fractures, muscle pain, and muscle weakness. Vitamin D deficiency in pregnant women is associated with a 400% increase in the probability of a Cesarean section (Wacker & Holick, 2013).

In addition to exposure to sunlight, there are benefits to being out in nature. Shinrin-yoku is a Japanese term that means "forest-bathing." The idea grew in popularity during the 1980s. Recognizing that the sensory overload associated with modern life in cities can make it difficult to relax and calm one's mind, spending time in nature was "prescribed" to help calm the mind. This idea is now practiced around the world for therapeutic and preventative health purposes. For good reasons! Recent work comparing a walk in the woods to a walk in an urban environment found a reduction in cortisol levels for those who walked in the forest but not among those walking in an urban environment (Kobayashi et al., 2019). There are clear psychological benefits as well. Walking in a forested area is associated with a reduction in depression, anxiety, anger, and increases in positive mood (Song et al., 2018). Moreover, a walk in the woods seems to be very beneficial for people with hightrait anxiety.

Therapy for Mental Wellness

Earlier in this text, we learned about conventional types of therapy. Traditional psychotherapy, also called talk therapy or counseling, helps people to identify and overcome thoughts, behaviors, and emotions that may be troubling them or interfering in their lives. Psychotherapy often helps clients to explore the root causes of psychological distress, address unhelpful, negative thought patterns, build coping resources, improve emotional resilience, and strengthen relationships and social support. In Table 9.2, we present an overview of specific mind-body approaches to therapy, which often include some traditional psychotherapy methods along with holistic and mind-body approaches.

Holistic Psychotherapy: The philosophy behind holistic psychotherapy is that the mind, body, and spirit are a single unit, operating in a way that seeks balance and harmony. Reduction in harmonious mutual action of mind, body, and spirit, and the resultant disharmony is what causes our experience of distress, affliction, and pain. What manifests as a physical symptom often reflects a mental or spiritual issue, and physical distress is not only experienced in the body. Most practitioners of holistic psychotherapy use techniques from traditional psychotherapy, like talking, discussing, and listening, alongside mind-body techniques like mindfulness, meditation, breathwork, yoga, spiritual support, and nutrition counseling. The idea is that if the therapy addresses the whole person, rather than one issue or problem, then integration of mind, body, and spirit becomes both the process and the goal.

Table 9.2 Other approaches to mind-body therapy

Modality	Description
Dance Therapy	The American Dance Therapy Association defines dance therapy as "... the psychotherapeutic use of movement to promote emotional, social, cognitive, and physical integration of the individual, for the purpose of improving health and well-being." For dance therapists, nonverbal language is as important as verbal communication, and the core components of dance are used in the therapeutic process
Music Therapy	According to the American Music Therapy Association, music therapy involves music-based interventions to help people achieve their individual goals. Under a therapeutic relationship, guided by a credentialed professional, music therapy interventions can address a variety of healthcare and educational goals
Animal-Assisted Therapy	As a therapeutic intervention, animal-assisted therapy includes animals in the treatment plan. This approach, based on the bond that develops between people and animals, is designed to help people develop a better sense of self-worth, understand and stabilize their emotions, improve communication, self-regulate, and develop socialization skills. Working with animals can provide more physical activity as well, especially out in nature
Eye Movement Desensitization Reprocessing Therapy (EMDR)	EMDR is a mental health treatment used primarily to help clients with trauma histories or PTSD/C-PTSD diagnosis to process their distressing memories. Specific movements of the eyes are used to help clients work through recollections of trauma. While the client briefly focuses on the memory, the repetitive eye movements help the person to unpack the emotion and change where it is stored in the brain, thereby reducing acute distress and vivid recall associated with the memory
Relaxation therapy	This approach helps reduce muscle tension and stress, lower blood pressure, and control pain. This therapy often involves tensing and then relaxing muscles throughout the body and may be used with guided imagery (focusing the mind on positive images) and meditation

Somatic Therapy (also called mind-body therapy): This type of therapy focuses on how emotions are experienced within the body, as well as how the mind and emotions interpret sensations from the body. Like holistic psychotherapy, traditional talk therapy techniques can be used, but the emphasis is on body awareness and healing. Somatic therapy has particularly been useful for trauma responses, PTSD, anxiety, depression, and complicated grief. The starting point for somatic therapy is to develop somatic awareness, which is the ability to intentionally and dependably interpret the signs and signals of the body. Somatic therapy also employs several specific techniques, including:

Grounding: The client utilizes techniques that help center themselves in the body sensations of the here-and-now.

Titration: The therapist guides the client to revisit a past traumatic event while monitoring and discussing the physical sensations (heavy breathing, crying, clenched hands, hunched shoulders) that occur in real time. This can be in concert with *pendulation*, where the therapist guides the client to the distressing sensations, then back again to a calm state.

Resourcing: Clients are guided to recall and discuss people (particularly protective or nurturing people) and places (safe or peaceful places) that promote bodily calm and relaxation in the present moment.
Sequencing: This is the process of following the movement of emotion-based tension around the body until it is released. The client is encouraged to observe and follow the tension, learning the pathways of emotion through their bodies.
Movement: Body movements through yoga, tai chi, dance, swaying, or other means enable positive bodily sensations and allow clients to tap into the natural potential of their body for pleasant sensations and healing.

Mindfulness-Based Cognitive Therapy (MBCT): Cognitive behavioral therapy (CBT) is a modality of psychotherapy that identifies negative, harmful, and unhelpful thoughts and behaviors and helps people to change them. A long history of research on CBT has shown that it is efficacious for a variety of mental health concerns, but its strongest effects seem to be in the treatment of depression, anxiety, eating disorders, and stress (Hofmann et al., 2012). MBCT combines CBT with mindfulness meditation and other mindfulness strategies in order to help teach people ways to intervene in their emotions before a negative spiral occurs, to change their negative and self-defeating way of thinking, and to manage stress in proactive and effective ways. Although MBCT was originally designed to help people cope with depression (e.g., Segal et al., 2012), it is now used with other mental health concerns like anxiety, addictive behaviors, and bipolar disorder.

Remember Your Growth Mindset

As we leave this chapter, remember the Wellness Tip from Chap. 1 to "mind your mindset." The shift in psychology that has moved toward promoting the positive aspects of our lives encourages a different type of mindset. That is, perceiving ourselves as able to continuously develop and improve is critical to flourishing. A growth mindset consists of a belief that our abilities and talents can be improved through putting effort into changing, learning new skills, and continuing even in the face of adversity. Through intentional activities, we can learn new talents and constantly work towards new goals. When we nurture these parts of ourselves, we benefit not only in all-around wellness, but we are also more satisfied with life, enjoy life more, and are more resilient when we encounter hardships. Figure 9.2 presents a helpful guide to other mind-body-based ways that we can enhance our ability to cope with and be resilient to challenges we may encounter in the course of everyday life. The essence of productive and healthful mind-body wellness is to devote ourselves to science-based paths of wellness in order to learn, grow, take a different perspective, persevere through obstacles, and engage our whole selves in the mental and physical joys of life.

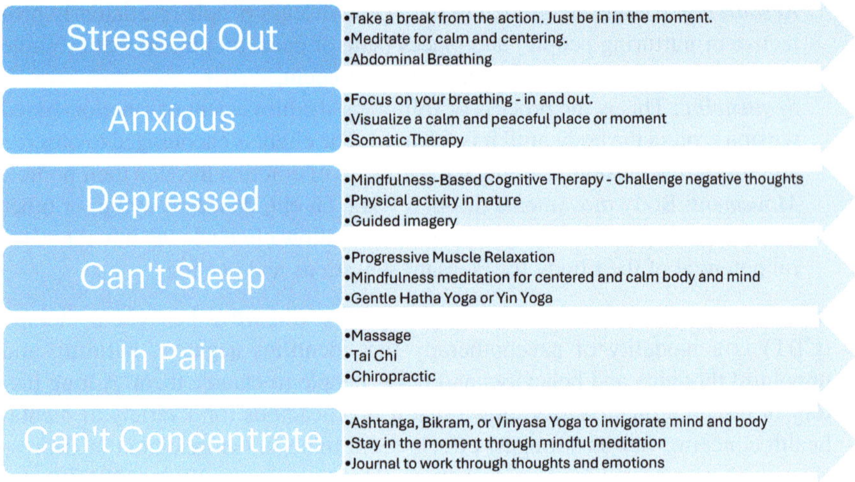

Fig. 9.2 "What Do I Do When I'm…" Mind-body approaches to common issues in everyday life

Wellness Tip—The Essential Practice of Self-Care

Self-care, a term gaining more attention and recognition in the academic world, on social media, and in the general population, reflects an acknowledgment that it is important for us to take time to ensure we are healthy and well. We have many responsibilities we juggle (e.g., work, family, friends, home, finances), and enacting a proactive plan to keep ourselves healthy and well increases our ability to more effectively manage these responsibilities. It is difficult to manage everything when we are not feeling well or not taking the time to improve our sense of well-being. The implications of self-care move beyond just personal benefits. When we feel well, healthy, and clear minded, we are better partners in our romantic relationships, better friends, better parents and caregivers, and more effective in our places of employment. Figure 9.3 presents self-care behaviors, practices, and techniques that are related to each of the eight dimensions of wellness.

Self-care has three key dimensions: self-care maintenance, self-care monitoring, and self-care management (Riegel et al., 2012). Self-care maintenance refers to our personal plan or program of actions we take regularly to maintain our health and wellness and prevent illness. This includes being knowledgeable about each dimension of wellness individually and also how they flow into and impact each other. For example, the physical health benefits of regular physical activity, including mind-body activities like yoga and tai chi, are well documented, and these physical activities help with weight management, improve brain health, reduce the likelihood of various diseases, and, importantly, improve ability to engage in everyday activities. But physical activity is not just about physical wellness—it impacts our mental

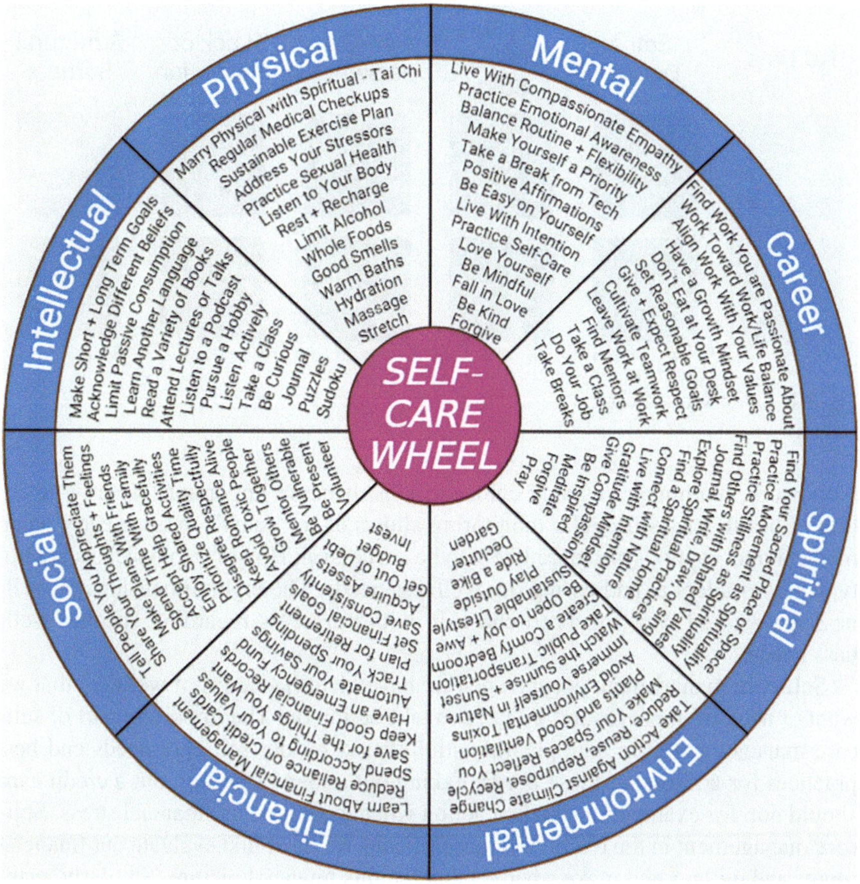
SELF-CARE WHEEL
Physical
Marry Physical with Spiritual - Tai Chi
Regular Medical Checkups
Sustainable Exercise Plan
Address Your Stressors
Practice Sexual Health
Listen to Your Body
Rest + Recharge
Limit Alcohol
Whole Foods
Good Smells
Warm Baths
Hydration
Massage
Stretch
Mental
Live With Compassionate Empathy
Practice Emotional Awareness
Balance Routine + Flexibility
Make Yourself a Priority
Take a Break from Tech
Positive Affirmations
Be Easy on Yourself
Live With Intention
Practice Self-Care
Love Yourself
Be Mindful
Fall in Love
Be Kind
Forgive
Career
Find Work You are Passionate About
Work Toward Work/Life Balance
Align Work With Your Values
Have a Growth Mindset
Don't Eat at Your Desk
Set Reasonable Goals
Give + Expect Respect
Cultivate Teamwork
Leave Work at Work
Find Mentors
Take a Class
Do Your Job
Take Breaks
Spiritual
Find Your Sacred Place or Space
Practice Movement as Spirituality
Practice Stillness as Spirituality
Find Others with Shared Values
Journal, Write, Draw, or sing
Explore Spiritual Practices
Find a Spiritual Home
Connect with Nature
Live with Intention
Gratitude Mindset
Give Compassion
Be Inspired
Meditate
Forgive
Pray
Environmental
Take Action Against Climate Change
Reduce, Reuse, Repurpose, Recycle
Make Your Spaces Reflect You
Plants and Good Ventilation
Avoid Environmental Toxins
Immerse Yourself in Nature
Watch the Sunrise + Sunset
Take Public Transportation
Create a Comfy Bedroom
Be Open to Joy + Awe
Sustainable Lifestyle
Play Outside
Ride a Bike
Declutter
Garden
Financial
Learn About Financial Management
Reduce Reliance on Credit Cards
Spend According to Your Values
Save for the Things You Want
Keep Good Financial Records
Have an Emergency Fund
Automate Your Savings
Track Your Spending
Plan for Retirement
Set Financial Goals
Save Consistently
Acquire Assets
Get Out of Debt
Budget
Invest
Social
Tell People You Appreciate Them
Share Your Thoughts + Feelings
Make Plans With Friends
Spend Time With Family
Accept Help Gracefully
Enjoy Shared Activities
Prioritize Quality Time
Disagree Respectfully
Keep Romance Alive
Avoid Toxic People
Grow Together
Mentor Others
Be Vulnerable
Be Present
Volunteer
Intellectual
Make Short + Long Term Goals
Acknowledge Different Beliefs
Limit Passive Consumption
Learn Another Language
Read a Variety of Books
Attend Lectures or Talks
Listen to a Podcast
Pursue a Hobby
Listen Actively
Take a Class
Be Curious
Journal
Puzzles
Sudoku

Fig. 9.3 Self-care wheel

health through lower rates of depression (Uebelacker et al., 2010) and improved emotional and mental well-being (e.g., Hassmén et al., 2000; Steptoe, 1992). Improved physical and mental wellness then flow into more positive approaches to relationships and enhanced mental clarity, ability to concentrate, and vitality at work and school. This is not to say that there are no barriers to self-care both within and among dimensions of wellness; both objective and subjective barriers to self-care exist, including financial constraints, physical and mental limitations, and lack of access to resources and support. Sometimes it helps to see self-care as an evolving process, rather than an event. Figure 9.4 describes some common barriers to self-care and some ways to address them.

Self-care monitoring consists of regularly assessing our health and wellness. Yearly physicals are an important way medical professionals assess changes in our health status over time. For example, as we age, certain tests and exams, such as

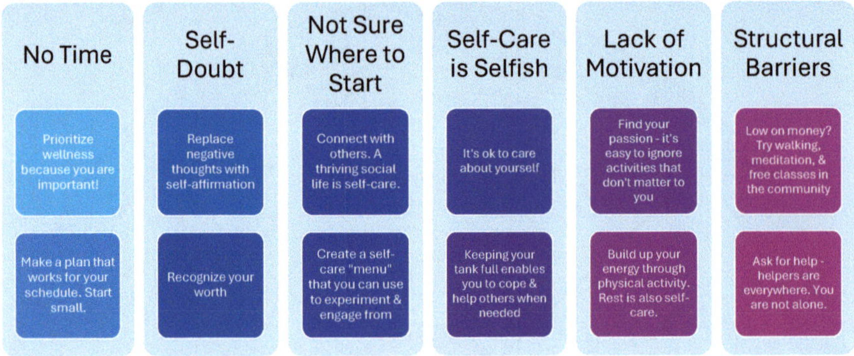
No Time
Prioritize wellness because you are important!
Make a plan that works for your schedule. Start small.
Self-Doubt
Replace negative thoughts with self-affirmation
Recognize your worth
Not Sure Where to Start
Connect with others. A thriving social life is self-care.
Create a self-care "menu" that you can use to experiment & engage from
Self-Care is Selfish
It's ok to care about yourself
Keeping your tank full enables you to cope & help others when needed
Lack of Motivation
Find your passion - it's easy to ignore activities that don't matter to you
Build up your energy through physical activity. Rest is also self-care.
Structural Barriers
Low on money? Try walking, meditation, & free classes in the community
Ask for help - helpers are everywhere. You are not alone.

Fig. 9.4 Barriers to self-care

bloodwork, mammograms, and colonoscopies, become important for early detection of health issues. Regular monitoring allows us to "catch" an issue early when medical interventions are more likely to be successful. However, physicians are not typically as adept at addressing our wellness needs. The eight dimensions of wellness are a good way for us to check in with ourselves regarding specific wellness needs.

Self-care management occurs when we have identified areas of wellness that we want or need to improve, and we need to take action on. The important part of self-care management is to take planful action, based on our self-care needs and best practices for addressing those needs. Taking out a loan or pulling out a credit card should not, for example, be the first action when experiencing financial stress. Self-care management in the realm of finances means we must first evaluate our financial inputs and outlays and make a budget that fits this financial picture. Similarly, managing our self-care in the area of career doesn't mean impulsively quitting our job when it is a consistent source of stress; instead, start searching for a better fit for you in terms of duties, workplace culture, and work-life balance.

Taken together, these three activities highlight the need for continuous self-care activities. It is important we are not just focusing on the care we need when we are not feeling well. Rather, it is essential this approach becomes a general process for how we maintain wellness. In *Outlive: The Science and Art of Longevity*, Dr. Peter Attia describes a shift to Medicine 3.0 (Attia & Gifford, 2023). This is a shift from being reactive, where intervention occurs once we know there is an issue, to a more proactive position, one where we are more involved in strategies to help ensure our well-being in the future. Living life with a well-being-conscious approach that centers our lifestyle choices encourages us to keep a focus on the balance between our mind and body. We should not wait for an issue to emerge before we decide to implement changes to improve our wellness. In contrast, making a self-care plan and implementing changes should be done prior to any health and wellness concerns forcing these behaviors.

References

Afonso, R. F., Kraft, I., Aratanha, M. A., & Kozasa, E. H. (2020). Neural correlates of meditation: A review of structural and functional MRI studies. *Frontiers in Bioscience, 12*(1), 92–115. https://doi.org/10.2741/S542

Arruda-Colli, M. N. F., Weaver, M. S., & Wiener, L. (2017). Communication about dying, death, and bereavement: A systematic review of children's literature. *Journal of Palliative Medicine, 20*(5), 548–559. https://doi.org/10.1089/jpm.2016.0494

Astin, J. A., Shapiro, S. L., Eisenberg, D. M., & Forys, K. L. (2003). Mind-body medicine: State of the science, implications for practice. *The Journal of the American Board of Family Practice, 16*(2), 131–147. https://doi.org/10.3122/jabfm.16.2.131

Association for Applied Psychophysiology and Biofeedback (n.d.). What is Biofeedback? https://aapb.org/#

Attia, P., & Gifford, B. (2023). *Outlive: The science & art of longevity*. Harmony.

Austin, J. H. (2013). Zen and the brain: Mutually illuminating topics. *Frontiers in Psychology, 4*, 784–784. https://doi.org/10.3389/fpsyg.2013.00784

Banushi, B., Brendle, M., Ragnhildstveit, A., Murphy, T., Moore, C., Egberts, J., & Robison, R. (2023). Breathwork interventions for adults with clinically diagnosed anxiety disorders: A scoping review. *Brain Sciences, 13*(2), 193.

Bishop, S. R., Lau, M., Shapiro, S., Carlson, L., Anderson, N. D., Carmody, J., Segal, Z. V., Abbey, S., Speca, M., Velting, D., & Devins, G. (2004). Mindfulness: A proposed operational definition. *Clinical Psychology: Science and Practice, 11*(3), 230–241. https://doi.org/10.1093/clipsy.bph077

Black, D. S., & Slavich, G. M. (2016). Mindfulness meditation and the immune system: A systematic review of randomized controlled trials. *Annals of the New York Academy of Sciences, 1373*(1), 13–24. https://doi.org/10.1111/nyas.12998

Bower, J. E., Woolery, A., Sternlieb, B., & Garet, D. (2005). Yoga for cancer patients and survivors. *Cancer Control: Journal of the Moffitt Cancer Center, 12*(3), 165–171. https://doi.org/10.1177/107327480501200304

Bronfort, G., Evans, R., Anderson, A. V., Svendsen, K. H., Bracha, Y., & Grimm, R. H. (2012). Spinal manipulation, medication, or home exercise with advice for acute and subacute neck pain: A randomized trial. *Annals of Internal Medicine, 156*(1 Pt 1), 1–10. https://doi.org/10.7326/0003-4819-156-1-201201030-00002

Büssing, A., Michalsen, A., Khalsa, S. B., Telles, S., & Sherman, K. J. (2012). Effects of yoga on mental and physical health: A short summary of reviews. *Evidence-based Complementary and Alternative Medicine, 165410*. https://doi.org/10.1155/2012/165410

Carmody, J., Baer, R. A., Lykins, E. L. B., & Olendzki, N. (2009). An empirical study of the mechanisms of mindfulness in a mindfulness-based stress reduction program. *Journal of Clinical Psychology, 65*(6), 613–626. https://doi.org/10.1002/jclp.20579

Creswell, J. D., & Lindsay, E. K. (2014). How does mindfulness training affect health? A mindfulness stress buffering account. *Current Directions in Psychological Science, 23*(6), 401–407. https://doi.org/10.1177/0963721414547415

Dasanayaka, N. N., Sirisena, N. D., & Samaranayake, N. (2021). The effects of meditation on length of telomeres in healthy individuals: A systematic review. *Systematic Reviews, 10*(1), 151. https://doi.org/10.1186/s13643-021-01699-1

Davis, M. C., Zautra, A. J., Wolf, L. D., Tennen, H., & Yeung, E. W. (2015). Mindfulness and cognitive–behavioral interventions for chronic pain: Differential effects on daily pain reactivity and stress reactivity. *Journal of Consulting and Clinical Psychology, 83*(1), 24–35. https://doi.org/10.1037/a0038200

Falkenberg, R. I., Eising, C., & Peters, M. L. (2018). Yoga and immune system functioning: A systematic review of randomized controlled trials. *Journal of Behavioral Medicine, 41*(4), 467–482. https://doi.org/10.1007/s10865-018-9914-y

Garland, E. L., Manusov, E. G., Froeliger, B., Kelly, A., Williams, J. M., & Howard, M. O. (2014). Mindfulness-oriented recovery enhancement for chronic pain and prescription opioid misuse: Results from an early-stage randomized controlled trial. *Journal of Consulting and Clinical Psychology, 82*(3), 448–459. https://doi.org/10.1037/a0035798

Goertz, C. M., Long, C. R., Vining, R. D., Pohlman, K. A., Walter, J., & Coulter, I. (2018). Effect of Usual Medical Care Plus Chiropractic Care vs Usual Medical Care Alone on Pain and Disability Among US Service Members With Low Back Pain: A Comparative Effectiveness Clinical Trial. JAMA network open, 1(1), e180105. https://doi.org/10.1001/jamanetworkopen.2018.0105

Gualano, M. R., Bert, F., Martorana, M., Voglino, G., Andriolo, V., Thomas, R., Gramaglia, C., Zeppegno, P., & Siliquini, R. (2017). The long-term effects of bibliotherapy in depression treatment: Systematic review of randomized clinical trials. *Clinical Psychology Review, 58*, 49–58. https://doi.org/10.1016/j.cpr.2017.09.006

Hassmén, P., Koivula, N., & Uutela, A. (2000). Physical exercise and psychological well-being: A population study in Finland. *Preventive Medicine, 30*(1), 17–25. https://doi.org/10.1006/pmed.1999.0597

Herman, P. M., Kommareddi, M., Sorbero, M. E., Rutter, C. M., Hays, R. D., Hilton, L. G., Ryan, G. W., & Coulter, I. D. (2018). Characteristics of chiropractic patients being treated for chronic low back and neck pain. *Journal of Manipulative and Physiological Therapeutics, 41*(6), 445–455. https://doi.org/10.1016/j.jmpt.2018.02.001

Herz, R. S. (2009). Aromatherapy facts and fictions: A scientific analysis of olfactory effects on mood, physiology and behavior. *International Journal of Neuroscience, 119*(2), 263–290. https://doi.org/10.1080/00207450802333953

Hofmann, S. G., Asnaani, A., Vonk, I. J., Sawyer, A. T., & Fang, A. (2012). The efficacy of cognitive behavioral therapy: A review of meta-analyses. *Cognitive Therapy and Research, 36*(5), 427–440. https://doi.org/10.1007/s10608-012-9476-1

Holmes, E. A., & Mathews, A. (2010). Mental imagery in emotion and emotional disorders. *Clinical Psychology Review, 30*(3), 349–362. https://doi.org/10.1016/j.cpr.2010.01.001

Jedel, S., Hoffman, A., Merriman, P., Swanson, B., Voigt, R., Rajan, K. B., Shaikh, M., Li, H., & Keshavarzian, A. (2014). A randomized controlled trial of mindfulness-based stress reduction to prevent flare-up in patients with inactive ulcerative colitis. *Digestion, 89*(2), 142–155. https://doi.org/10.1159/000356316

Jensen, R. K., Lillesø, S., Jensen, J. S., & Stochkendahl, M. J. (2023). Patient expectations and levels of satisfaction in chiropractic treatment for lumbar radiculopathy. A mixed methods study. *Chiropractic & Manual Therapies, 31*(1), 13. https://doi.org/10.1186/s12998-023-00486-0

Kabat-Zinn, J. (1994). *Wherever you go, there you are: Mindfulness meditation in everyday life.* Hyperion.

Kabat-Zinn, J. (2003). Mindfulness-based interventions in context: Past, present, and future. *Clinical Psychology: Science and Practice, 10*(2), 144–156. https://doi.org/10.1093/clipsy.bpg016

Killingsworth, M. A., & Gilbert, D. T. (2010). A wandering mind is an unhappy mind. *Science, 330*(6006), 932–932. http://www.jstor.org/stable/40931861

Kobayashi, H., Song, C., Ikei, H., Park, B.-J., Kagawa, T., & Miyazaki, Y. (2019). Combined effect of walking and forest environment on salivary cortisol concentration. *Frontiers in Public Health, 7*, 376–376. https://doi.org/10.3389/fpubh.2019.00376

Koschwanez, H. E., Kerse, N., Darragh, M., Jarrett, P., Booth, R. J., & Broadbent, E. (2013). Expressive writing and wound healing in older adults: A randomized controlled trial. *Psychosomatic Medicine, 75*(6), 581–590. https://doi.org/10.1097/PSY.0b013e31829b7b2e

Kumar, V. M. (2010). Sleep is neither a passive nor an active phenomenon: Sleep is neither passive nor active. *Sleep and Biological Rhythms, 8*(3), 163–169. https://doi.org/10.1111/j.1479-8425.2010.00445.x

Lemay, V., Hoolahan, J., & Buchanan, A. (2019). Impact of a yoga and meditation intervention on students' stress and anxiety levels. *American Journal of Pharmaceutical Education, 83*(5), 7001. https://doi.org/10.5688/ajpe7001

Lindqvist, E., Östling, R., & Cesarini, D. (2020). Long-run effects of lottery wealth on psychological well-being. *The Review of Economic Studies, 87*(6 (317)), 2703–2726. https://doi.org/10.1093/restud/rdaa006

Ma, S. H., & Teasdale, J. D. (2004). Mindfulness-based cognitive therapy for depression: Replication and exploration of differential relapse prevention effects. *Journal of Consulting and Clinical Psychology, 72*(1), 31–40. https://doi.org/10.1037/0022-006X.72.1.31

Malarkey, W. B., Jarjoura, D., & Klatt, M. (2013). Workplace based mindfulness practice and inflammation: A randomized trial. *Brain, Behavior, and Immunity, 27*(1), 145–154. https://doi.org/10.1016/j.bbi.2012.10.009

McCoy, H., & McKay, C. (2006). Preparing social workers to identify and integrate culturally affirming bibliotherapy into treatment. *Social Work Education, 25*(7), 680–693. https://doi.org/10.1080/02615470600905895

Morone, N. E., Greco, C. M., Moore, C. G., Rollman, B. L., Lane, B., Morrow, L. A., Glynn, N. W., & Weiner, D. K. (2016). A mind-body program for older adults with chronic low back pain: A randomized clinical trial. *JAMA Internal Medicine, 176*(3), 329–337. https://doi.org/10.1001/jamainternmed.2015.8033

Moynihan, J. A., Chapman, B. P., Klorman, R., Krasner, M. S., Duberstein, P. R., Brown, K. W., & Talbot, N. L. (2013). Mindfulness-based stress reduction for older adults: Effects on executive function, frontal alpha asymmetry and immune function. *Neuropsychobiology, 68*(1), 34–43. https://doi.org/10.1159/000350949

Neff, K. D., & Germer, C. K. (2013). A pilot study and randomized controlled trial of the mindful self-compassion program. *Journal of Clinical Psychology, 69*(1), 28–44. https://doi.org/10.1002/jclp.21923

Nelis, S., Vanbrabant, K., Holmes, E. A., & Raes, F. (2012). Greater positive affect change after mental imagery than verbal thinking in a student sample. *Journal of Experimental Psychopathology, 3*(2), 178–188. https://doi.org/10.5127/jep.021111

Pearson, J., Naselaris, T., Holmes, E. A., & Kosslyn, S. M. (2015). Mental Imagery: Functional Mechanisms and Clinical Applications. Trends in cognitive sciences, 19(10), 590–602. https://doi.org/10.1016/j.tics.2015.08.003

Petrie, K. J., Fontanilla, I., Thomas, M. G., Booth, R. J., & Pennebaker, J. W. (2004). Effect of written emotional expression on immune function in patients with human immunodeficiency virus infection: A randomized trial. *Psychosomatic Medicine, 66*(2), 272–275.

Philippot, P., Chapelle, G., & Blairy, S. (2002). Respiratory feedback in the generation of emotion. *Cognition and Emotion, 16*(5), 605–627. https://doi.org/10.1080/02699930143000392

Riegel, B., Jaarsma, T., & Strömberg, A. (2012). A middle-range theory of self-care of chronic illness. *Advances in Nursing Science, 35*(3), 194–204. https://doi.org/10.1097/ANS.0b013e318261b1ba

Saeed, S. A., Antonacci, D. J., & Bloch, R. M. (2010). Exercise, yoga, and meditation for depressive and anxiety disorders. *American Family Physician, 81*(8), 981–986.

Segal, Z., Williams, M., Teasdale, J., & Kabat-Zinn, J. (2012). *Mindfulness-based cognitive therapy for depression* (2nd ed.). Guilford Publications.

Smith, D., Nyarwath, O., Abuya, P. A., & Presbey, G. M. (2002). *Thought and practice in African philosophy*. Konrad Adenauer Stiftung.

Smyth, J. M., Stone, A. A., Hurewitz, A., & Kaell, A. (1999). Effects of writing about stressful experiences on symptom reduction in patients with asthma or rheumatoid arthritis: A randomized trial. *Journal of the American Medical Association (JAMA), 281*(14), 1304–1309. https://doi.org/10.1001/jama.281.14.1304

Sohal, M., Singh, P., Dhillon, B. S., & Gill, H. S. (2022). Efficacy of journaling in the management of mental illness: A systematic review and meta-analysis. *Family Medicine and Community Health, 10*(1), e001154. https://doi.org/10.1136/fmch-2021-001154

Song, C., Ikei, H., Park, B.-J., Lee, J., Kagawa, T., & Miyazaki, Y. (2018). Psychological benefits of walking through forest areas. *International Journal of Environmental Research and Public Health, 15*(12), 2804. https://doi.org/10.3390/ijerph15122804

Steptoe, A. (1992). Physical activity and psychological well-being. In N. G. Norgan (Ed.), *Physical activity and health* (pp. 207–229). Cambridge University Press.

Strauss, C., Cavanagh, K., Oliver, A., & Pettman, D. (2014). Mindfulness-based interventions for people diagnosed with a current episode of an anxiety or depressive disorder: A meta-analysis of randomised controlled trials. *PLoS One, 9*(4), e96110. https://doi.org/10.1371/journal.pone.0096110

Taylor, A. G., Goehler, L. E., Galper, D. I., Innes, K. E., & Bourguignon, C. (2010). Top-down and bottom-up mechanisms in mind-body medicine: Development of an integrative framework for psychophysiological research. *Explore, 6*(1), 29–41. https://doi.org/10.1016/j.explore.2009.10.004

Torkan, H., Blackwell, S. E., Holmes, E. A., Kalantari, M., Neshat-Doost, H. T., Maroufi, M., & Talebi, H. (2014). Positive imagery cognitive bias modification in treatment-seeking patients with major depression in Iran: A pilot study. *Cognitive Therapy and Research, 38*(2), 132–145. https://doi.org/10.1007/s10608-014-9598-8

Uebelacker, L. A., Epstein-Lubow, G., Gaudiano, B. A., Tremont, G., Battle, C. L., & Miller, I. W. (2010). Hatha yoga for depression: Critical review of the evidence for efficacy, plausible mechanisms of action, and directions for future research. *Journal of Psychiatric Practice, 16*(1), 22–33. https://doi.org/10.1097/01.pra.0000367775.88388.96

Wacker, M., & Holick, M. F. (2013). Sunlight and vitamin D: A global perspective for health. *Dermato-Endocrinology, 5*(1), 51–108. https://doi.org/10.4161/derm.24494

Chapter 10
Wellness and Our Humanity: Mind, Body, and Soul

There are many paths to becoming the best version of ourselves, but in all cases creating our best self requires a sense of wholeness and a perception that all parts of ourselves are working in harmony. In some ways, it is easier to "work on" the parts of ourselves that are both obvious (to us and/or to others) and regular topics of conversation and attention, such as our physical selves, social selves, and mental/emotional selves. However, there are parts of us that sometimes get less attention or, for some people, might be easier to neglect in favor of other pursuits. These facets of us are just as important as our corporeal selves. We will start by discussing our spiritual selves and move to a topic that many people don't think too much about—our experience of pain and how we cope with suffering. Pain and suffering are weighty topics, but they are part of what makes us human and part of what we share with all of humanity. Then we will end with how our intellectual wellness enriches our life and how we produce great things through human creativity and ingenuity.

Defining Spiritual Wellness

Spiritual wellness is perhaps the most difficult aspect of wellness to define. Spirituality means so many things to diverse people and cultures across the world, but the one commonality to spirituality throughout time is that it embodies the virtue of hope. Hope keeps us going through the hard times; it helps us to cope, be resilient, and to bounce back from adversity. Hope gives us a reason to act and to keep moving toward our goals, and it contributes deeply to our sense of well-being and happiness. Spiritual wellness can be defined as uniting our sense of our life's meaning and purpose with our morality to guide our choices and behaviors. Spiritual wellness often includes a connection with something greater than oneself, which can include deities, nature, the universe, ancestors, or even a cause or creed. To put it simply, spiritual wellness encompasses our needs to "do good, feel good, and be

S. M. Henney, J. D. Hackett, *Mind-Body Wellness*,
https://doi.org/10.1007/978-3-031-91611-3_10

good." This is distinct from the definition of religion, which is an organized system of beliefs, customs, and practices that centers around the doctrines of a distinct faith. Religion typically involves worship of a god or multiple gods, and belief in supernatural being(s) of different types. Religiosity is how closely a person adheres to the belief system and follows the required practices of the religion; a person high in religiosity is a committed follower of the religion, both in beliefs and behaviors.

Although there is a body of research on the effects of spirituality and religiosity on physical and mental health, much of it focuses on specific religious traditions (such as Judeo-Christian beliefs) and many studies conflate spiritual practices with religious doctrine. Koenig et al. (2012) reviewed the existing literature surrounding the link between spiritual practices and health. They found a wide range of physical health benefits of spirituality and religiosity, including lowering risk factors for hypertension, heart disease, dementia, and endocrine problems, while raising the ability to cope with pain and sickness. In the realm of mental health, they review evidence that religiosity helps people cope with and/or work through anxiety, depression, substance abuse, and problems in relationships. They do note, importantly, that religiosity can also have negative effects and outcomes related to instilling irrational fears and paranoia, oppressive and authoritarian control tactics, guilt, anxiety related to sin and punishment, and a rigid, inflexible approach to life.

Spiritual Wellness Check-In

Pause for a moment here to think about your current spiritual wellness. You might start by considering these questions:

1. What gives me hope?
2. What is my purpose in life?
3. What makes life meaningful?
4. What are my personal values and where did they come from?
5. What helps me to cope when things get hard?
6. What (or who) comforts me the most when I am low or feeling ill?

Your answers to these questions can help you to check in with yourself spiritually, but they can also guide you toward practices and approaches that you can use to enhance your spiritual wellness in areas of personal value to you. Common spiritual wellness practices include prayer, meditation, spending time in nature, music, volunteerism, and sitting quietly with your own thoughts.

What Practices Are Used to Promote Spiritual Wellness?

Prayer is a spiritual communication with a higher power and is central to almost all religious traditions. As a devotional practice, prayer is a way people consistently set aside time to genuinely express their desire to be in relationship with the spiritual. There are many different purposes for and types of prayer: prayers of thanksgiving are for expressing gratitude for our blessings; intercessory prayer is when we pray for others; penitent prayer expresses regret for mistakes; supplication or petition prayers humbly ask for help or fulfillment of a need; and prayers of praise are worshipful prayer reminding us of the goodness and power of the object of praise. A daily devotional refers to both a time we set aside to pray or reflect on the holy and also a book or reading that guides us in this activity. Devotionals can help people to consistently and regularly maintain and grow their spirituality. For example, daily prayer is one of the Five Pillars of Islam, a devotional practice that connects Muslims together and expresses their religious devotion.

In addition to prayer, other traditions have practices that are designed to enhance our spiritual wellness. Examples include:

Mandala (from the Sanskrit, meaning "circle"). A symbol in some Asian cultures that is typically a symmetrical design with a circular shape. The mandala can be used to guide meditation, as a sacred space, to call the sacred to us, or as self-expression.

Mantra. This is a repeated sound, word part, word, or group of words that focuses the mind on a spiritual purpose. Some mantras do not have a literal meaning, while others do. Mantras induce a stillness and relaxation that create a receptive and open state of mind so that the spiritual can be recognized and received.

Sacred walking or labyrinth walking. Labyrinths have a long history as a spiritual discipline that nurtures reflection and contemplation. As a practitioner walks the labyrinth toward the center, they focus on a spiritual purpose (prayer, supplication, problem-solving, etc.) and gain insight as they walk and think. The goal is to exit the labyrinth with new clarity of thought and understanding.

Fasting. Spiritual fasting is not only about food; it is about abstaining from certain things for a period of time in order to focus the mind and body on a purpose or to purify the mind and body. An example of a nonfood fast is a "social media fast" or "technology fast" in which we voluntarily restrict our use of technology to relieve us of distractions and to allow us to pay attention to other important facets of our well-being. Fasting can also increase our sense of personal control and agency over our behaviors, which has benefits far beyond the time limits of the fast.

Retreats and pilgrimages. These popular pursuits combine spiritually purposed spaces/places with spiritual programms and activities. They typically provide important spaces for dedicated reflection where one can focus on personal growth and mission without the hassles and distractions of daily life. Retreats often focus on a certain aspect of healing or spiritual growth (mindfulness, trauma work, leadership development, closer connection to a higher power, etc.), whereas pilgrimages are seen as sacred journeys (either voluntary or obligatory to a religion) in which the person treks or travels to a landmark, site, or geographical location that holds great significance to one's spiritual path. This journey's purpose is transformative and profound to understanding one's relationship to the divine.

Giving of ourselves. Giving of our time, talents, and assets is a concrete expression of compassion for others. It can nurture connections with others, provide a sense of happiness and pleasure, increase life satisfaction, and lower negative moods and thoughts (Aknin et al., 2019). Alfred Adler (1870–1937), a pioneer in psychotherapeutic techniques, introduced the concept of *Gemeinschaftsgefühl*, which can be translated as a "social interest" or "community feeling" that underlies good mental health. Success in social relationships and positive feelings about self and others rests on purposeful and consistent investment in building better relationships, communities, and society.

Technology. Although it is not everyone's preference, for some people there is a role for technology in their spiritual wellness journey. There are a wide variety of free and paid apps, including religion-specific apps, which offer inspiring messages and affirmations, verses from sacred texts, structured journaling, tracking of spiritual activities like meditation, prayer, or fasting, planning for regular spiritual habits/routines, and techniques for mindful living. Also available on the internet are classes, films, articles and blogs, podcasts, and how-to help for getting started with or maintaining a spiritual journey. Finally, video streaming services can be a great way to start learning about the range of spiritual practices, as they can provide a short and to the point introduction to a technique or approach.

I Don't Have Time for Spiritual Wellness!

Not everyone has the time or resources to go on a spiritual retreat or to fast from an important activity of life. However, we do not have to "think big" to make time for our spiritual practices—we can start small by simply being purposeful about spiritual time. Whatever spiritual practices we observe, we should make sure to:

- Designate a specific place or space.
- Set aside a defined time each day, even a small amount of time, to focus on our spiritual practice.
- Make it part of our daily routine by connecting with something we already do, like eating breakfast.
- If it fits with our worldview, let technology help in the forms of e-readers, apps, or guided lessons and activities.

Prioritize Personhood

Whatever spiritual practices one observes should enhance wellness, a sense of place in the greater scheme, and awareness of the positive aspects of human existence. In fact, spiritual wellness practices can have self-affirming, other-affirming, and life-affirming results that, if practiced regularly in both actions and behaviors, can improve physical and mental health. Some of the elements of human experience that can benefit from spiritual wellness practices include:

Purpose. Spiritual practices can help people to recognize and define what motivates and moves them forward toward their goals—a "driving force." Spiritual practices often include self-examination, which allows people to put words to their greatest hopes, greatest fears, and the personal assets that will allow them to live their best life. Of course, these practices also help identify those parts of a person that are not benefiting themselves or others and that they wish to change; thankfully, spiritual traditions allow people to have the space to change and to grow and to remake themselves. Using a set of diverse and cross-cultural samples, Willroth et al. (2021) found that both having a sense of purpose and retaining it in midlife are important to experiencing better physical health as we age.

Gratitude. Relatively simple habits of thankfulness and thanksgiving, such as telling others we appreciate them, returning a kind favor, and gratitude journaling, are deeply beneficial to our physical and mental well-being. Gratitude not only makes us feel good, be more optimistic, and be more resilient, but it also reduces negative emotions, like frustration, depression, and anxiety. The foundational work of Emmons and McCullough (2003) showed not only improved subjective well-being for those who practice gratitude but also that others in relationships with participants noticed these improvements! This brings to light an important part of expressing gratitude—by being appreciative, humble, and authentic, we improve not only ourselves, but we improve our social and romantic relationships, gain more friends, and enjoy a larger social network (Emmons, 2007).

Forgiveness. Forgiveness is a gift we give ourselves when we release our hurt, resentment, and bitterness about wrongs done to us by others. The act of forgiving brings a reduction in anger, frustration, anxiety, and depression, and an increase in feelings of subjective wellness. To be clear, unforgiveness can be conceptualized as both a contributor and reaction to poor mental health, whereas forgiveness is a strategy for maintaining and improving good mental health (Toussaint et al., 2015). Lack of forgiveness and the associated negative psychological states can contribute to allostatic load, which in turn impacts our long-term physiological health. There are a variety of spiritual wellness techniques that focus on letting go of past hurts, including prayer, meditation, journaling, and inner child work.

Compassion and empathy. Empathy is the ability to understand and relate to the suffering of others, whereas compassion is acting to ease their suffering. In essence, empathy is cognitive ("I understand what you are going through") and emotional ("I have felt your pain—I've been through this before"), whereas compassion is behavioral ("I can see you are stressed—Let me help"). The combination of empathy and compassion is the basis for The Golden Rule (to treat others as you would like to be treated), which is at the heart of many faith traditions. Spiritually, empathy encourages us to feel in community with all humanity, as the human experiences of joy, contentment, and suffering can be universally shared. Similarly, the spiritual practice of compassion is enacted through acts of service, cultivating kindness toward self and others, and being a force for good in our environment.

Lovingkindness and kindheartedness. Lovingkindness is an expression of affection and tenderness that arises from positive feelings of love and thoughtfulness. Kind people make the world a better place just by living their truth; everyone remembers acts of kindness and the people who walk the world in a spirit of lovingkindness. Spiritual growth in every tradition trends toward kindheartedness to people, other living beings, and the natural world and away from selfishness, pettiness, and malice.

The Loneliness Epidemic

A major impediment to wellness is loneliness, which makes us feel hopeless, useless, and broken. A quarter of people worldwide report feeling very or fairly lonely, but the loneliest people are young adults, ages 19–29 (Meta-Gallup, 2022). Being lonely does not mean being alone all the time; even when with others, lonely people are immersed in a mental state where they feel separate, apart, and cut off from the benefits of the social world. This is distinct from social isolation, which is the absence of contact with others and low or no social support, because people can be lonely without being socially isolated. Overcoming loneliness is a big task, one that takes the use of psychological and social assets and a great deal of courage. Advice to just "be with people" or "get out and have fun" is seldom helpful, as the problem with loneliness is emotion and mindset, rather than just being in the presence of others.

Thus, the primary ways to address loneliness have to do with increasing authentic connections and creating a sense of belonging. Here are some ideas to get started:

- Volunteer with a focus that you feel passionate about or invested in. If you are passionate about animal welfare, volunteering at a shelter already gives you something in common with the other volunteers and a basis for belonging.
- Take advantage of activities designed for your age group. Your college or community has activities designed for you—identify the activity that is the "most you" and start connecting there.
- Identify internet-based opportunities to connect. Sometimes it just feels exhausting or overwhelming to jump into a new in person social activity. Instead, start with a Zoom game night, online gaming, or e-sports to build connections based on shared interests and shared enjoyment.
- Get an animal companion. One of the greatest sources of unconditional love, shared joy, and companionship are our pets. Pets increase our capacity to connect, reduce stress and anxiety, and provide structure to our days.

Human Suffering

Human suffering and spirituality have been linked together through human history, so much so that spiritual renewal and/or deepening of spiritual life can be triggered by an intensely painful experience. Hearing the news that one has cancer, the loss of a loved one, or being the victim of a crime can all lead one to seek spiritual comfort. Spiritual practices, including religion, can help some people to find meaning and purpose through their pain. Indeed, there is a philosophy called the "spirituality of suffering," which is not seeking suffering for the sake of suffering, but rather using our spiritual strengths and a relationship with a higher power to confront the painful challenges life brings and to come out with deeper faith at the end.

The possibility of resilience in the face of experiences of pain, trauma, and suffering has led to interest in the concept of post-traumatic growth. Post-traumatic growth means that we can acquire positive transformation and constructive change after any type of trauma (like abuse, illness, victimization, natural disaster, and war) as long as we are able to work through and process our thoughts, feelings, and other consequences of these experiences. Thus, we do not only "survive" these experiences, but by putting trauma in the context of meaning, learning, and personal development, we can grow and change in a positive way from them. The process of restoring meaningful social relationships and personal goals, together with the ability to recognize and process the trauma, are all part of post-traumatic growth. Tedeschi and Calhoun (1996) identified five core aspects of post-traumatic growth: appreciation for life, positive relationships, openness to new possibilities, personal resilience, and spiritual change.

A significant source of stress and reduction of subjective feelings of wellness occurs around illness and pain. When we feel physically unwell or perceive pain in some part or parts of our bodies, our mental and emotional interpretation of that pain is key to how we cope with it. For most people, pain or physical feelings of being sick are related to stress, distress, unhappiness, fatigue, depression, and/or anxiety. Pain is a persistent and universal cause of human suffering across all times and places. We cannot legitimately talk about wellness in mind and body without addressing the fact that people are or will be in pain at some point in their lives, sometimes severely or chronically so.

Pain Versus Suffering

Let's start by defining pain and then suffering. Pain is an unpleasant or even unbearable sensation or perception. Pain typically results from some form of bodily dysfunction or disorder, such as from injury, illness, or disease. It can be localized or generalized, can be relatively simple (my foot hurts) or complex (I hurt all over), and can be perceived as mild to very severe. Pain can be acute (or immediate), short-term (such as after a broken arm that heals well), or chronic (persistent in duration over time). Chronic pain is an entity all to itself. Figure 10.1 presents the pain cycle that can result when we experience long-lasting or persistent pain. Chronic pain is really a cycle of hurt and distress that has components of emotion, thought, and behavior baked into it.

Persistent pain: When a person starts experiencing chronic pain over time due to illness, injury, or disease.

Reduced activity: Pain tells us to slow down. We desire to not experience pain, so we decrease our activity level in response.

Emotional distress: As we become less active, we evaluate our health and wellness negatively and we feel tired and defeated by our pain.

Withdrawal: We withdraw from our normal activities in order to avoid pain.

Impairment of function: We experience a loss of normal functioning and even disability.

Remember, there is some truth to the idea of "use it or lose it." The key to exiting the chronic pain cycle is engagement with appropriate activities and therapies that preserve movement and activity levels while minimizing pain.

Suffering, on the other hand, is our interpretation or impression of pain and the consequences of pain. Suffering involves our distress, specifically our subjective understanding of the painful sensations we experience. "Suffering" is a heavy word. It means to consciously endure pain, illness, poverty, or loss, and it implies extremity and misery, even agony. The word "consciously" is important, because suffering occurs in the present and we are aware of it. In some ways, this heightens our awareness of our own pain—it is right there in our faces, so to speak, and it is difficult to ignore or escape.

Fig. 10.1 The pain cycle

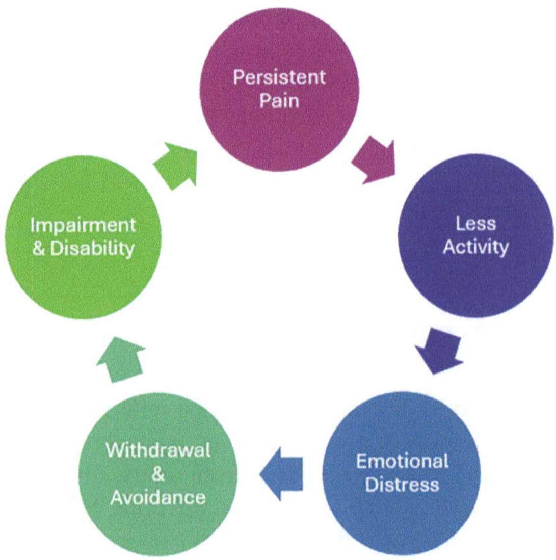
Persistent Pain
Less Activity
Emotional Distress
Withdrawal & Avoidance
Impairment & Disability

It's important to note that we can't say that there is only a one-way causality from pain to suffering, meaning that feeling pain causes us mental and emotional pain. It is true that this is one causal pathway, but it is equally true that mental and emotional pain can cause us to feel physical pain and that mental and emotional pain can enhance the perception of physical pain. This is the philosophy behind a mind-body approach. In fact, the dynamic interaction between physical pain, thoughts, and emotions is complex and not completely understood. We know, though, that pain, emotion, and cognition feed each other. Our pain history, social situation, expectations, beliefs, predisposition to anxiety and/or depression, and many other factors also influence the relationship between pain and our reaction to it.

We can do a lot with our emotions, thoughts, and behaviors to both increase our own suffering and also to decrease our suffering. Jon Kabat-Zin (n.d.) says that one of the most important things we can do is to "stop compounding suffering"—we have to disentangle the sheer physical sensation of pain from the emotional component (this pain is making me anxious) and cognitive component (I can't handle this) in order to make our suffering less. We uncouple cognition and emotion from physical sensation to liberate ourselves from the suffering of pain—none of our thoughts or feelings are actually the pain itself. Since suffering is within our awareness in the now, we can also learn to cope with it and adopt strategies to mitigate our suffering. We can take advantage of the resources that are available to us to alleviate our suffering, such as conventional medicine, therapy, guided meditation, and more. Many options are available at the college or university and in the community.

Treatment of Pain

It is very clear that we underestimate and undertreat pain. Some people go through much or all of their lives in pain, resulting in great suffering, without effective treatment or intervention. Sometimes this is from a lack of effective treatments or lack of knowledge about how to deploy treatments effectively, but other times people simply are not believed about their own self-reports of pain. Why are we so bad at treating pain or even acknowledging the need to?

- Doctors, nurses, and other health professionals themselves do not know enough about the correct assessment and management of pain. For example, some years ago the family of a nursing home patient was awarded $15 million after the patient died a painful death from terminal metastatic prostate cancer. Even though the man rated his pain as 10 (unbearable), a nurse refused to administer an opioid pain reliever based on her belief that he would become addicted. Note that this was a significant deviation from typical standard of care, as addiction is not a major factor in cancer pain relief, particularly for terminal patients.
- Failure to make pain relief a priority or even to acknowledge that pain relief is an essential component of patient care.

- There is no one and no entity to enforce accountability in providing adequate pain relief.
- Doctors are worried about being scrutinized by regulatory agencies regarding their prescribing habits for controlled medications.
- Race and/or gender may play a role in how reports of pain and requests for pain relief are received by healthcare professionals. For example, from labor to postpartum, Hispanic and Black mothers were found to have higher reports of pain, but were provided with lower doses of opioid pain relief than their White counterparts (Greene & Kilpatrick, 2024).
- The widespread and persistent myths about addiction, tolerance, and side effects related to opioids and related drugs. The US war on drugs and our concerns about addiction and misuse of opioids and similar analgesics can also be seen as a significant contributor to a decrease in willingness to address pain and an increase in human suffering.

Highlight on Nondrug Treatments for Pain

Although the world is full of suffering, it is also full of the overcoming of it.—Helen Keller

Drug-based treatments for pain should be discussed within a doctor-patient relationship and the benefits vs risks carefully considered. Although a comprehensive assessment of these methods is beyond the scope of this text, Table 10.1 presents some of the broad categories of drug-based treatments for pain along with several nondrug treatments. In this section, we will focus on several types of nondrug treatments that can be used within a mind-body framework.

Mindfulness. Mindfulness-based interventions (MBI) have been found to improve the well-being of fibromyalgia (Kaplan et al., 1993) and cancer (Carlson et al., 2001) patients, reduce perceptions of suffering in chronic pain patients, and reduce relapse (a notoriously difficult task) for substance abuse disorders

Table 10.1 Drug and nondrug treatments for pain

Drug treatments	Nondrug treatments
Over the counter (OTC) drugs, such as aspirin, acetaminophen, ibuprofen, etc. OTC topicals, such as Aspercreme, IcyHot, etc. Prescription oral drugs, such as corticosteroids, opioids, antidepressants, anticonvulsants (anti-seizure medications) Prescription non-oral drugs, such as lidocaine patches, suppositories, creams, lotions Injections, such as nerve blocks, trigger point blocks, etc.	Physical therapy Nerve stimulation, such as TENS or spinal stimulation Biofeedback Meditation and mindfulness techniques Chiropractic Massage Prayer Counseling/psychotherapy Surgery

(Bowen et al., 2014). One example of a mindfulness-based approach to pain reduction is an 8-week program called Mindfulness-Based Stress Reduction (MBSR; Kabat-Zinn, 2013), which is designed to enable people to develop mindfulness skills and practices that will help them cope with anxiety, depression, and pain. MBSR is a true mind-body technique in that it combines body scanning (head-to-toe self-inventory of the body to identify areas of tension or pain), meditation, and simple yoga positions. Although much of MBSR is experienced in a group setting, there are also homework and activities to make sure that the techniques are used in everyday life.

Physical therapy (PT). The goal of PT is to return patients to the level of functioning and pain status that is achievable within the context of their current health concerns. People come to PT with a variety of injuries, diseases, disorders, and disabilities, some of which will ultimately resolve back to full wellness, but other patients will have to learn ways to live with and live through ongoing medical treatments and associated pain. The interventions used by physical therapists can include exercise, heat or cold, massage, electrical stimulation (such as TENS), and stretching. The gains in strength, flexibility, movement, and mobility will help relieve pain and encourage appropriate return to functional activities.

Counseling/psychotherapy. Pain can be associated with feelings of loss of control, depression, frustration, and negative thoughts, and therapy can help people cope with these mental and emotional consequences of pain. One mind-body-based therapy is called Mindfulness-Based Cognitive Therapy (MBCI). Traditional cognitive therapy assists clients to identify and challenge negative, nonproductive, and self-defeating thought patterns and to replace them with more positive and favorable ways of thinking. MCBI pairs this with meditation, focused breathing, visualization, present moment awareness, and other methods that help patients defocus from and divert negative thought processes by replacing them with a calm, peaceful, and positive mental state.

Prayer. Prayer has been used over human existence to ask for intercession by a higher power to eliminate the causes of pain, to ask for relief or release from pain, and as a strategy to cope with pain. The use of prayer increases with the onset of pain (Dezutter et al., 2011), and it can reduce perception of pain intensity and discomfort versus those who do not pray (Jarego et al., 2023).

Remember that all treatments have consequences and side effects. One could argue that there are certain treatments more likely to result in side effects than others, but there is no intervention that we do with human beings that has an effect without a cost. Sometimes this cost is worth paying—for example, meditation has a cost in time and substitution for other activities, but it greatly improves quality of life for many people. Yet sometimes the side effects are not worth the reduction in pain; in other words, the treatment makes life worse than the original pain. It is absolutely necessary for professionals and patients alike to do a cost-benefit analysis: (1) Is the treatment effective; (2) Does the treatment increase or decrease suffering; (3) Is it affordable and available; and (4) Does the benefit outweigh the cost? In the end, it is only in conjunction with our healthcare provider that we can decide what pain management interventions are to our benefit.

Feeding Our Intellectual Selves

Part of what makes us human and unique is our intellect in all of its forms and expressions. Intellectual wellness is a facet of overall wellness that includes creativity, ingenuity, curiosity, problem-solving, reasoning, and an openness to intellectual growth, expanding knowledge, and new experiences. Like all aspects of wellness, intellectual wellness looks different for different people, and it is not at all centered on being "book smart," having a lot of formal education, or having a high IQ. Expressions of intellectual superiority are often the antithesis of intellectual wellness, as confidence and trust in our intellectual capacities—whatever they are—is part of true wellness. Indicators of intellectual wellness can include:

- Choosing both work and recreational activities that challenge one to grow in knowledge and understanding.
- Being willing and able to engage in solving the problems and addressing the issues of life.
- Engaging in opportunities to express creativity, ingenuity, and imagination.
- Expressing intellectual autonomy by developing ideas and opinions through reading, research, and curiosity.
- Active efforts to improve the ability to critically analyze, memorize, concentrate on, evaluate, and comprehend information.
- Openness to new experiences, ideas, and people.

Brain Training

People have often associated intellectual wellness with being "sharp" or with cognitive/mental fitness and agility. Crossword puzzles, sudoku, puzzles, brain teasers, and memory games are all commonly understood ways to "exercise the brain." Brain training or cognitive training technologies, which are specifically marketed to improve mental dexterity and quickness as well as to stave off mental decline, are a huge industry to the tune of almost $2 billion. However, the ability of these programs and apps to substantively improve mental functioning and delay the cognitive issues associated with aging is an open question, with some studies showing improvement and others showing little benefit to brain training programs. George and Whitehouse (2011) state, "these products are sociocultural objects deeply imbued with the values and ideologies of our age" (p. 591), which implies that we value a specific type of intellectual activity centered around speed, memory, autonomy, and technology uptake. These authors persuasively argue that a reductionist view of brain health that focuses narrowly on brain games misses the real gains in intellectual wellness to be found in human interaction and community engagement.

Health Literacy and Intellectual Wellness
Health literacy involves being able to navigate all of the steps necessary to find, understand, evaluate, and engage with healthcare information in order to use the information to live a healthful life. The skills of health literacy include using technology, reading, critical thinking, listening, communicating, and self-advocacy. We can see that these skills are all related to our definition of intellectual wellness. Health literacy, just like intellectual wellness, can be developed via concerted effort and partnership with healthcare professionals. People can study, research, observe their health symptoms and signs, organize their health information (appointments, test results, diagnoses, treatments, etc.), and learn to ask the right questions. The National Library of Medicine (n.d.) states that people with better health literacy practice many important wellness-related behaviors, including obtaining needed preventive services (like vaccinations), manage their chronic and acute illnesses more capably, have better physical health outcomes, and make fewer medication efforts.

Creativity

Creativity is notoriously hard to define. We typically look at new, imaginative, and distinctive creations, particularly in the arts, as the result of a creative process. However, creativity is at work in every field and aspect of human effort—science, business, engineering, and politics are also hubs of creativity. One way to understand creativity is that it is based on a person in context approaching a particular task, problem, or activity in a unique and productive way. Sternberg and Lubart's (1991) investment theory of creativity uses a "buy low, sell high" metaphor, in which creative people seek out unknown, unrealized, or unpopular ideas (buy low) and work diligently to develop, refine, and promote these ideas until they are broadly accepted and "popular" (sell high). Such people utilize six assets to their advantage when working through creative activities: intellectual capacity, knowledge, cognitive approach, personality, motivation, and environment. However, the dynamic that brings forth creativity not only rests on how something is done or thought about (the "creative process"), but also on why and under what conditions of knowledge, time, and expertise the creativity occurs (e.g., Csikszentmihalyi, 2014).

How do we develop creativity? Creativity has a small genetic component, so creativity is not necessarily something we are "born with." Rather, it is an approach or mindset that can be cultivated and nurtured with the right experiences and support. As Sternberg (2023) says, "creativity is not so much an innate ability as it is an attitude toward life," and he makes the point that living a life of creativity takes courage, integrity, and wisdom. In this context, it is important to note the difference between creative potential, the latent ability to be creative that can be developed via effort and environment, creative activity, the act or action of creating, and creative output, the product of creativity that can be seen, read, heard, experienced, and so forth.

Creative activities reflect and impact both the physical operations of the brain and the functional processes of the mind and emotions. Creativity is not centered in one part of the brain exclusively; Katz (1997) argues that the idea that creativity is "located in" the brain's right hemisphere should be discarded. Rather, creativity emerges from various parts of the brain and pathways/connections within the brain (e.g., Dietrich & Kanso, 2010). For example, the hippocampus helps to process, store, and retrieve memories and the amygdala helps manage emotion, both of which are important to imagination, interpretation, and ingenuity. Additionally, the prefrontal and frontal lobes, temporal lobe, neurotransmitters, neurocircuitry, and other neuroanatomy have in various ways been implicated in the processes of creativity (e.g., Weir, 2024). This strongly implies that there is no established "right way" to be or become creative or even to impact the capacity for creativity. Thus, it is good to maintain a healthy skepticism when we hear advertising or view social media posts about products, apps, or supplements "guaranteed" to improve our thinking, expand our minds, and stimulate peak creativity.

The Art of Becoming

The process of "becoming" is a creative process—becoming more satisfied, more fulfilled, more "you" is an artistic act that people bring to reality through their individual thoughts, feelings, and behaviors. As a person moves through life, they create themselves, their present, and their future. Some people do this over and over again in an ongoing creative process, others reach a balance where they are content and satisfied, while others get "stuck" on their path to becoming through fear, trauma, lack of resources, and lack of support. Consider this poem and what it tells us about overcoming fear on our path to becoming:

Fear by Khalil Gibran.
It is said that before entering the sea.
a river trembles with fear.
She looks back at the path she has traveled,
from the peaks of the mountains,
the long winding road crossing forests and villages.
And in front of her,
she sees an ocean so vast,
that to enter.
there seems nothing more than to disappear forever.

But there is no other way.
The river cannot go back.

Nobody can go back.
To go back is impossible in existence.

The river needs to take the risk.
of entering the ocean.
because only then will fear disappear,
because that's where the river will know.
it's not about disappearing into the ocean,
but of becoming the ocean.

On the other hand, we have plenty of evidence that stress is a killer of creativity, meaning that stress negatively impacts intellectual wellness just as it does for other domains of wellness. In a meta-analysis of studies that examined the effects of creative arts interventions, Martin et al. (2018) found that treatments focused on creative activities were impressively consistent in producing positive stress-reduction outcomes, including lowered perceived stress, increased ability to manage stress, reduced anxiety, and improved mood. In another systematic review of creative arts interventions, Stuckey and Nobel (2010) found that, although there were methodological limitations in some studies, in general "creative engagement can decrease anxiety, stress, and mood disturbances" (p. 261). In their words, the improvements observed in physical and psychological health within the context of creativity are evidence for the "healing power of the arts."

Capitalizing on the wellness benefits of creativity does not mean that we need to become an artist, writer, or musician. Creativity can be expressed in the activities of everyday life, such as daydreaming, cooking, gardening, journaling, doodling, hobbies, and even creation-oriented gaming. Studying the relationship between everyday creativity and flourishing, Conner et al. (2018) found that their subjects reported "more enthusiasm and higher flourishing following days when they were more creative than normal" (p. 186). In the workplace, employees who are high in excitement and interest in the work and low in loneliness and depressed mood are likely to be rated as creative by their managers (Wright & Walton, 2003). There is a very interesting link between daydreaming and creativity in day-to-day life, as it appears that certain types of daydreaming are related to specific domains of creativity. For example, Zedelius et al. (2021) studied adult college students both in the lab and via experience sampling (providing prompted information about daydreaming throughout the day, prompted by their cell phones). They found that daydreaming about something personally meaningful was related to artistic creativity and daily inspiration, whereas fantastical daydreaming was related to creative writing and daily creative activities.

Curiosity

One of the hallmarks of intellectual well-being is a healthy sense of curiosity about self, others, and the world around us. There are different types of curiosity. For example, epistemic curiosity refers to curiosity that motivates us to learn and to know, specific curiosity is wanting to know particular information, social curiosity is our interest in how people think, their emotions, and why they behave as they do, and diversive curiosity is the intense desire to explore new sources of knowledge (novelty) and to escape boredom. These different types of curiosity might be related to people's choices and behaviors, such as socially curious people being highly interested in what makes people tick and choosing psychology as a major or people high in diversive curiosity endlessly scrolling through social media in search of something new that sparks humor or interest.

Curiosity is a key driver of both learning and retaining what is learned (Gruber et al., 2014). Students, in particular, benefit from a keen sense of curiosity and inquisitiveness. Von Stumm et al. (2011) describe a "hungry mind" as a foundational element of academic success and note that, not only do intellectually curious students perform better in college, but also "intellectually stimulated students are likely to be more satisfied with their university experience and to enjoy their studies." Studying a sample of university students, Gallagher and Lopez (2007) found curiosity to be "associated with a broad range of continuous indicators of psychological, social, and emotional well-being" via developing a "focus on, contact with, and engagement in novel or challenging situations" (p 246–247). These authors make the point that flourishing in many aspects of life, not only in academics, is possible for students who exhibit the trait of curiosity.

Albert Einstein said that curiosity drives us to persistently ask questions and described himself as "passionately curious." Curiosity can be cultivated in a variety of ways. Goldstein (2013) suggests that curiosity is an essential part of mindfulness practices in that mindfulness allows the mind to pay attention to possibilities and potentials, and also directs us to let our minds be free to explore what we know and don't know. Curiosity can also be fostered by committing to lifelong learning, embracing a growth mindset, engaging in positive and nurturing social relationships, and being open-minded enough to challenge our own assumptions and to welcome novel ideas.

Improving Intellectual Wellness

Intellectual wellness distinctly focuses on our thoughts, knowledge, insight, and wisdom in ways that other domains of wellness do not. However, these aspects of ourselves can feel very intangible and hard to influence. Here are some ideas for improving your intellectual well-being:

- Have an active social life where you are surrounded by interesting and diverse people.
- Read for pleasure, interest, and knowledge.
- Do puzzles and games, including board games, card games, video games, gaming, and esports.
- Write out your thoughts, feelings, and insights in a journal or as a creative writing project.
- Experience the arts in a variety of ways to broaden your thinking and knowledge about artistic expression; art is not only found in a museum, the opera, or a symphony, it is also taking a photography class, playing an instrument, going to a concert, or walking a curated garden.
- Challenge yourself to try new things, explore new skills and hobbies, have new experiences, and meet new people. It is comforting and safe to stay within our purview, but intellectual growth must be accompanied by content, meaning you must provide experiences and material for your intellect to work with.

- Broaden your knowledge base through lifelong learning—take a class on anything you are interested in!
- The brain needs stimulation but also must rest to have time for reflection and imagination. Take the time to be outdoors, meditate, exercise, or listen to music.
- Reduce your stress, as stress interferes with all aspects of well-being.

Openness to Experience

The term openness to experience is often used to describe a personality trait (defined by the Five-Factor Model of Personality) whereby a person is inclined to experience new things, meet new people, and accept new ideas. In regard to intellectual wellness, however, openness to experience is more of a cognitive approach or cognitive style that denotes the ability to be flexible, adaptable, open to nontraditional approaches/environments, understanding of feelings, and eager to learn. Personal growth is linked to openness to experience in that those who are more open, particularly those who are also extroverted, seek out opportunities for exploration and understanding of self (Schmutte & Ryff, 1997). Additionally, openness to experience is associated with post-traumatic growth (Prasad & Johnston, 2024), effective coping and coping mechanisms (McCrae & Costa Jr, 1986), health-related quality of life (Pereira-Morales et al., 2018), and satisfaction with life (Stephan, 2009). In contrast, people who are not open to experience are resistant to change, prefer routines and schedules, have a narrow band of interests, and tend to be more traditional in their lifestyles and behaviors.

Consider for a moment how quickly things change in terms of technology, popular culture, and social expectation over a person's lifetime (picture your grandparents learning how to use a smartphone). For example, technology uptake refers to the ability to accept and use novel technologies in the course of one's daily life. As people age through the lifespan, technology uptake will be more attainable for those who have the cognitive flexibility to adapt and learn how to utilize new technologies. McElroy et al. (2007) found that openness to experience predicts Internet use, stating that "Curious and open-minded people are more likely to use the Internet to seek information" (p. 817). There are many apps that assist us with our physical, mental, and cognitive well-being (and other apps that are just plain fun to use!) and also technology that keeps us connected to family, friends, and interest groups. People who can engage with these technologies can maintain important relationships, have information at their fingertips, and make their lives more productive, enjoyable, and satisfying.

Wellness Tip—The Power of Purpose

Purpose is an intention to achieve a personally meaningful goal, often having to do with causes or pursuits that positively impact the lives of others. A "sense of purpose" means that we are aware of this goal, what it means to us to pursue it, and what it will mean to achieve it. Purpose-laden goals do not have to be big or change lives in epic ways, but we do perceive them as having the potential to change things for the better, enrich life, and make life easier. Our sense of purpose should motivate us to act and help us to cope through challenges, but, most of all, it should inspire us. A happy side effect of a vibrant sense of purpose is that it appears to lower the incidence of problematic physical symptoms, such as sleep issues, obesity, and sedentary lifestyles (e.g., Kim et al., 2022) and also impacts aspects of mental wellness like less reactivity to stress and greater resilience (e.g., Sutin et al., 2023).

Our sense of purpose is not a one-time choice but rather will change over our lives as we grow into our sense of self and gain autonomy and socioemotional assets. Cotton Bronk et al. (2009) found that from adolescence into adulthood, having identified a purpose in life is positively related to life satisfaction. They also note the benefits of a developmental focus on purpose and state, "During adolescence and emerging adulthood young people need to be encouraged to engage in a broad and varied search for purpose, and they should also be encouraged to focus on how they plan to make progress toward their purposes in life." This highlights the fact that finding and engaging with our sense of purpose is a process and a practice—a journey, if you will, to achieve our goals and fulfill our purpose. It also suggests that there are ways to help ourselves and others grow into a sense of purpose. These can include:

Self-reflection, including meditation, can help identify the things that matter to you.
Find your passion, as this intensity is needed to push through barriers and challenges.
Set goals that are achievable; these can be stretch goals, but they should be within the realm of possibility.
Learn what you need to know to pursue your purpose.
Connect with people who support your vision and can help you reach your goal.
Mentor others to fulfill their purpose and be a positive role model for them.

References

Aknin, L. B., Whillans, A. V., Norton, M. I., & Dunn, E. W. (2019). Happiness and prosocial behavior: An evaluation of the evidence. In J. F. Helliwell, R. Layard, & J. D. Sachs (Eds.), *World happiness report* (pp. 67–86). Sustainable Development Solutions Network.

Bowen, S., Witkiewitz, K., Clifasefi, S. L., Grow, J., Chawla, N., Hsu, S. H., Carroll, H. A., Harrop, E., Collins, S. E., Lustyk, M. K., & Larimer, M. E. (2014). Relative efficacy of mindfulness-based relapse prevention, standard relapse prevention, and treatment as usual for substance use disorders: A randomized clinical trial. *JAMA Psychiatry, 71*(5), 547–556. https://doi.org/10.1001/jamapsychiatry.2013.4546

Carlson, L. E., Ursuliak, Z., Goodey, E., Angen, M., & Speca, M. (2001). The effects of a mindfulness meditation-based stress reduction program on mood and symptoms of stress in cancer outpatients: 6-month follow-up. *Supportive Care in Cancer: Official Journal of the Multinational Association of Supportive Care in Cancer, 9*(2), 112–123.

Conner, T. S., DeYoung, C. G., & Silvia, P. J. (2018). Everyday creative activity as a path to flourishing. *The Journal of Positive Psychology, 13*(2), 181–189. https://doi.org/10.1080/17439760.2016.1257049

Cotton Bronk, K., Hill, P. L., Lapsley, D. K., Talib, T. L., & Finch, H. (2009). Purpose, hope, and life satisfaction in three age groups. *The Journal of Positive Psychology, 4*(6), 500–510. https://doi.org/10.1080/17439760903271439

Csikszentmihalyi, M. (2014). *The systems model of creativity*. Springer.

Dezutter, J., Wachholtz, A., & Corveleyn, J. (2011). Prayer and pain: The mediating role of positive re-appraisal. *Journal of Behavioral Medicine, 34*(6), 542–549. https://doi.org/10.1007/s10865-011-9348-2

Dietrich, A., & Kanso, R. (2010). A review of EEG, ERP, and neuroimaging studies of creativity and insight. *Psychological Bulletin, 136*(5), 822–848. https://doi.org/10.1037/a0019749

Emmons, R. A. (2007). *Thanks!: How the new science of gratitude can make you happier*. Houghton Mifflin Harcourt.

Emmons, R. A., & McCullough, M. E. (2003). Counting blessings versus burdens: An experimental investigation of gratitude and subjective Well-being in daily life. *Journal of Personality and Social Psychology, 84*, 377–389. https://doi.org/10.1037/0022-3514.84.2.377

Gallagher, M. W., & Lopez, S. J. (2007). Curiosity and well-being. *The Journal of Positive Psychology, 2*(4), 236–248. https://doi.org/10.1080/17439760701552345

George, D. R., & Whitehouse, P. J. (2011). Marketplace of memory: What the brain fitness technology industry says about us and how we can do better. *The Gerontologist, 51*(5), 590–596. https://doi.org/10.1093/geront/gnr042

Goldstein, E. (2013). *The now effect: How a mindful moment can change the rest of your life*. Atria.

Greene, N. H., & Kilpatrick, S. J. (2024). Racial/ethnic disparities in peripartum pain assessment and management. *Joint Commission Journal on Quality and Patient Safety, 50*(8), 552–559. https://doi.org/10.1016/j.jcjq.2024.03.009

Gruber, M. J., Gelman, B. D., & Ranganath, C. (2014). States of curiosity modulate hippocampus-dependent learning via the dopaminergic circuit. *Neuron, 84*(2), 486–496. https://doi.org/10.1016/j.neuron.2014.08.060

Jarego, M., Ferreira-Valente, A., Queiroz-Garcia, I., Day, M. A., Pais-Ribeiro, J., Costa, R. M., Pimenta, F., & Jensen, M. P. (2023). Are prayer-based interventions effective pain management options? A systematic review and meta-analysis of randomized controlled trials. *Journal of Religion and Health, 62*(3), 1780–1809.

Kabat-Zin, J. (n.d.). *Mindfulness, pain, and suffering*. MasterClass. https://www.masterclass.com/classes/jon-kabat-zinn-teaches-mindfulness-and-meditation/chapters/mindfulness-pain-and-suffering

Kabat-Zinn, J. (2013). *Full catastrophe living: Using the wisdom of your body and mind to face stress, pain, and illness* (2nd ed.). Random House.

Kaplan, K. H., Goldenberg, D. L., & Galvin-Nadeau, M. (1993). The impact of a meditation-based stress reduction program on fibromyalgia. *General Hospital Psychiatry, 15*(5), 284–289. https://doi.org/10.1016/0163-8343(93)90020-o

Katz, A. N. (1997). Creativity in the cerebral hemispheres. In M. A. Runco (Ed.), *Creativity research handbook* (pp. 203–226). Hampton Press.

Kim, E. S., Chen, Y., Nakamura, J. S., Ryff, C. D., & VanderWeele, T. J. (2022). Sense of purpose in life and subsequent physical, behavioral, and psychosocial health: An outcome-wide approach. *American Journal of Health Promotion, 36*(1), 137–147. https://doi.org/10.1177/08901171211038545

Koenig, H. G., King, D. E., & Carson, V. B. (2012). *Handbook of religion and health* (2nd ed.). Oxford University Press.

Martin, L., Oepen, R., Bauer, K., Nottensteiner, A., Mergheim, K., Gruber, H., & Koch, S. C. (2018). Creative arts interventions for stress management and prevention-a systematic review. *Behavioral Sciences, 8*(2), 28. https://doi.org/10.3390/bs8020028

McCrae, R. R., & Costa, P. T., Jr. (1986). Personality, coping, and coping effectiveness in an adult sample. *Journal of Personality, 54*(2), 385–404. https://doi.org/10.1111/j.1467-6494.1986.tb00401.x

McElroy, J. C., Hendrickson, A. R., Townsend, A. M., & DeMarie, S. M. (2007). Dispositional factors in internet use: Personality versus cognitive style. *MIS Quarterly, 31*(4), 809–820. https://doi.org/10.2307/25148821

Meta-Gallup (2022). *The global state of social connections.* https://www.gallup.com/analytics/509675/state-of-social-connections.aspx

National Library of Medicine (n.d.). *An introduction to health literacy.* https://www.nnlm.gov/guides/intro-health-literacy

Pereira-Morales, A. J., Adan, A., Lopez-Leon, S., & Forero, D. A. (2018). Personality traits and health-related quality of life: The mediator role of coping strategies and psychological distress. *Annals of General Psychiatry, 17*, 25. https://doi.org/10.1186/s12991-018-0196-0

Prasad, A. R., & Johnston, K. L. (2024). Embracing "COVID-normal": Positive personality and posttraumatic growth in the COVID-19 pandemic. *Personality and Individual Differences, 228*, 112744. https://doi.org/10.1016/j.paid.2024.112744

Schmutte, P., & Ryff, C. (1997). Personality and well-being: Reexamining methods and meanings. *Journal of Personality and Social Psychology, 73*(3), 549–559. https://doi.org/10.1037/0022-3514.73.3.549

Stephan, Y. (2009). Openness to experience and active older adults' life satisfaction: A trait and facet-level analysis. *Personality and Individual Differences, 47*(6), 637–641. https://doi.org/10.1016/j.paid.2009.05.025

Sternberg, R. J. (2023). Eight lessons from my research on creativity. *Greater Good Magazine.* https://greatergood.berkeley.edu/article/item/eight_lessons_from_my_research_on_creativity

Sternberg, R. J., & Lubart, T. I. (1991). An investment theory of creativity and its development. *Human Development, 34*(1), 1–31. https://doi.org/10.1159/000277029

Stuckey, H. L., & Nobel, J. (2010). The connection between art, healing, and public health: A review of current literature. *American Journal of Public Health, 100*(2), 254–263. https://doi.org/10.2105/AJPH.2008.156497

Sutin, A. R., Luchetti, M., Stephan, Y., Sesker, A. A., & Terracciano, A. (2023). Purpose in life, stress mindset, and perceived stress: Test of a mediational model. *Personality and Individual Differences, 210*, 112227. https://doi.org/10.1016/j.paid.2023.112227

Tedeschi, R. G., & Calhoun, L. G. (1996). The posttraumatic growth inventory: Measuring the positive legacy of trauma. *Journal of Traumatic Stress, 9*(3), 455–471. https://doi.org/10.1007/BF02103658

Toussaint, L., Worthington, E., & Williams, D. R. (2015). *Forgiveness and health: Scientific evidence and theories relating forgiveness to better health.* Springer. https://doi.org/10.1007/978-94-017-9993-5

von Stumm, S., Hell, B., & Chamorro-Premuzic, T. (2011). The hungry mind: Intellectual curiosity is the third pillar of academic performance. *Perspectives on Psychological Science, 6*(6), 574–588. https://doi.org/10.1177/1745691611421204

Weir, K. (2024). The science behind creativity. *Monitor on Psychology, 53*, 3. https://www.apa.org/monitor/2022/04/cover-science-creativity

Willroth, E. C., Mroczek, D. K., & Hill, P. L. (2021). Maintaining sense of purpose in midlife predicts better physical health. *Journal of Psychosomatic Research, 145*, 110485–110485. https://doi.org/10.1016/j.jpsychores.2021.110485

Wright, T. A., & Walton, A. P. (2003). Affect, psychological well-being and creativity: Results of a field study. *Journal of Business and Management, 9*(1), 21–32. https://doi.org/10.1504/JBM.2003.141098

Zedelius, C. M., Protzko, J., Broadway, J. M., & Schooler, J. W. (2021). What types of daydreaming predict creativity? Laboratory and experience sampling evidence. *Psychology of Aesthetics, Creativity, and the Arts, 15*(4), 596–611. https://doi.org/10.1037/aca0000342

Chapter 11
Day-to-Day Wellness

We often perceive improvements or reduction in wellness in terms of big changes, like changing jobs, ending or starting a relationship, birth of a child, and so forth. These are important life events, for sure, but even the smaller things we do on a daily basis and our regular daily environments have an impact on our wellness. In this chapter, we will cover specific issues that affect our wellness every day, like the impact of daily hassles and how to manage conflict.

Defining Daily Hassles

Each and every day humans all over the world cope with internal and external occurrences that challenge our wellness in small but noticeable ways. The nuisances that occur every day in our lives persistently impact our feelings of wellness, and these nuisances have largely unacknowledged, and definitely underappreciated, negative effects on our lives. These nuisances are called daily hassles, and although they may not be objectively stressful or stressful to everyone, they are stressful because people perceive them that way (Lazarus & Folkman, 1984). Examples of daily hassles include both frequent and infrequent occurrences, like being late to work, the kids missing the bus, forgetting to get bread for sandwiches at the store, not having time to get a prescription refilled, and so many others (see Fig. 11.1). We are so used to having these daily issues, hassles, and roadblocks in our lives that we often don't stop to take stock of what they are or what is causing them, and this makes a solution hard to pinpoint. First, let's define daily hassles, which tend to have the following characteristics:

S. M. Henney, J. D. Hackett, *Mind-Body Wellness*,
https://doi.org/10.1007/978-3-031-91611-3_11

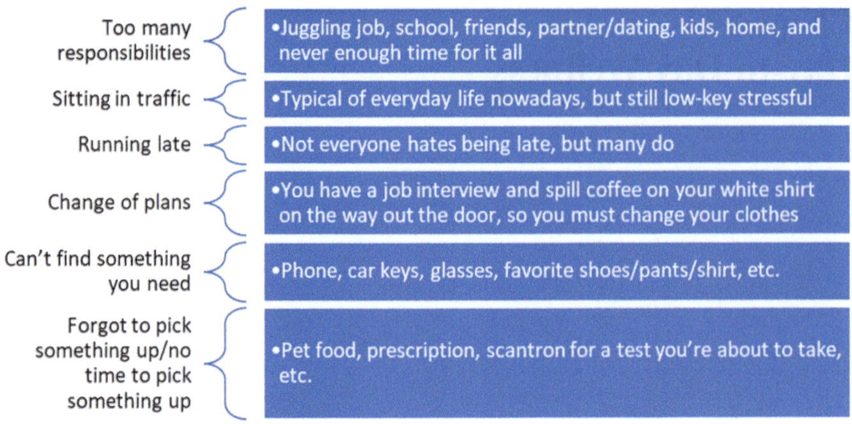

Fig. 11.1 Examples of daily hassles

1. Daily hassles are **unexpected**. This continues to be true, even though it might seem as if we should be able to anticipate them, since they keep occurring.
2. Daily hassles are **difficult to avoid**. We have certain requirements of life that are legitimately our responsibility, and avoiding engaging with these responsibilities results in more substantial problems.
3. Daily hassles are **objectively small or "minor."** In the moment we are dealing with them, however, they may elicit a stress reaction.
4. Daily hassles are **disruptive** to our routine. In other words, they interrupt the flow of our day and so are noticeable. They can even require a change of plans (for example, if you have a flat tire before an important client presentation and must call an expensive rideshare to get to work).

Reaction to Daily Hassles

Remember that a daily hassle is not, individually, a major stressor in that it is a small or minor event. Our immediate reactions tend to match this level of importance, as we tend to react with irritation, annoyance, and/or frustration instead of more intense emotions. However, it is also clear that daily hassles have an additive and amplification effect over time and with repeated experience. The additive or accumulation effect occurs when the effects of the hassles build up and, when put together, become a more substantial source of stress. This is especially true if the hassles are spaced close together in time and recur regularly. As stress accumulates in this way, we react repetitively, and the hassles contribute to a chronic, low-level stress state. Once people have accumulated hassles and minor stressors, it doesn't take much additional stress to tip them over into being overwhelmed.

It's important to note that the more stressors people accumulate, the "heavier" they can feel psychologically because they amplify each other. This can happen with the accumulation of many repetitive daily hassles or in the aftermath of a major life event. For example, in the aftermath of divorce, single parents may struggle to cope with daily hassles like making time for children's activities, housework, grocery shopping and food preparation, work obligations, and self-care. The distress of the divorce can "prime" the stress reactivity system to react more strongly to minor daily hassles; for example, instead of reacting with irritation to traffic, we feel anger or escalate to road rage.

Research on Daily Hassles

Traditionally, research has tended to focus on the big "life events" that occur over most people's lifespan, such as birth, death, marriage, divorce, conflict, disability, and so forth. There is no doubt that these can impact our well-being, with research indicating that we can have substantial and long-lasting impacts on our cognitive and emotional well-being for years after a particularly stressful life event (Kettlewell et al., 2019). Overall, life events perceived as negative have more impact on well-being than do life event uplifts, but the good news is that most people return to a baseline level of wellness over time. It is in the past couple of decades that researchers have started to recognize that the small and frequent inconveniences of life are consistently diminishing our well-being. In fact, there is evidence that the higher the occurrence of daily hassles, the lower our sense of subjective well-being. This is a negative correlation, which means as our hassles increase, our well-being goes down and vice-versa.

Daily hassles can affect our psychological well-being, including increasing our susceptibility to anxiety and depression and decreasing our sense of self-worth and self-efficacy (McIntosh et al., 2010). For students, the changes associated with starting college can bring a new range of daily hassles associated with independence, taking initiative, time management, and organization. These additional sources of hassles can be related to increased reporting of depressive symptoms (Bouteyre et al., 2007). Finally, as daily hassles accumulate, a person might start to focus on what they don't get done, instead of what they do accomplish. This can make them feel worthless and can make their attempts to "get things done" seem hopeless. Finding a positive and productive way to deal with daily hassles will promote positive mental wellness, as these skills both decrease our potential for stress-related symptoms of depression and anxiety and also increase our sense of agency and efficacy.

Defining Uplifts

Uplifts are the good things that happen to us during the day. In other words, they are positive occurrences that notably improve our feelings of well-being. Functionally, uplifts are the counterbalance to daily hassles. Like daily hassles, any individual uplift can occur rarely or regularly, and they don't have to be uplifting to everyone,

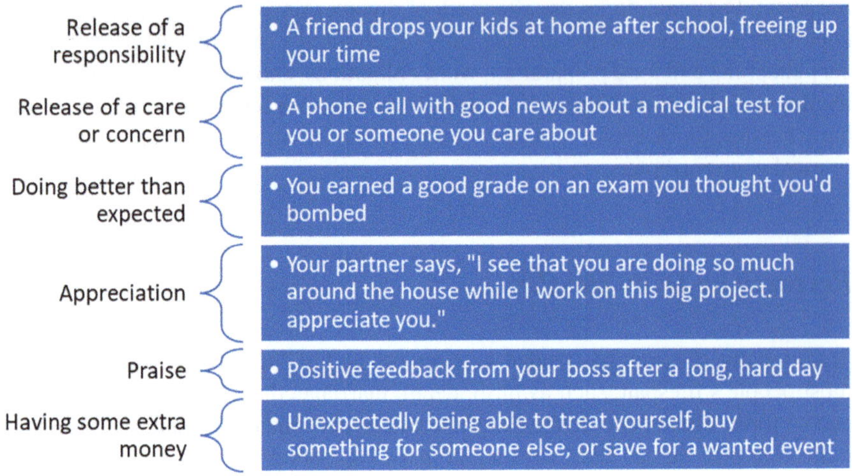

Fig. 11.2 Examples of uplifts

just to us! Examples of uplifts include receiving an unexpected accolade or praise at work or school, completing a task that had been put off, having a great evening out with friends, a fun day with one's partner, or receiving a gift of something one really wanted. Figure 11.2 presents additional examples of uplifts in daily life.

Uplifts have the following characteristics:

1. Daily uplifts are perceived as **positive**. They can be affirming of one's worth, relationship-affirming, make us smile or laugh, or just plain make one feel good.
2. Daily uplifts are primarily **unexpected or unpredictable**, but some can be foreseen.
3. Daily uplifts are **objectively minor or slight**. This is not finishing a marathon or getting a promotion, rather a simple gesture, sentence, or moment.
4. Daily uplifts **lighten our "stress load"** in that they are often perceived or experienced as a release of tension, relaxation of concern, and a moment of peace.

Research about Uplifts

Experiencing uplifts appears to be important to maintaining our physical and mental well-being. Many of the studies on hassles and uplifts use what is called a diary method for collecting data. Using this method, study participants record their own behaviors, feelings, and experiences related to the study topic every day over a period of time. For example, if we were interested in finding out the number of hassles and uplifts experienced by students living in dorms and how it relates to their mental health, we would ask students to make a daily record in a structured way of a variety of potential hassles, uplifts, and mental health symptoms.

There are relatively few studies that focus only on uplifts, rather it is common for research to include both hassles and uplifts or focus on the balance of hassles to uplifts. It is not only the presence of too many daily hassles to cope with that affect people negatively, but also *deficits in uplifts* that affect our well-being. There is evidence, for example, that people who experience a deficit in uplifts have more inflammatory markers than do those with more regular personal and social uplifts (Strawbridge et al., 2019). As we know from previous chapters, inflammation is implicated in illness and disability progression for many diseases. Also, people suffering from depression tend to report more hassles and fewer uplifts, but successful treatment for depression reduces reports of hassles and increases experiences of uplifts (Panaite et al., 2021). These types of findings are hopeful and positive; by purposefully increasing our uplifts and decreasing our hassles, either through an intervention like therapy or through our own goal-directed behavior, we can be more well in both body and mind.

Coping with Daily Hassles and Maximizing Uplifts

In our young and middle adulthood, we are very susceptible to the negative effects of daily hassles. The things we must accomplish during the day seem to multiply over the years each time we add something to our lives—relationships, children, pets, home ownership, student loans, career, and more. However, as we age into later life, we experience both fewer uplifts and fewer daily hassles. Life becomes simpler as children move out, we downsize our living spaces, and we are ensconced in productive work and, later, in our retirement.

One of our most impactful wellness achievements is to minimize the consequences of daily hassles and maximize the opportunity to receive uplifts. This is important because negative events and stressors impact us more profoundly than do positive events and uplifts; the negative is more salient, noticed more promptly, and processed more quickly than is the positive (Baumeister et al., 2001). The goal is to control our reactivity in both mind and body to daily hassles, while remaining fully open to partaking in uplifting experiences. Here are some ways that we can diminish our sensitivity to hassles and improve our awareness of uplifts:

Breathe. Breathing is an entry point to controlling the body's reactivity. Breathwork is a go-to technique for these situations, as it is portable, can be done in any situation, and is not bound by the environment. However, breathing through a stressful situation takes practice, as it is not just a process of normal breathing (although focusing on breathing in the moment is a great start). Practice by both slowing down breathing [count slowly 5-4-3-2-1 while breathing in] and quickening breathing [count quickly 1-2-3-4-5 while breathing out]. The goal is to give oneself control over the body's reaction, wherever one is, and whatever one is doing.

Go positive, seek solutions. How people think about things is a key to how they react to them. Reroute the process of thinking—stop focusing on the problem and start looking at solutions. For example, instead of thinking "My house is a complete wreck," instead focus on, "I'm going to empty the dishwasher so I can have a clean sink." Also, instead of thinking, "My commute is a disaster," instead focus on, "I'm going to leave 5 minutes earlier tomorrow to see how that goes."

Be prepared. Yes, it's the Boy Scout motto. And also yes, it's really good advice! Preparation increases control, increases the ability to respond rather than react, and increases the opportunity for important needs to be met during a stressful experience.

Identifying our parts and our responsibility. We sometimes create the very situations that stress us out. For example, we procrastinate, do not study enough or regularly, party too much or stay up too late so that we are grumpy, irritable, and not thinking clearly. People expect others and the environments around them to change for them (like loud roommates or barking dogs next door). An important life lesson is that the only person we can change or control is ourselves, including their own situation and their own reactions. Learning how to deal with people who won't change their behaviors to suit us is a very, very tough thing to do, but it is possible and worthwhile.

Target what we can change. First, we need to look closely at a hassle we are experiencing right now—Is this a recurring hassle? If so, we should change something! Keeping on doing the same things and reacting in the same ways makes us stuck in a stress loop. We can neither stop caring nor keep being stressed…if a person can't find the stuff they need to take to work in the morning, they should start laying it out the night before in a defined location. If a person is stressed by their roommate's noise, they could try headphones, earplugs, or a white noise machine or app. People have more options than they think.

Accept what we cannot change. Some daily hassles are just a part of living, and we cannot completely eliminate the hassles of our lives. The mindfulness technique of nonjudgmental acceptance is when we do not analyze our stressful experience, nor do we hold it tightly or push it from us; rather, we are aware of it and accept it as a part of life in this moment (Mahlo & Windsor, 2021). This helps us to address our stressful moments with calm and inner quiet, rather than reactivity.

Look for the good! We get so caught up in how hard life is that we forget that there is beauty and connection and opportunity for happiness and growth all around us. We can keep our eyes and hearts open. Most of all, we can keep our sense of wonder and awe—if we don't, we will miss all the things that make this life lovely and worthwhile.

Again, changing the ways that we create and interpret stress in our lives can have a truly transformative impact on our stress levels. Sometimes a person can do this themselves by establishing new routines, better time management, or a more realistic sleep schedule. Sometimes the issues might seem insurmountable and help from a counselor or therapist is necessary…that's ok! People don't have to have, or think they have, mental health diagnoses to see a counselor. Problems of daily living are legitimate reasons to seek professional help.

Race and Ethnicity in the Wellness Space

Wellness culture is not egalitarian. It targets people who either are or feel they are excluded from or underserved by the practices and institutions of conventional medicine. Marginalized people of every description are vulnerable to the unsubstantiated claims of wellness marketing, which prey on their historical trauma and lack of access to established healthcare systems. Yet, wellness culture is dominated by the majority culture, and often marginalized communities do not find that wellness culture is any more responsive to their unique needs than is traditional health care.

Do wellness concepts hold up across cultures? Different functions and practices of wellness are valued differently across and between different cultures. Well-being is not only based on what people have (their assets of every kind) but also on what they think or feel, their attitudes and beliefs, and their social expectations and traditions, which will differ across cultures and the wealth of their country. How people adapt over time to their conditions must be considered at both the population and individual levels, as communities or individuals might change their common or internal standards of well-being over time.

Racism can and does occur in the wellness space, including race-based disparities in access to wellness practices and spaces, lack of representation of people of color in wellness spaces, the framing of wellness around majority culture, and the centering of white bodies as models or ideals of wellness. Furthermore, there is a distinct lack of culturally relevant wellness products and wellness supports for communities of color. Overall, this means that programming and marketing heavily target white audiences, continuing the marginalization of people of color into the wellness space and reinforcing systemic inequality.

The mind-body wellness space also is vulnerable to various forms of cultural appropriation, which occur when culture-specific practices are adopted and/or marketed without respecting the cultural traditions and beliefs behind the practices. For example, cultural healing practices are contextual, specific to the belief system, and often spiritually based. The assumption that they can be conveyed to and legitimately practiced by nonparticipants in the culture can be perceived as arrogant and disrespectful and is the very reason that the term cultural appropriation exists. If wellness seekers are thinking about a shamanistic retreat or a healing ritual in a culturally relevant space (like a sweat lodge), they should reflect on whether they belong there and what they hope to take away from the experience.

Finally, wellness narratives tend to focus on personal responsibility and an individual accountability for illness and lack of well-being. This minimizes the effects of institutional racism and systemic factors like poverty, lack of access to healthcare, and low health literacy, which make it difficult or impossible for some people of color to engage in wellness culture.

What do we do when we identify a group that is unwell in some facet(s), and we find that these issues can be traced, at least in part, to disparities created by historical trauma, prejudice, and/or inequitable access to resources? We can design interventions and programs to address the disparities and remedy them in a culturally relevant way. For example, Barlow et al. (2015) describe the "Family Spirit" program designed by the Johns Hopkins Center for American Indian Health as a program designed to help Indigenous parents of babies and toddlers develop skills that promote a positive developmental trajectory for their children. The program is designed to be culturally and community relevant by: (1) acknowledging and addressing risks associated with historical ethnic trauma and loss of cultural traditions, especially parenting traditions, (2) listening to the community members, who said the best place to intervene in the cycle of health vulnerability was with young parents, and (3) using health educators from the Indigenous community. Acknowledging trauma, listening to the community, and using change agents and professionals from within the community are key ways that health and wellness can be competently addressed in ethnic communities.

Wellness as a Student

As a group, college students describe themselves as remarkably stressed and as tired, worn out, overwhelmed, depressed, and anxious. According to the Healthy Minds Study, which includes data from 373 colleges in the United States, more than 50% of students met the criteria for at least one mental health issue in 2020–21 (Lipson et al., 2022). This is a substantial increase from prepandemic levels. Additionally, utilization of mental health services by college students is low overall, and there is evidence of considerable inequity in using mental health services for students of color. Although tests, assignments, and getting to class are important potential stressors for college students, college students' problems are not, of course, just about college. Relationships, roommates, housing, homesickness, work, money, debt, and family are just a few of the other stressors that may weigh heavily on a college student. College students have many sources of distress, but they also have helping resources as well as many potential sources of uplifts. The bottom line is that universities and colleges are key contexts for student wellness, and students can both achieve academic success and thrive personally when they are healthy and well.

Supporting Student Wellness

Success in the classroom is a component of wellness that is specific to the student experience. The top five barriers to academic success reported by students include: (1) faculty teaching style, (2) exceedingly difficult coursework, (3) balancing schoolwork with family, home, work, and social obligations, (4) unclear academic expectations, and (5) mental health challenges (Flaherty, 2023). Students want to decrease their stress overall and increase the quality and quantity of sleep. Universities and colleges should provide resources that support student wellness at all levels of the institution. A whole-student approach to wellness at a university addresses student functioning in several core areas: relationships, capacity-building, communication, behavior, emotions, and leadership/community (McCallum & Price, 2016). Figure 11.3 describes some of the many things that colleges and universities can do to support student academic achievement through wellness.

It is important to acknowledge that the sources and severity of distress change as students move through their college careers. For example, homesickness or problems associated with dorm living may only be an issue for the first year or two of college, and then adaptation to the new environment and/or moving to a more congenial, less stressful environment may occur. Also, most students during or after their first year cobble together time management, organization, and study strategies that work for them within their academic and social contexts. Thus, many students (but not all) experience a reduction in problems related to managing and balancing workload, or at least an increase in coping, over time. However, things can always happen to challenge this adaptation. A new job, a loss in the family, a change in living circumstances to something that is less appealing, mental health challenges, and many other situations can upset the status quo and re-introduce high levels of stress, poor adaptation, and ineffective coping.

As they move through the college years, students' perceptions of what college means can also change. In the first few years, students are often decoding how college works, making friends, and figuring out how to get things done. As they move toward the end of college, students often find that other things having to do with school seem to matter more. GPA may become a big concern, as does finding internships, making choices about career path, and applying to jobs or graduate school. All of these may create anxiety and uncertainty, and it may seem like so much to do and so many decisions to make. A reliable way of perceiving and responding to the challenges inherent in determining postcollege pathways is a necessary coping skill in these later years. Students may respond to these challenges with a variety of healthy and unhealthy behaviors, such as:

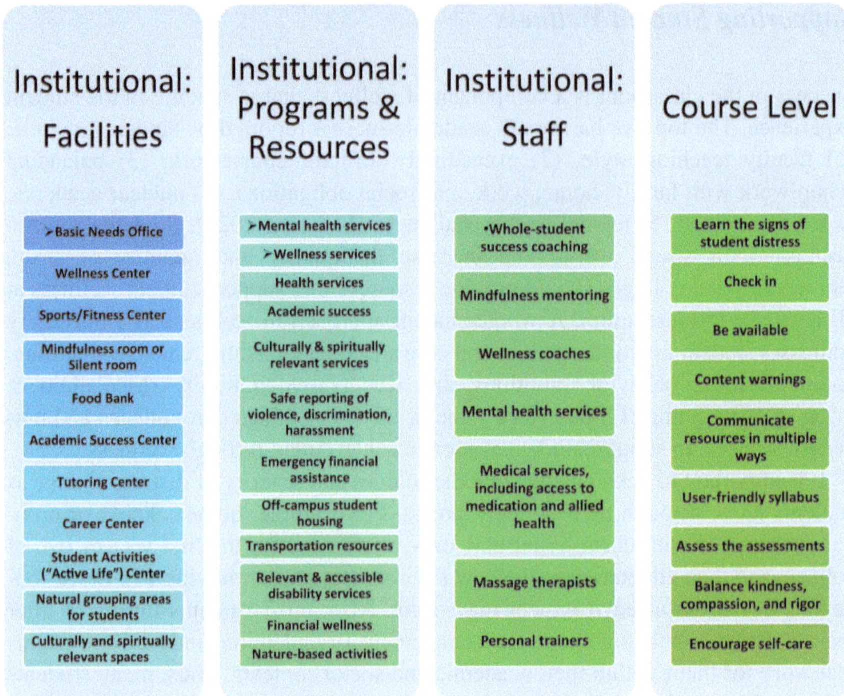

Fig. 11.3 University supports for student wellness

Healthy Coping

Spend time with loved ones. People should surround themselves with others whom they like to spend time with and enjoy their company. Being around others who make us feel comfortable can relieve a great deal of stress, even if we don't talk about what's troubling us.

Take a break. Between classes, homework, and other obligations, students may find most of their days booked solid with plans, activities, and tasks that need to be done. If students feel overwhelmed by all that they need to do, they should take a break. Schedule an afternoon where there is nothing to do but read a favorite book or watch a movie.

Communicate. Instead of silently suffering when assignment instructions are unclear or when the course content is difficult to understand, reach out! The vast majority of college professors want to hear from students when they are struggling (and when they are not!). It may sound old-fashioned, but it is true that, "The only way to know is to ask." If a student needs help with a class, tutoring, assistance with registration, or information about campus mental health services, they should ask until they get an answer that helps.

Sleep. When students feel rested, they are more motivated, remember what they have learned, make better decisions, get along better with others, and are less reactive to stress. Indeed, developing healthful sleep patterns is a foundational aspect of wellness, as it affects every area of life positively. When students make sleep a priority, they find that other aspects of wellness improve as well.

Take care of our bodies. This includes both eating well and exercising regularly. One of the most important things that a college student can do is to make a plan for healthful eating. This includes knowing where healthy food can be found at school or on the way to/from school and bringing food from home. Similarly, scheduling time to exercise is key to success; often, this can be done on the way to or from class.

Identify a personal go-to stress reliever. There are a thousand lists on the internet about how to relieve mental, emotional, and behavioral stress, but there is only one *you*. Maybe music or gaming is a reliable stress outlet for you, but maybe your best friend benefits most from a nap. Perhaps you have not yet found what consistently relieves your stress, but you should keep trying until you do!

Unhealthy Coping

Ignore the problem. Ignoring, running from, or withdrawing from the problem typically won't make them go away and, in fact, they can worsen or morph into different problems. Step back and look at the problem directly in order to find a solution—one is out there. If a busy schedule creates anxiety, people should evaluate what they are doing versus what they can do and see what they can change.

Online procrastination. Procrastinating online with social media, other internet sources, gaming, and streaming is common at all ages but is particularly prevalent for young people. There is no shortage of digital distractions we can lose ourselves in to avoid problems. While it's healthy to find a balance between work and relaxation, it's important to place limits on the use of digital media. The more time we spend streaming content or scrolling through socials, the more chance of falling behind in schoolwork. This, of course, adds to the overall stress burden we experience, which will feed this negative cycle of avoidance.

Substances. Smoking, drinking, or using drugs may offer relief in the short-term but after their effects wear off, people may find themselves feeling more stressed than before. For instance, drinking alcohol even moderately interferes with healthy sleep, leaving one tired, lethargic, and down.

Relying on stimulants. One might be surprised to know that caffeine addiction is the single most common legal drug addiction. Drinking coffee and energy drinks to fuel a late-night study session will inevitably lead to a crash later on. This can multiply problems in daily life, if the aftereffects interfere with other responsibilities. Also, stimulants boost cortisol levels in the body, which can increase physical consequences like inflammation, headache, and gastrointestinal distress.

Over- or undereating. When stressed, people can either crave comfort food or find that their appetite is gone altogether. In either case, food stops being a source of nutrition and becomes a way to address emotions. People sometimes experience a "break-up diet," which occurs when someone stops or reduces eating during the emotionally difficult post-relationship phase. It is possible, through therapy or structured intervention (like eating diaries or replacement activities) to move eating away from the emotional world and back into its functional role.

Wellness Tip—Overcoming Barriers to Wellness

Why is wellness sometimes a struggle? We all want to be happy and well, so it seems like it should be easy to achieve optimal well-being. Anything that gets in the way of our well-being and self-care can be called a "wellness barrier." Figure 11.4 presents a variety of barriers to well-being that people typically experience; some of the most common barriers from this list are lack of time, lack of resources, and too many obligations. For example, as much as someone might want to eat better, exercise, and manage their weight, if they work three jobs (time) that barely cover food and rent (resources) and have children to get to school, help with homework, feed, and get to bed (obligations), then any ability to focus on self-care seems like a distant dream. Each of these barriers also contributes to stress reactions, such as feelings of overwhelm, anxiety, depression, and physical manifestations of stress and distress. These are often (but not always) tied to age and/or life stage. Managing our own wellness becomes more complicated the more demands that are placed on our time—work, school, children, paying bills, and so forth.

What do we do when we encounter barriers to our well-being? First, assess the barrier and note if it is something that is new or has been happening for a long time, if changing it is a small tweak or a large/lengthy process, and what solutions come to mind. Then seek programs, apps, and social support that will help you to address the barrier. Remember that change can be difficult, and monitoring your mindset, keeping a positive outlook, and keeping your goals at the front of your mind are necessary parts of success. Finally, eliminate perfectionism from your expectations by recognizing that imperfection is part of being human and we learn by embracing our missteps as opportunities to improve. Here are some common barriers to wellness and some workable solutions that you could try:

Barrier: No Time to Exercise

Solutions:

1. *Walk and Talk*. Instead of sitting to take phone calls, instead walk while you talk. Take a lap around the hallways at work and go around the block at home. If you can, invest in earpods that make walking and talking easy and hands-free.

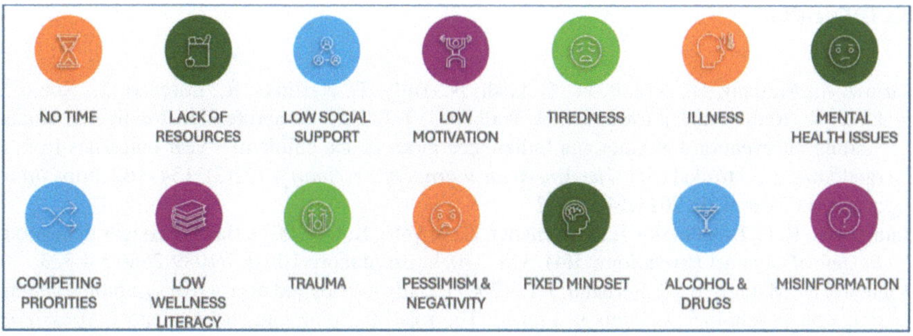

Fig. 11.4 Barriers to well-being

2. *Plan ahead.* Keep a work-out bag in your car. You will be much more likely to stop at the gym on the way home from work/school or take a short walk at lunch if your sneakers are readily available.

Barrier: Lack of Motivation

Solutions:

1. *Tap into your unique needs.* Wellness gurus may like to believe that everyone has a "drive to be fit," but some people work out to be attractive, rather than caring about their health. That's ok…use whatever gets you started as your own personal (and valid) reason to start your wellness journey.
2. *Your first goal should be small and realistic.* Don't revamp everything at once. Set a small, achievable goal at first—even eating one apple a day is better than no fruit at all.

Barrier: Competing Priorities

Solutions:

1. *Use the buddy system.* It is more fun to hang out with friends or to sleep in than go to the gym. Make the most of your wellness time by doing your activities—meal prep, gym time, volunteering—with a friend or family member.
2. *Integrate, don't separate.* Build wellness into your daily routines and spaces. Take a walk while your kids are at practice. Pick up right-sized containers for meal prepping next time you are out shopping. Get a walking pad so you can watch TV and walk at home.

References

Barlow, A., Mullany, B., Neault, N., Goklish, N., Billy, T., Hastings, R., Lorenzo, S., Kee, C., Lake, K., Redmond, C., Carter, A., & Walkup, J. T. (2015). Paraprofessional-delivered home-visiting intervention for American Indian teen mothers and children: 3-year outcomes from a randomized controlled trial. *The American Journal of Psychiatry, 172*(2), 154–162. https://doi.org/10.1176/appi.ajp.2014.14030332

Baumeister, R. F., Bratslavsky, E., Finkenauer, C., & Vohs, K. D. (2001). Bad is stronger than good. *Review of General Psychology, 5*(4), 323–370. https://doi.org/10.1037/1089-2680.5.4.323

Bouteyre, E., Maurel, M., & Bernaud, J. L. (2007). Daily hassles and depressive symptoms among first year psychology students in France: The role of coping and social support. *Stress and Health: Journal of the International Society for the Investigation of Stress, 23*(2), 93–99. https://doi.org/10.1002/smi.1125

Flaherty, C. (2023, February 13). *Survey: Students cite barriers to success, seek flexibility*. Inside Higher Ed. https://www.insidehighered.com/news/student-success/academic-life/2023/02/13/survey-top-five-barriers-student-success

Kettlewell, N., Morris, R. W., Ho, N., Cobb-Clark, D. A., Cripps, S., & Glozier, N. (2019). The differential impact of major life events on cognitive and affective wellbeing. *SSM—Population Health, 10*, 100533. https://doi.org/10.1016/j.ssmph.2019.100533

Lazarus, R. S., & Folkman, S. (1984). *Stress, appraisal, and coping*. Springer.

Lipson, S. K., Zhou, S., Abelson, S., Heinze, J., Jirsa, M., Morigney, J., Patterson, A., Singh, M., & Eisenberg, D. (2022). Trends in college student mental health and help-seeking by race/ethnicity: Findings from the national healthy minds study, 2013–2021. *Journal of Affective Disorders, 306*, 138–147. https://doi.org/10.1016/j.jad.2022.03.038

Mahlo, L., & Windsor, T. D. (2021). State mindfulness and affective well-being in the daily lives of middle-aged and older adults. *Psychology and Aging, 36*(5), 642–659. https://doi.org/10.1037/pag0000596

McCallum, F., & Price, D. (2016). *Nurturing wellbeing development in education: From little things, big things grow*. Routledge.

McIntosh, E., Gillanders, D., & Rodgers, S. (2010). Rumination, goal linking, daily hassles and life events in major depression. *Clinical Psychology & Psychotherapy, 17*(1), 33–43. https://doi.org/10.1002/cpp.611

Panaite, V., Devendorf, A. R., Kashdan, T. B., & Rottenberg, J. (2021). Daily life positive events predict well-being among depressed adults 10 years later. *Clinical Psychological Science, 9*(2), 222–235. https://doi.org/10.1177/2167702620956967

Strawbridge, R., Sartor, M. L., Scott, F., & Cleare, A. J. (2019). Inflammatory proteins are altered in chronic fatigue syndrome—A systematic review and meta-analysis. *Neuroscience and Biobehavioral Reviews, 107*, 69–83. https://doi.org/10.1016/j.neubiorev.2019.08.011

Chapter 12
Career and Financial Wellness

Career Wellness

We cannot discuss wellness without talking about work, as we spend so much of our lives in the workplace. Career or occupational wellness includes identifying a career path that reflects our values, lifestyle goals, and financial needs. It involves engaging in meaningful work that fits our interests, skills, and talents in a workplace that is supportive, enriching, and satisfying. Most adults, including students, work either within the home or outside of the home. In fact, we will ultimately spend one-third of our lives working, or an average of 90,000 h over the course of our lifetime. That's a lot of investment of time, but work is also an investment of effort.

Work is necessary for us in a very practical sense, enabling us to acquire food, shelter, and basic necessities. However, work is also beneficial to us in a variety of other ways. Although it is probably strictly true that "money can't buy happiness," there is abundant evidence that a baseline amount of money is needed to purchase or source the foundational elements of life satisfaction—shelter, warmth in winter and shade in summer, clothing, food, and clean water. Thus, the monetary benefits of work cannot be underestimated, as it is related to our functional wellness as well as our subjective life satisfaction. Work is more psychologically fulfilling for us when we feel like we have the tools, community, and autonomy we need to thrive in our workplace, but also when we have the ability to provide for our families and benefit socially (Hagler et al., 2016).

Espousing the benefits of work is not to say that it is all positive, as work can also be stressful, emotionally difficult, physically harmful, and can challenge our feelings of adequacy and worth. Poor workplace culture, lack of management and peer support, workplace harassment, job insecurity, inactivity, and lack of control over schedule and work activities have all been related to stress, mental distress, and burnout (Stansfeld et al., 2013). Burnout is a significant concern for many workers and occurs when workers perceive that the stressors of their job far outweigh the

S. M. Henney, J. D. Hackett, *Mind-Body Wellness*,
https://doi.org/10.1007/978-3-031-91611-3_12

benefits, which puts them in an emotionally, physically, and mentally exhausted and depleted state (Edú-Valsania et al., 2022). Brownout is typically seen as the beginning stages of burnout and is characterized by increasing loss of motivation and enthusiasm about work. Burnout and the processes that lead to it can be associated with low productivity, aversion to work tasks, increased absenteeism, fatigue, inability to concentrate, and detachment from work and colleagues. The solutions to burnout are best conceptualized as a partnership between the employer (who can address leadership development, work–life balance, and work climate) and the employee (who can use time management strategies, exercise, therapy, and mindfulness) with the goal of improving work conditions both individually and collectively. It's worth noting that burnout and brownout are not specific to the workplace, but rather can be experienced in many aspects of daily life where the demands placed on us exceed our coping resources, including school, parenting, volunteerism, and sports, to name a few.

Work also involves an opportunity cost, which is the cost to us of choosing one option over another. We spend so much time at work that opportunity costs are inevitable. For example, to succeed at work and fulfill our work obligations, we sacrifice time with our partners and children, our friends, valued recreational activities, and other avenues of personal growth and fulfillment (Vander Elst et al., 2016). Finally, although work itself can be stressful and dissatisfying at times, it is unemployment that is most distressing to people at almost every level. In addition to financial strain and increased risk of homelessness and hunger, unemployed people suffer more from depression (including suicidality), anxiety, pessimism, self-blame, relationship problems with friends and family, and divorce than do employed persons. Thus, just the state of being employed has some mental and physical benefits and protective factors (e.g., Wood & Burchell, 2018). This may be, at least in part, because work is a source of meaning, usefulness, and efficacy for many people, and, even though stressful, has benefits to subjective well-being. Kaplan (1995) states, "Looking back on a life of purpose and productivity, even if one experienced some stress along the way, might well be more satisfying than looking back on a stress-free life in which little was accomplished" (p. 180).

In addition to the factors discussed above, our mindset about work and our appraisals of the benefits and costs of work are key to our perception of career well-being. The Challenge–Hindrance Stressor Framework (CHSF) suggests that there are certain aspects of work called *challenge demands* that support our career and personal development in positive ways, such as autonomy, leadership, workload, and even reasonable time pressures (Podsakoff et al., 2023). On the other hand, there are *hindrance demands* that cause us stress and strain and that negatively impact our physical, emotional, and mental well-being, such as workplace politics, unclear expectations, impossible deadlines, and responsibility without authority. To be clear, both challenge and hindrance demands are stressors, but challenge demands are closer to eustress in their effect on us, and hindrance demands are closer to chronic or episodic stress, leading to distress at work.

Work–Life Balance and Integration

Most people are familiar with the term work–life balance, which assumes that our work life and personal life should be fully separate with a strong boundary in between, and yet completely in balance with equal meaning, effort, and investment for each. The assumption is that we are required to invest wholly in both work and home to be successful in both spheres. However, we can see how it could easily become a source of stress for us to constantly be worried about balancing time between work and home or leisure activities. To address this stress, workplaces have offered a variety of work–life benefits, including flexible schedules, remote working, onsite or subsidized childcare, and wellness benefits (like fitness, smoking cessation, weight management, yoga, and many more). In general, these programs are very popular with workers and have been found to be related to greater employee satisfaction and retention (Scribner et al., 2020), improved mental health and reduced burnout (Ernawati et al., 2022), and better metabolic health (such as weight, blood pressure, and cholesterol), particularly in high-risk groups (Neville et al., 2011). However, there has also been some concern about whether the cost of these programs is commensurate with the benefits derived by the employees and the employer (for example, would this money be better spent on raises or other concrete incentives?). Indeed, we are seeing some workplaces pull back from their flexible schedules and remote working programs due to concerns about productivity, communication, accountability, and loss of office culture.

A different philosophy about the relationship between work and nonwork is called work–life integration. Figure 12.1 illustrates the different presentation of work–life balance versus work–life integration. The assumption behind work–life integration is that we all have many roles, one of which is work, and it is largely impossible to achieve "balance" between these roles in any meaningful sense. This is because our roles expand and contract over time and for a variety of reasons, sometimes even on a daily basis. For example, if a child or elderly parent is sick, the family role expands and the work role must contract, even in the short run until the child or parent is well or another can take over responsibility. Work–life integration

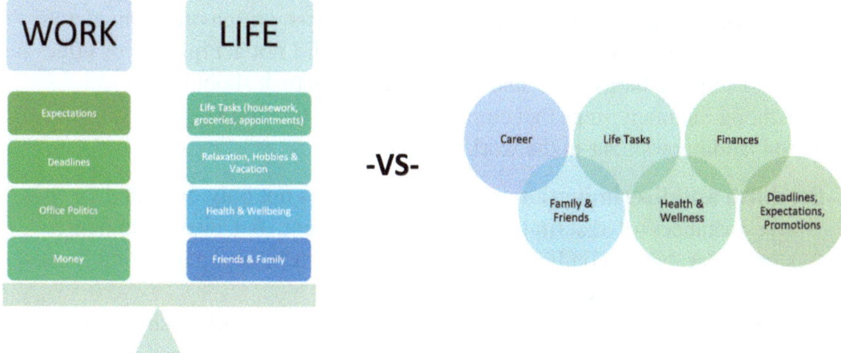

Fig. 12.1 Work–life balance vs work–life integration

assumes that work and nonwork can act in harmony or at least in cooperation with each other, but this requires trust, accountability, and open communication between the employee and the workplace. The main work–life integration strategies used today are flexible work hours and flexible schedules. The assumption is that an employee's optimum productivity could be achieved working from home, without the daily stress of commuting, and that home obligations do not always sync with a traditional 9–5 schedule. Employees are given autonomy and trust to manage their personal and professional time in ways that suit them while still maintaining productivity and meeting performance expectations. A Pew Research Center study shows that just over a third of US workers with jobs that can be done at home are working at home 100% of the time (Parker, 2023). This same study indicates that the main benefit these workers see from working from home is a better work–life balance, but they also believe working from home helps them to get their work done within their deadlines. Finally, work–life integration may be even more relevant to today's gig economy workers, where there is not a reliance on a traditional workplace or employer, so the boundary between work and home life is even less distinct. There is some evidence that gig economy workers may prefer this type of work–life integration and may perceive greater satisfactions deriving from it (e.g., de Janasz et al., 2023).

Discrimination in the Workplace

Race- and ethnicity-based inequitable treatment in the workplace is relatively common. For example, a 2023 Pew Research Center report indicates that more than 40% of Black workers reported experiencing unfair treatment in the hiring process, promotions, and/or pay, far more than their White, Hispanic, and Asian counterparts. Workplace racism can be experienced via the range of racist behaviors and assumptions from implicit bias to microaggressions to explicit harassment and discrimination (Horowitz & Parker, 2023). Not only is this morally wrong and socially reprehensible, it is a liability risk for the companies that allow it to continue. For example, the EEOC filed and won a lawsuit against a paper company where racial slurs were broadcast over the company's intercom, a makeshift noose, and swastikas were displayed, and "long live the confederacy" was written on a confederate flag displayed in a common area. The company did not act quickly or effectively to stop the harassment and paid the price, as they should have.

Among the many steps that employers can take to eliminate bias, discrimination, and harassment in the workplace are:

Establish antidiscrimination policies that address not only overt and extensive instances of discrimination and harassment, but also microaggressions, race-based conflict, and discrimination in hiring, pay, promotions, and other employment benefits.

Enforce antidiscrimination policies at all levels and in all instances. There is no "harmless joking" concerning race in the workplace, nor should the executive suite be immune to antidiscrimination policies.

Focus on employee buy-in via diversity and inclusion training for both new and existing employees as well as soliciting employee feedback. If employees are turned off by or bored during training or, most importantly, if they do not understand the purpose and need for the training, then the opportunity for knowledge gain and personal growth has been missed.

Provide a safe and anonymous way for employees to speak up about workplace discrimination and harassment. Few people who feel that they are at risk of losing their job will speak up, so procedures to ensure safe reporting increase the likelihood that problems will be identified and addressed expeditiously.

Employee Assistance Programs that feature both trauma-informed therapy and culturally relevant therapy play a crucial role in supporting victims of workplace discrimination, crisis management, and promoting growth and positive change in all employees.

Requiring culture change is perhaps the most important of all employer actions. Employers are required by law and by decency to protect employees from discrimination and harassment, and the most sure and lasting way to do this is culture change—to promote equity and inclusion for every employee at all times by changing hearts and minds to embrace an inclusive mindset.

Career Readiness Pathways

The track to professional fulfillment and associated satisfaction is one with known processes and pathways. The purpose of following a career readiness pathway is to both increase employability and to improve our chances of acquiring a meaningful career that fulfills us and enhances our well-being. Consider these steps (also displayed in Fig. 12.2) on the path to career wellness:

Self-Assessment. The first career planning task is to take stock of one's interests, skills, and values related to work. What is highly motivating and breeds excitement about a future career? What life priorities are at the top of the list—family, status, money, travel, free time? What is one good at, and what needs improvement? There are many career readiness and career aptitude resources available through the counseling or career services office at most schools, or it is easy to find resources online. However, remember to put the results in context—individuals are the final judge of what their career path should be, not a test, teacher, or family member.

Research career options. There is abundant information available at our fingertips about industry job forecasts, the ins and outs of various work settings, and the specific job requirements for different career paths. The internet is a valuable source of information, but it should not be the only one. Talking to a wide variety

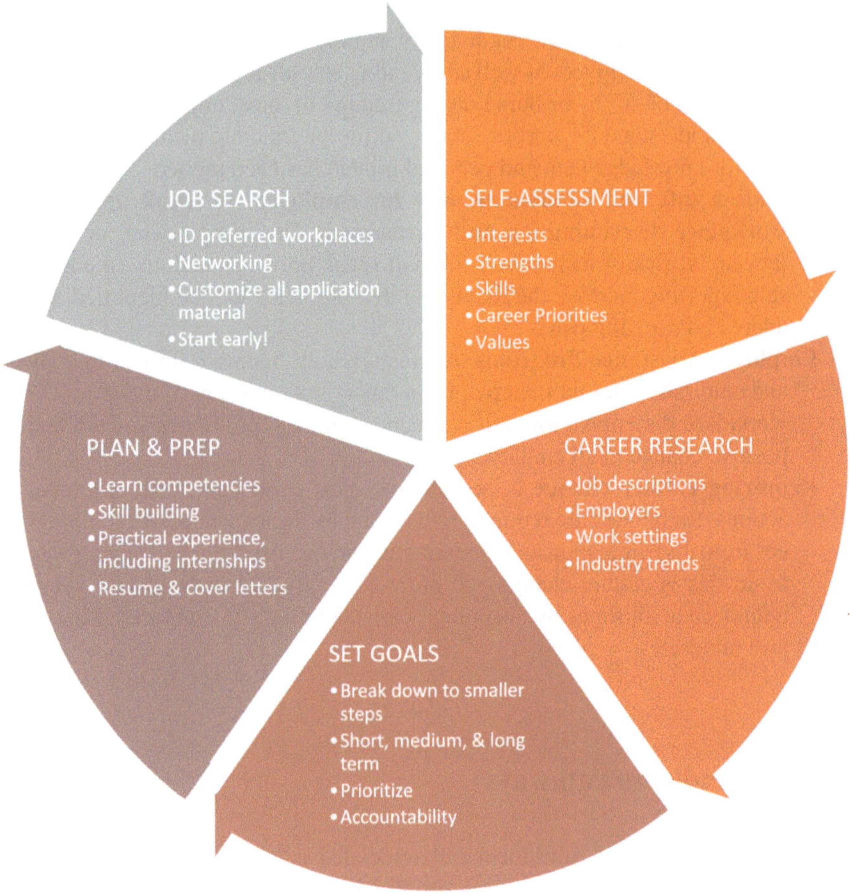
JOB SEARCH
• ID preferred workplaces
• Networking
• Customize all application material
• Start early!
SELF-ASSESSMENT
• Interests
• Strengths
• Skills
• Career Priorities
• Values
CAREER RESEARCH
• Job descriptions
• Employers
• Work settings
• Industry trends
SET GOALS
• Break down to smaller steps
• Short, medium, & long term
• Prioritize
• Accountability
PLAN & PREP
• Learn competencies
• Skill building
• Practical experience, including internships
• Resume & cover letters

Fig. 12.2 Steps to career wellness

of people about things we are interested in—family, friends, teachers/professors, even people out in the world (at a sports game or restaurant or concert)—is a great way to gain knowledge about career paths and to make connections. People can find out about jobs that they never knew existed or about a twist on a career path that fits them better than the one they were considering. Internships are also a proven way to explore career pathways and, eventually, to get a job. The 2023 National Association of Colleges and Employers (NACE) nationwide survey indicated that employers value job-relevant internship experience more than major, GPA, or general work history. This is because industry-specific experience matters, so students should make sure they get this type of experience before pursuing their professional career.

Goal setting should start early. In order to succeed professionally while maintaining well-being, goal setting is necessary. Remember that we are not just setting one goal, rather people should have both broad life goals (i.e., to "be a doctor") and many specific goals (i.e., to score competitively on the SAT). People will also have short-, medium-, and long-term time frames for goals. Without goals, people don't know where they are, where they want to be, and how to get where they want to go. So many people are stuck in jobs they don't like on a career path that is not meaningful to them, but this is less likely if they set meaningful and achievable goals. Success in meeting career goals is also related to setting up accountability goals, such as having a career coach, writing down goals and checking them regularly, and/or having an accountability partner (someone who knows our goals in detail and will monitor and support us). In addition to the SMART goal process discussed in Chap. 4, Mark Murphy (2010) refers to HARD goals, which move us out of our comfort zone and motivate us to achieve. HARD goals are:

Heartfelt: A goal should be something you care about. You should be able to answer what the goal means to you.

Animated: The goal should be something that occupies your thoughts. It should be clear in your mind, and you should be consistently processing and thinking about achieving your goal.

Required: The goal should be something you need to do; if you don't need it, you won't do it.

Difficult: A goal isn't a simple task that can be checked off a list. Goals should challenge us, make us resilient to barriers, and enhance personal and professional growth.

Make a concrete plan. A goal is a result or desirable outcome, while a plan is the process to be followed to achieve this outcome. Career planning typically requires the goal to be broken down into achievable steps, which makes the goal manageable and helps to avoid procrastination. For example, an early part of a career plan is to determine what education or training is needed for a chosen field. Some jobs require degrees and/or graduate work and/or certification, while others do not. The plan should also include career readiness activities, like perfecting customizable templates for the resume and cover letter, gaining practical experience through internships or volunteering, and building soft skills, such as teamwork, professional communication competencies, and collaboration.

Search wisely for jobs. The modern employment landscape requires attention to detail, persistence, and a very early start, as hiring timelines are often months long and involve multiple rounds of interviews. First, understand the target industry via internships, networking, and reading trade publications and news. Build relationships with people who have the preferred job or work at the target companies; these are the people who have already done what the job seeker is trying to do! When actively identifying job vacancies, expand the parameters of the search by not being confined to one big job aggregator, as not all companies post on all job sites; a better strategy is to search multiple aggregators as well as company websites. Finally, never use the same resume and cover letter for every job. Tailor the resume and, particularly, the cover letter with keyword-rich customizations from the position's job description.

Financial Wellness

One of our biggest sources of daily stress is money—making it, spending it, and not having enough of it. Financial stress and strain make us physically, mentally, and emotionally ill. It can also have significant impacts on relationships, with finances being one of the major sources of marital conflict (Papp et al., 2009). Going through financial stress can be related to poor spending habits, low income, low financial literacy, and lack of impulse control. However, it is also true that we can have times when events hit us hard in our pocketbook and, even if we do have some emergency savings, it is not enough to cover the cost. Hospitalizations and extended illness, unexpected job loss, home or car repairs, and unaffordable housing costs (i.e., increase in rent or electricity) are all key sources of financial crises for many households. This can make people feel overwhelmed and unable to cope, resulting in depression, anxiety, and even ignoring the problem completely in order to fight off panic. Financial wellness occurs when we are currently able to capably manage our finances, meet our financial obligations, and feel secure in our financial future. Financially well people know their financial situation in detail and are able to describe both how and why they manage their finances in order to meet both current and future financial needs.

An important aspect of starting a financial wellness journey is to clarify our own values about money. Saying one "wants to be rich" is not a value, although it may be a goal one has. Financial values include concepts like freedom, safety, independence, fun, adventure, quality of life, and charity. Values around money are core parts of a personal belief system—how does money serve our personal wants and needs, and how will we deploy our money to meet our goals? In simple terms, personal financial values drive what we believe we should and should not spend money on and how much we should save. Questions we can ask ourselves to clarify our financial values include:

- What does money mean to me?
- What satisfies me or makes me happy?
- What scares me or makes me anxious?
- What activities and experiences am I most passionate about?
- What activities and experiences give our life meaning and purpose?
- How much do I think I need safety and stability versus fun and good times?

Our financial goals and behaviors are an extension of our values. *Values awareness* is knowing our values and aligning our daily activities and behaviors with those values. For most people, the foundational habits and decisions that reflect their values center around: (1) spending less than they earn, (2) budgeting, (3) saving, and (4) eliminating or reducing debt. In the context of financial wellness, values awareness means that we have the ability to make good decisions in line with our values, which can result in a purposeful approach to money and a happier, more contented life.

Achieving Financial Wellness

Financial assessment. The first step to financial wellness is to document how much is coming in and where the money being spent is going. While it is true that some people have a fixed/stable monthly paycheck, this doesn't hold true for hourly workers and those in the gig economy, so it is just as important to be clear about the money that is coming in as what is going out. Many people have a laissez-faire attitude toward their bank balance; they keep track of it in their heads or by frequently checking their balance and then spend until the account is close to zero. Track the money in and out for at least one month by using a free app or by creating a spreadsheet or table (phones are useful for this) including income and all spending, even the iced coffee or bag of chips. It is very easy to lose track of things that are bought with credit/debit, online, or with our phone, so make sure to log the food delivery or gas purchase as soon as it is made.

Create a budget. Many people do not have a budget because they do not know how to design one. In addition to the many free or low-cost budgeting apps and programs, our financial institutions are likely to have a budgeting program or a simple spreadsheet that can be used. An easy rule of thumb for budgeting is making spending adhere to the 50-30-20 rule (see Fig. 12.3). First, 50% of income should go toward essential needs, like housing, utilities, transportation, and food. Within this category are two types of expenses—fixed and flexible. Fixed expenses don't change month-to-month, such as rent/mortgage, car payment, and insurance. Flexible expenses, such as utilities, groceries, and gas, can vary by quite a bit on a monthly or seasonal basis. Flexible expenses in the needs category should be averaged over time or over a season for a budgetary entry; otherwise, they can be budget busters (such as unusually high utility prices in the summer or winter, depending on where one lives). Second, 30% of income should go to the things that make life enjoyable and livable, such as entertainment, travel, shopping, and charity. One great way not to overspend in this category is to take this money out

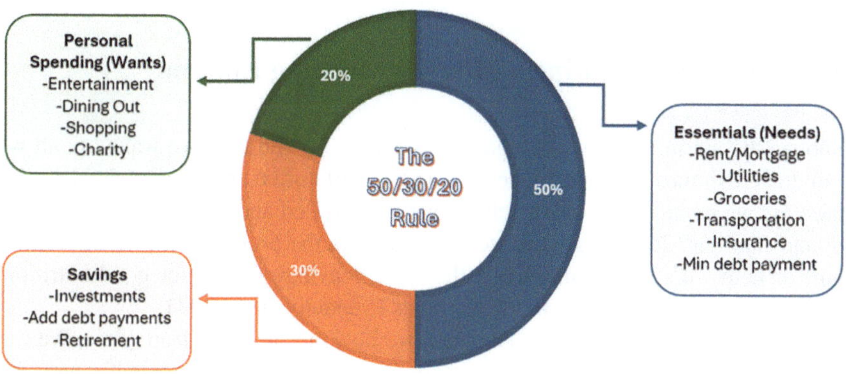

Fig. 12.3 The 50/30/20 budget

of our bank account in cash each month—once the money has been spent, there is no more personal spending for the month. Finally, 20% of income should always go to savings, which includes saving for specific long-term purchases (like a car or down payment on a house), saving for future security (like retirement savings), and paying down consumer debt (making extra or larger payments).

Emergency fund. Up to that 44% of adults report that they can't afford a $1000 emergency. This means they likely don't have savings (or very low savings) and are living paycheck-to-paycheck. The minimum emergency fund for adults should be one month's take home pay. Of course, people can't just save one month's pay all at once, so they should stick to the 20% per month recommendation until they have a full month's emergency fund. Then start working toward a three-month emergency fund, which is typically recommended for optimal ability to respond to life's crises.

Pay off Debt: Debt is a tool that can be used productively and is sometimes necessary to reach our goals; examples of "good debt" could be a reasonable mortgage or business start-up debt. However, consumer debt composed of credit card debt, student loans, car loans, and personal loans is a prison that traps people in a cycle of financial captivity; they have less freedom, more financial burden, and less ability to adapt to crises or changing financial circumstances. In order to be financially well, individuals must remove the fear and stress of consumer debt and claim the liberty to pursue their financial goals.

Life will always throw stressors and challenges at us. Learning how to effectively manage or confront these will improve our day-to-day wellness. We cannot predict exactly what stressors we will encounter or when we may experience them. Developing coping mechanisms and maintaining a positive outlook will improve our ability to manage hassles when they arise. As John Lennon said, "Life is what happens when you're busy making other plans." Being prepared allows us to cope with the unexpected.

Wellness Tip—Creating a Mindful Morning Routine

Snooze the alarm, then snooze again, and again…by the time we wake up, all we can do is rush through basic hygiene, grab a cup of coffee, and run out the door. By the time we make it to work or school, we are frazzled and feeling behind already. Sound familiar? It's not the snooze button that is the problem—snoozing doesn't hurt or help—it's the rushing that's the issue, leaving no time for good nutrition, mindfulness, or comfortable morning rituals (Sundelin et al., 2024).

How our day starts sets the foundation for how our day goes from there. We can help ourselves to get the best possible start to our day by creating a mindful morning routine. Routines help us feel like our lives are predictable and orderly, which in turn reduces anxiety and stress and increases cognitive functioning and emotional regulation (e.g., Medved, 2004). This is true not only for the individual, but for social units like a family—all members of a family benefit from structure, but it is a developmental asset for adolescents and young adults to have predictable sleeping, eating, and activity schedules (Barton et al., 2019). In *My Morning Routine*, Spall and Xander (2018) interviewed 64 successful people, from CEOs of major companies to authors to influencers. They found that, while the specific order or composition of morning routines can differ, successful people do have morning routines that they value and that they feel contribute to their success. Successful people understand that beginning our day with morning routines is part of living with intention—we set our plan or intentions for the day and routine helps us to bring them to life.

In sum, this all means that we create a positive mindset by starting the day mindfully, which then fosters a calm and clear emotional and mental approach to the challenges of the day. In order to enact a mindful morning routine, it is important to embrace the fact that a good morning starts the night before, with a consistent bedtime and good sleep hygiene. Here are more steps to designing a mindful morning routine:

1. **Set an alarm for the same time every day**. You don't have to "wake up early" for a successful day, but you should be consistent about whatever time works best for you.
2. **Don't immediately reach for your phone**. Relax in bed for a moment and take stock, mentally and physically.
3. **Hydrate**. Your body has been without water for a long time. Have water by your bed, and before your feet hit the floor, drink some water.
4. **Enjoy small/brief rituals** (i.e., comfy slippers, pleasant aroma, stretching). Making your bed, for example, sets a tone of productivity for the day, since you have already completed one complete task!
5. **Pick a mindful practice that works for you** on this day. Journal, meditate, reflect, exercise, or stretch—listen to your body and mind for what you need.
6. **Nourish your body** with a high-protein breakfast.
7. **Feed your mind** as well as your body with a short activity, such as art, a crossword, sudoku, a short podcast, or a page of a book.
8. **Make routine tasks more mindful**, such as breathwork while getting dressed or making breakfast.

References

Barton, A. W., Brody, G. H., Yu, T., Kogan, S. M., Chen, E., & Ehrlich, K. B. (2019). The profundity of the everyday: Family routines in adolescence predict development in young adulthood. *Journal of Adolescent Health, 64*(3), 340–346. https://doi.org/10.1016/j.jadohealth.2018.08.029

de Janasz, S. C., Kim, S., Schneer, J. A., Beutell, N. J., & Wong, C. (2023). Work-family integration and segmentation in the gig economy: An exploratory study on Airbnb hosts' experiences. *Tourism and Hospitality Research, 23*(1), 60–71. https://doi.org/10.1177/14673584221085211

Edú-Valsania, S., Laguía, A., & Moriano, J. A. (2022). Burnout: A review of theory and measurement. *International Journal of Environmental Research and Public Health, 19*(3), 1780. https://doi.org/10.3390/ijerph19031780

Ernawati, E., Mawardi, F., Roswiyani, R., Melissa, M., Wiwaha, G., Tiatri, S., & Hilmanto, D. (2022). Workplace wellness programs for working mothers: A systematic review. *Journal of Occupational Health, 64*(1), e12379. https://doi.org/10.1002/1348-9585.12379

Hagler, M., Hamby, S., Grych, J., & Banyard, V. (2016). Working for Well-being: Uncovering the protective benefits of work through mixed methods analysis. *Journal of Happiness Studies: An Interdisciplinary Forum on Subjective Well-Being, 17*(4), 1493–1510. https://doi.org/10.1007/s10902-015-9654-4

Horowitz, J. M., & Parker, K. (2023). *How Americans view their jobs*. Pew Research Center. https://www.pewresearch.org/social-trends/2023/03/30/how-americans-view-their-jobs/

Kaplan, S. (1995). The restorative benefits of nature: Toward an integrative framework. *Journal of Environmental Psychology, 15*(3), 169–182. https://doi.org/10.1016/0272-4944(95)90001-2

Medved, C. E. (2004). The everyday accomplishment of work and family: Exploring practical actions in daily routines. *Communication Studies, 55*(1), 128–145. https://doi.org/10.1080/10510970409388609

Murphy, M. (2010). *HARD goals: The secret to getting from where you are to where you want to be*. McGraw Hill.

National Association of Colleges and Employers (2023). *Job Outlook 2024*. https://www.naceweb.org/docs/default-source/default-document-library/2023/publication/research-report/2024-nace-job-outlook.pdf

Neville, B. A., Bell, S. J., & Whitwell, G. J. (2011). Stakeholder salience revisited: Refining, redefining, and refueling an underdeveloped conceptual tool. *Journal of Business Ethics, 102*(3), 357–378. https://doi.org/10.1007/s10551-011-0818-9

Papp, L. M., Cummings, E. M., & Goeke-Morey, M. C. (2009). For richer, for poorer: Money as a topic of marital conflict in the home. *Family Relations, 58*(1), 91–103. https://doi.org/10.1111/j.1741-3729.2008.00537.x

Parker, K. (2023). *About a third of U.S. workers who can work from home now do so all the time*. Pew Research Center. https://www.pewresearch.org/short-reads/2023/03/30/about-a-third-of-us-workers-who-can-work-from-home-do-so-all-the-time/

Podsakoff, N. P., Freiburger, K. J., Podsakoff, P. M., & Rosen, C. C. (2023). Laying the foundation for the challenge–hindrance stressor framework 2.0. *Annual Review of Organizational Psychology and Organizational Behavior, 10*, 165–199. https://doi.org/10.1146/annurev-orgpsych-080422-052147

Scribner, M., Sasso, P. A., & Puchner, L. (2020). Stress management and coping strategies in undergraduate students at a Midwestern State University. *New York Journal of Student Affairs, 20*(1), 4.

Spall, B., & Xander, M. (2018). *My morning routine: How successful people start every day inspired*. Penguin. ISBN: 9780735220287.

Stansfeld, S. A., Shipley, M. J., Head, J., Fuhrer, R., & Kivimaki, M. (2013). Work characteristics and personal social support as determinants of subjective well-being. *PLoS One, 8*(11), e81115. https://doi.org/10.1371/journal.pone.0081115

Sundelin, T., Landry, S., & Axelsson, J. (2024). Is snoozing losing? Why intermittent morning alarms are used and how they affect sleep, cognition, cortisol, and mood. *Journal of Sleep Research, 33*(3), e14054–e14054. https://doi.org/10.1111/jsr.14054

Vander Elst, T., Cavents, C., Daneels, K., Johannik, K., Baillien, E., Van den Broeck, A., & Godderis, L. (2016). Job demands-resources predicting burnout and work engagement among Belgian home health care nurses: A cross-sectional study. *Nursing Outlook, 64*(6), 542–556. https://doi.org/10.1016/j.outlook.2016.06.004

Wood, A. J., & Burchell, B. (2018). Unemployment and well-being. In A. Lewis (Ed.), *The Cambridge handbook of psychology and economic behaviour* (2nd ed., pp. 234–259). Cambridge University Press. https://doi.org/10.1017/9781316676349.008

Chapter 13
The Environment and Our Wellness

Environmental wellness is living all parts of life in environments that are healthful, stimulating, pleasant, and that support well-being. This includes experiencing safe and clean environments, free from threat of bodily or emotional harm, and also with abundant access to clean water, healthy food, and fresh air. Environmental wellness also encompasses having ecological awareness, which means being informed about how our actions and inactions impact both the world's ecology and our local ecosystems. Within this framework, it is important to take stock of the strengths and deficits of our environments and to be aware of how our environment is affecting us, both daily and in the long term.

The many environments that surround us can be enriching and healthful, enhancing both physical and mental well-being. Consistent involvement with the natural world is associated with reduced stress, better mood, and increased emotional regulation (Bratman et al., 2012). Clean environments with minimal toxins and health risks not only promote wellness in all our dimensions, but they can also help restore us to better mental and physical health after stress, illness, or disability (e.g., Kaplan, 1995). Our well-being is intricately interconnected with the health of our environment, and supporting a healthy, clean, and wholesome environment creates the conditions in which human flourishing is possible (World Health Organization, 2018).

Environments can also be barriers to flourishing and sources of economic and social disadvantage. People who live in areas with abundant crime, inadequate affordable housing, poor educational systems, high unemployment, and environmental toxins and pollutants experience handicaps and obstacles to success and flourishing that people in less problematic environments do not have. Ideally, all people should be able to control their environments to the extent that they can choose settings that are most conducive to their personal wellness. However, it is a fact of life that geography, socioeconomics, ability and disability, family history, age, race, and trauma or disaster can seriously impact our ability to influence our environment. Lack of control over our own environmental setting is a stressor in and

S. M. Henney, J. D. Hackett, *Mind-Body Wellness*,
https://doi.org/10.1007/978-3-031-91611-3_13

of itself and can lead to unhappiness and dissatisfaction, fear and anxiety, and a variety of physical symptoms.

The World Health Organization (n.d.-a, -b) has stated that about one out of every four (24%) deaths worldwide are "due to modifiable environmental risks." The environmental conditions that support healthy living include:

- Clean air.
- Safe drinking water.
- Access to healthy food.
- Sanitation (including waste management and access to hygiene).
- Protection from chemicals, chemical waste, and radiation.
- Competent agricultural practices.
- Built environments that support health (including housing, transportation, city planning, etc.)
- Safe places of work.
- Natural/green spaces and ample biodiversity.
- Stable climate.

Environmental Stressors

From a wellness perspective, environmental stressors are aspects of or occurrences in the environment that cause stress, strain, and distress. If these environmental conditions become chronic, they can lead to psychological and physical symptoms and diseases. Environmental stressors can be daily hassles (which we discussed in Chap. 11), chronic ambient conditions (like air or water pollution), conflict and war, or disasters/catastrophes (like a severe earthquake or hurricane). Predictability and control are important to how we perceive environmental stressors. If an event is predictable (an extreme heat wave in the south in summer), we perceive it as less stressful because we can prepare for it. On the other hand, a catastrophic weather event, such as the effects of an inland tropical storm (like Helene in 2024), can cause untold stress, suffering, and misery——people do not think it could be so devastating (never having seen or heard of such an event), and so do not prepare as if it will be. Although each of these environmental stressors has the potential to create varying degrees of negative impact on our minds and bodies, not all effects of environmental stress are bad. Environmental stress also creates conditions where we must adapt, change, and grow to meet the challenges of the environment. Adaptation happens over time, and if we can't adapt and grow, then we tend not to flourish in the new environmental reality.

> One can choose to go back toward safety or forward toward growth. Growth must be chosen again and again; fear must be overcome again and again. —Abraham Maslow

The Nature of Risk

Humans are pretty bad at evaluating their risk from different environmental hazards. A hazard is some aspect of the environment that could potentially harm us. Environmental hazards include infection/disease, sanitation, water and air quality, toxins, transportation, and so forth. In addition to the presence of hazardous conditions, the lack of certain things can cause hazards. For example, lack of sanitation infrastructure can cause disease, lack of access to healthcare can delay necessary or life-saving care, and lack of appropriate oversight and regulation can cause toxic and dangerous conditions. Examples of our problems with assessing risk are driving and sun exposure. Fear of flying is much more pervasive than fear of driving, yet flying is far safer than driving (driving is 96 times as dangerous as flying). In fact, driving is one of the most risky voluntary activities people do on a daily basis—we are more likely to die driving to the airport than flying on a plane. Sun protection is another source of faulty risk assessment. People believe that because it is good for them to be in nature, then "getting a base tan" (or worse, a "base sunburn") or "having a healthy tan" is good for us. In fact, tanning is the skin's response to sun damage, and risk of skin cancer increases with every burn (childhood burns being particularly harmful), and photoaging (wrinkles, spots/blotches, loss of skin tone) is attributable to sun exposure.

What causes us to falter in evaluating risk? The first reason is our cognitive biases. People display an optimistic bias when they believe that they are less likely than other people to experience a negative event. For example, people think "I am a good driver, so I'm not as at risk for a bad accident as other people," but this underestimates how much other drivers can impact our outcomes. We also have a tendency toward confirmation bias, in which we pay the most attention to information that confirms our existing beliefs and knowledge. For example, when we seek information on a treatment, product, or approach to a health, we tend to look in places where we have found information we "liked" before and to listen to like-minded people. We hardly ever seriously consider opposing views, and we underestimate the role of algorithms and AI in feeding us the information we want to hear. Humans also have a risk perception gap, which is the difference between how we perceive risk and the actual consequences of risk exposure. This gap is the result of the impact of emotions on our risk perception, but also of a lifetime's worth of experience that hones our frame of reference and our mental shortcuts (Brown, 2014). Thus, it's not only that we "ignore" information that we don't like, it's that we lack the frame of reference to even consider it reasonably.

Why does all of this matter? The end result of our deficient assessment of risk is poor decision-making. We treat our faulty perception of risk as if it was actual risk. A good example of faulty risk perception is vaccine hesitancy. For the overwhelming majority of people, vaccines are safe and effective because they are rigorously tested and closely monitored, with the benefits outweighing the risk of mild reactions. An example of the global benefit of vaccination is the fact that we do not have to live with the threat of smallpox. The smallpox eradication story is an extraordinary public health triumph, which included global collaboration at a previously unheard-of level, scientific innovation, the power of vaccination, and the willingness of individual people to be vaccinated. Nonetheless, vaccine-preventable diseases, such as measles and whooping cough (pertussis), are on the rise worldwide. We also are able to virtually eliminate cervical cancer worldwide via immunization, if we have the will to do so. Misinformation and myths about vaccine safety, often disseminated via the internet and social media, decrease our ability to accurately assess the benefits vs risks of vaccination. The more we believe the misinformation, the more confirmation bias comes into effect, leading to an information silo that leads us to discount good science and even our own experience (i.e., most anti-vaccination advocates benefit themselves from vaccination). By accessing a wide range of information from a variety of sources, seeking expert guidance, and taking opportunities for practicing critical thinking, people can become better at assessing risks. This fosters a culture of informed decision-making, effective prevention efforts, and health and wellness awareness, which can significantly enhance personal well-being as well as healthier communities.

The Physical Environment

The physical environment includes the quality of air, water, and land that surrounds us. Clearly, a living environment that is clean, safe, and toxin-free is important for physical health. While certain single exposures to environmental toxins can be detrimental to health (i.e., nuclear radiation), more commonly the issue is repeated or continuous exposure. This results in cumulative effects over time, which can exacerbate negative health risks and increase the potential for disease and ill health (Sexton & Hattis, 2007). Lest we forget that we are whole beings, however, a low-quality environment that is high in toxicity also contributes to mental health problems. Zu et al. (2020) make the important point that while clean environmental conditions (like good air quality) may not reduce mental illness (or produce good mental health) on their own, dirty and polluted environmental conditions can increase chances of poor mental health. Here are some key areas of concern for environmental wellness:

Outdoor Air Quality: Airborne pollutants can be caused by natural processes, such as dust storms, wildfires, pollen, and mold, or man-made processes, like transportation, agriculture, and industry. These create pollutants like carbon monoxide, particulate matter (dust, ash, industrial emissions), and biological agents, which can cause lung disease and impaired breathing (e.g., Pope et al., 2009). The primary ways to improve outdoor air quality involve community, social, and political action, such as government and industry regulation and community health and sustainability practices.

Indoor Air Quality: The indoor air environment can be very different from what we experience outside. In some ways, it is even more important to our well-being, because, for example, Americans spend about 90% of their time indoors (Environmental Protection Agency, n.d.). Some of the threats to indoor air quality at home include dust, mold, volatile organic compounds (VOCs), air freshening products, and cleaning products, while air quality threats at work are largely dependent on type of employment, but can include asbestos, particulate matter, VOCs, and industrial by-products. In our indoor environments, we can improve air quality with air purifiers, good ventilation, and choosing eco-friendly cleaning and personal products.

Water Quality: Runoff or poor management processes by industry and agriculture, improper disposal of chemicals and pharmaceuticals, poor wastewater/sewage management, urbanization, and oil/chemical spills are just some of the ways the quality of our water is negatively impacted. The types of toxins involved include heavy metals, nitrogen and phosphorus fertilizers, pesticides, all types of drugs, PCBs, dioxins, microbes, and microplastics. We can reduce exposure to water pollutants by using filtered water, checking water quality, and not swimming in contaminated water.

Soil Quality: Like water pollution, some primary sources of soil contamination are industrial waste, agricultural runoff, waste/sewage, improper disposal of chemicals, and urban development. Pesticides and herbicides in agriculture can have endocrine-disrupting effects that are associated with reproductive health problems and developmental delays (e.g., Gore et al., 2015). This impacts human health primarily through the food chain, as contaminated soil impacts the safety of crops and food animals.

Sensory Quality: Taken together, light and noise pollution are called multisensory pollution. Light pollution is artificial light that disrupts or inhibits natural darkness, such as city lights, street/highway lights, billboards, and external household lighting. Light pollution inhibits human sleep, animal migration, the activities of nocturnal animals, and viewing of the night sky. We can address light pollution through specific public policy interventions that limit light proliferation and skyglow and by using low-wattage bulbs, downward-facing fixtures, motion sensors, and darkout window coverings. Noise pollution is a disruption of the natural acoustic environment through loud, excessive, or repetitive noises. It can have both subtle and obvious effects on human well-being, including hearing loss, tinnitus, sleep disruption, stress, and anxiety. Many solutions to noise pollution involve government and community regulation, including the construction of sound barriers (such as along highways), implementation of restrictions on allowable noise levels for industrial and construction areas, zoning that separates industrial from residential areas, and the use of soundproofing to make workplaces and homes less noisy.

What Is Oxidative Stress and Why Is it Important?

Many people may not have heard of oxidative stress, but it plays a crucial role within the body in the development of ill health and disease. Oxidative stress occurs when the body has an excess of molecules called reactive oxygen species (ROS, sometimes called free radicals) and insufficient antioxidants to neutralize them. ROS are unstable and highly reactive molecules that can damage cells and DNA. Antioxidants are used by the body as a defense against ROS damage and can be made by the body (endogenous) or obtained from foods or supplements (exogenous).

While lifestyle factors like smoking, alcohol consumption, and poor diet can contribute to oxidative stress, some of the main factors are environmental. For example, exposure to air pollution, contaminated water, UVB radiation (sun exposure), pesticides, heavy metals, ionizing radiation, and household or industrial chemicals or solvents are all associated with ROS production in the body (Bhattacharyya et al., 2014). The results of this process include damage to the components of our cells, including DNA, proteins, and lipids, which then disrupt normal cellular function and contribute to disease. Additionally, increased oxidative stress activates inflammatory responses and impairs immune function, leaving us vulnerable to infection and disease. Inflammation in the body is particularly concerning, as it can contribute to insulin resistance (leading to type 2 diabetes), hardening of the arteries (atherosclerosis), autoimmune diseases (multiple sclerosis and rheumatoid arthritis), inflammatory bowel disease, and asthma. Furthermore, chronic oxidative stress and persistent inflammation can result in cellular changes and mutations that increase risk for cancer. The accumulation of oxidative damage over time is a key driver of the aging process, damaging DNA, impairing cellular function, and contributing to age-related diseases.

There are two main ways to reduce oxidative stress: avoid the causes of excessive ROS and increase antioxidants. For the former, not smoking, reducing or eliminating alcohol consumption, and limiting exposure to toxins involve lifestyle changes that most people can make. Increasing antioxidants to battle oxidative stress can be accomplished via antioxidant-rich food choices:

- Vitamin C: Citrus fruit, berries, broccoli, bell peppers.
- Vitamin E: Seeds and nuts (sunflower, almonds), avocado, salmon.
- Carotenoids: Carrots, leafy greens, tomatoes.
- Flavonoids: Berries, green and black tea, citrus, whole grains.
- Selenium: Shellfish, meat, dairy, Brazil nuts.
- Zinc: Oysters, red meat, pumpkin seeds, rolled oats.

Diet and the Environment

Our environment impacts our diet via the types and variety of foods we have readily available to us and our ability to afford them. In the bigger environmental picture, the healthfulness of our diet is a function of farming techniques (such as use of chemicals and pesticides), how food is cleaned or sanitized, modes and timeframes of transportation, the availability of locally sourced foods, and the retail environment. However, even in our modern world, there are still people who lack regular access to nutritious food. In 2023, 13.5% (18.0 million households) were food insecure, and many Americans (up to 39 million people) live in food deserts (Rabbitt et al., 2024). We can envision how being constantly hungry or having low/no access to healthy food would impact our overall wellness. In his Hierarchy of Needs, Maslow (1954) places food in the most basic of human needs and motivations; if a person is hungry, all other aspects of wellness go out the door in the quest to obtain food.

Some people believe that the answer to the environmental and food safety problems of conventional farming is buying organic food. However, buying organic is not in the budget of many people, and the variety of local organic foods may be lacking. People who live in food deserts have challenges sourcing affordable conventional food, let alone pricey organic foods that are less likely to be available in corner stores or low-cost grocery stores. The good news is that it is possible to source healthy nonorganic food on a budget. Each year the Environmental Working Group (n.d.), a nonprofit concerned with agriculture research and advocacy, publishes its' Green Fifteen (TM) list of produce with the lowest tested pesticide level. In 2023, this list included common staple items like corn, frozen peas, and onions, along with more specialty items like avocados and mangoes.

Avoiding or limiting foods known to be high in toxins is necessary for any healthful diet. These include foods and drinks like fish that are high in mercury (typically larger/older fish like marlin, shark, king mackerel, etc.), cherry pits and apple seeds (contain high concentrations of cyanide), and unpasteurized foods and drinks (like raw milk). It is particularly important to avoid such products for children, pregnant women, and immune-compromised individuals. However, many of the "avoid this TOXIC food" messages that we hear on social media or from friends and family are simply fear mongering, attempts to generate followers, and/or the result of misinterpretation of information. For example, the message that "sugar is evil" abounds from all sources, and so we go Keto or prevent our children from having a slice of cake at a birthday party. However, sugar itself is not toxic, rather overuse of it and reliance on it in the average diet can be bad for our health. Similarly, the message that "chemicals in our food are poisoning us" alongside pointing at a list of long, scary-sounding words on a food label, misses the point that all food is composed of chemicals, many of which are natural to the food. This doesn't mean that we shouldn't be concerned about chemical additives to our food—we should be—but not all additives are toxic, and how much we consume of the additive is typically related to how dangerous it is. A diverse diet that includes a variety of foods limits our exposure to toxins associated with specific foods.

In addition to the act of choosing specific foods, there are other actions we can take to make our diet safer. Spoiled and mishandled food can spread diarrheal disease and Hepatitis A, so good food storage practices, appropriate cooking temperatures, avoiding cross-contamination, and ensuring proper hygiene (including hand washing and gloves) for anyone who handles food are imperative. Staying mindful of cooking methods (charring and overcooking create harmful chemicals), thoroughly washing fruits and vegetables, limiting additives (even sugar and salt), and sourcing local food or growing food are ways to monitor and maintain a safe diet, protecting individual and public health.

Using the Environment as a Cue for Wellness

October Theory (sometimes called Octobering) refers to purposefully using the fall as a time of self-examination and introspection, with the goal of personal transformation. The idea is that we transition along with nature—as nature begins its autumnal transformation with the vibrancy of fall foliage, cooler temperatures, and shorter days, this engages us in contemplation of the necessity of change, the passage of time, and the cycles of life. Life slows down in the fall, and so should we. It is, figuratively speaking, a time to "gather"—to gather with friends and families to celebrate holidays, to cook and eat together, and to approach the challenges of the winter months in community with others.

April Theory is the springtime companion to October Theory and refers to a time of renewal, growth, and emotional rebirth that accompanies the arrival of spring. As the spring unfolds, the symbolism of growth and rejuvenation abound—flowers bloom, trees bud, and animals and birds are out-and-about. The rains of April can also be viewed as a time of spiritual cleansing, and the April sunshine invigorates and inspires our optimism and vitality. The symbolism of April includes new beginnings and rebirth, meaning that we have the opportunity to evaluate our goals and aspirations to find motivation to stay on track or to start anew.

What do the transitions of the seasons mean to you? What are the ways that you can embrace the changing seasons as part of an intentional approach to evaluating your well-being within the context of your environment?

Consumer Products

Many everyday products that we buy for our homes and for personal care contain toxins that we should avoid. Everyone should be particularly careful about products that are used by children and pregnant women. For example, older toys and some imported toys may contain high levels of lead, phthalates, and other toxins, which can be associated with developmental delays and learning disabilities. This means carefully vetting not only the safety but also the potential toxicity and harmfulness of products that we buy or allow to come into our homes and workplaces. Some common sources of problematic ingredients include:

Plastics: Many plastic containers as well as the lining of food and beverage cans contain Bisphenol A (BPA), which can leach out over time or with heating and cause hormone disruption and other health issues. Alternatives include glass, stainless steel, and bioplastics.

Personal Care Products: Lotions, cosmetics, hair care products and dyes, body wash, and nail polish and remover can contain formaldehyde, parabens, phthalates, and sulfates. These are related to allergic reactions, respiratory effects, endocrine dysfunction, and even cancer. In order to avoid these toxins, check labels for "paraben-free," "phthalate-free," and "SLS-free" ingredients, prioritize natural oils (like coconut oil) and plants (like aloe vera), and consider making homemade products from ingredients like baking soda, apple cider vinegar, and essential oils.

Household Cleaning Products: Everything from glass cleaner to detergent to disinfectants contain harsh chemicals like ammonia, bleach, and VOCs. These can cause respiratory issues, allergic reactions, and skin irritation.

Cookware: Nonstick pans should not be used at high temperatures and should be replaced if damaged or peeling. Also, plastic cutting boards can be a source of microplastics in food.

Furniture and Home Decorating: Flame retardants, drywall, paints, varnishes, solvents, and lead paint or accents on decor can be sources of VOCs (like formaldehyde, toluene, and xylene) and polybrominated diphenyl ethers (PBDEs). These can cause respiratory problems, headaches, hormone disruption, and neurological damage.

Significantly reducing exposure to harmful consumer products has obvious health benefits. Making informed choices about these products includes reading labels for nontoxic ingredients, and remembering that just because something sounds like a chemical does not necessarily mean that it is bad for us. Also opt for eco-friendly, sustainable products when possible, including making our own cleaning products (always remember to label homemade products with a list of ingredients). For example, vinegar diluted with water (1 cup of each) makes an excellent household cleaner, and a couple of drops of essential oil make it smell better, too! Baking soda also has many uses as a household cleaner and deodorizer.

Infectious Disease

We don't have to look very far for an example of how devastating infectious disease can be for human wellness. Covid-19 has killed upwards of three-quarters of a billion people worldwide (World Health Organization, n.d.-a, -b), and this is just one of the many infectious diseases that impact humans. Infectious disease is a significant risk not only to human lifespan, but also to increased physical and mental disability, heightened pain and suffering, and decreased quality of life. Infectious diseases hit all ages and socioeconomic classes, but the hazards are not experienced equally—not many know that the infections behind pneumonia and diarrhea kill upwards of a million young children a year, even though they are readily preventable through vaccination and treatable with antibiotics (UNICEF, n.d.). Let's not forget the economic impacts of infectious disease, which both drive up healthcare costs and reduce economic productivity and workplace participation. Covid-19 spotlighted how quickly infectious diseases can spread globally, and it underlined the need for worldwide scientific cooperation and investment in research and public health.

From a wellness perspective, one part of addressing infectious disease is prevention. Simple acts of hand washing, safe food handling, practicing safer sex, and staying away from people who are ill (and staying home when we are the ones who are ill) are everyday practices that lower the risk of contracting and spreading disease (Drexler and Institute of Medicine, 2010). Other relatively straightforward methods of reducing exposure to infectious disease are to pay attention to good ventilation (open a window) and airflow indoors and to spend time daily outdoors (but practice good bug bite prevention). On the other hand, practices like aromatherapy, while pleasant, do not prevent or counteract infectious disease, and neither does the pseudoscience of homeopathy.

Good health and wellness literacy includes improving understanding of how infectious diseases are transmitted and prevented, which empowers people to make informed choices about their health. For example, people with high health literacy will push back against narratives that insist that childhood exposure to diseases like chickenpox in childhood "strengthens the immune system." This is pure anti-science rhetoric and ignores the risk of acute and chronic health problems that result from disease. In the case of chickenpox, although the infection is often mild, risks include bacterial infection, infections of the lungs or brain, and bleeding problems. The virus that causes chickenpox also stays in the body on the nerve roots as a latent infection, later emerging to cause shingles. Shingles is a painful, often debilitating, disease that can result in long-term nerve pain. Simply put, safe and effective vaccinations can take chicken pox and shingles off the table for most people who use them—getting the disease isn't better for us.

Wellness Tourism

The global market for medical tourism was 47 billion US dollars in 2024, and a large portion of this was specifically wellness, beauty, and antiaging tourism. The destinations favored in wellness tourism can be found worldwide and include resorts, spas, camps, thermal and mineral springs, fitness centers, and retreat centers. The typical programs, activities, and practices that people seek in wellness tourism include:

Spa Treatments: Practices that promote relaxation, stress relief, and rejuvenation, such as massage therapy, body treatments like exfoliation, scrubs, and wraps, facials, manicures, pedicures, heat therapy (sauna, steam, hot water), and cryotherapy.

Mindfulness: Offerings can include guided or individual meditation and mindfulness exercises, either by themselves or in conjunction with other activities. Nutrition/eating, nature, fitness, movement, music, creative work, journaling, and therapy/counseling can all include mindfulness components.

Fitness Programs: Activities that promote physical health and enhance awareness of the mind-body dynamic, including yoga, tai chi, hiking, running, strength and cardio workouts, dance, and Pilates.

Nutrition and Diet: Programs can include structured diet options, nutrition and healthy eating workshops, cooking classes, detox activities, and weight loss (if desired).

It is not only the immersive and whole-person nature of wellness retreats and spas that contribute to well-being, but also the travel aspect of wellness tourism has benefits in and of itself. Detaching from daily routine, separating from the stress of work, improvement in perceived happiness, and enhanced life satisfaction are all benefits from the act and experience of traveling and tourism (Chen & Petrick, 2013). The added benefits of wellness tourism include improved fitness levels, reduced stress, enhanced relaxation, improved mental wellness, and being in community with like-minded people. Responsible tourism, ecologically friendly travel, and building the capacity for a sustainable lifestyle are also often a part of wellness tourism. Ultimately, wellness tourism is an industry and a money-making enterprise, but one that reaps benefits in personal well-being and also environmental awareness and sustainability.

Environmental Safety

All people deserve a safe environment, free from threats of bodily harm, mental and emotional damage, and exposure to toxins and carcinogens. When we implement environmental safety measures, the goal is to eliminate or mitigate hazardous conditions and to reduce preventable injuries and accidents. Such measures and regulations can address issues like air and water quality, waste disposal, transportation safety, and hazardous materials. These regulations can address immediate problems, but they often also lead to sustainable practices that benefit people in the long term, such as clean air and smog mitigation initiatives leading to reductions in respiratory issues (Brunekreef & Holgate, 2002). However, it is important to remember that not all environmental safety measures are broad and complex. Environmental safety can be as simple as checking smoke detector batteries, tying or hiding cords and cables so they are not a trip hazard, using motion-activated lights, installing nonslip mats and grab bars in showers and tubs, and securing firearms separate from ammunition.

Environmental threats can, of course, be deadly, but it is much more likely that we will be injured by an environmental hazard. Below we will discuss two major sources of harm to which people are regularly exposed and that pose significant risk of injury and disability—sometimes severe and permanent disability.

Transportation. Traffic is a significant source of both death and disability, with 45,000 Americans dying in car accidents every year and almost 2.5 million injured. Transportation is actually a highly regulated sector, and safer road construction, driving regulations (speed limits, seatbelt laws), and vehicle safety requirements all have reduced fatal motor vehicle accidents. Stringent and high-visibility enforcement of motor vehicle laws related to speeding, distracted driving, and impaired driving also lowers the number of traffic accidents (Taylor et al., 2022). However, the human factor remains a key piece in the risks of driving, with people vastly underestimating their risk from driving and also having the propensity to flexibly follow or ignore traffic safety regulations, which increases their risk of accidents. Sustainable transportation alternatives include public transit, biking, carpooling, park and ride, hybrid and electric cars, but even though these alternatives may have less environmental impact, they still have the safety risks inherent in transportation.

Workplace Safety: Workplace safety involves measures to maintain safe working conditions by minimizing hazardous physical conditions, reducing exposure to hazardous substances, maintaining air quality, ensuring appropriate ergonomics, and eliminating workplace violence. Part of enhancing workplace safety is administrative and structural, such as enforcing rules about appropriate use and storage of chemicals and making sure that equipment and machinery are regularly inspected and maintained in good working order. Another part is the human factor, such as regular training, participation in safety initiatives, and creating a culture of safety. Why is this important to our wellness? In the United States, there are more than 5000 workplace deaths every year, and 4.5 million workplace injuries requiring medical evaluation. Not only is this injurious to our bodies, but the dangers of the workplace affect our mental health, motivation, and stress levels.

Improving Environmental Wellness

Emphasizing a connection to the environment fosters a sense of responsibility and care for the world around us. At the individual level, we can address our environmental wellness via where we live, our lifestyle choices, and the car, food, and consumer products we purchase. However, there is a larger picture to environmental wellness, wherein our choices in the areas of politics, activism, and volunteerism speak to our commitment to preserving the natural world and building a sustainable future.

Environmental Policies. It's important for individuals to understand how local, national, and global environmental policies affect their wellness. Our society and communities have many laws, regulations, and policies addressing the environment, the goal of which is primarily to protect the natural world and humans' interactions with it. However, environmental policies can come into conflict with economic interests and, unfortunately, nature is often on the losing end of that equation.

National Parks

The US National Park Service (NPS) was established in 1916 as part of the Department of the Interior. This was the result of a conservation movement with the goal of preserving and protecting the USA's natural and cultural heritage for future generations. The awe-inspiring vistas of the Grand Canyon, the majesty of Yellowstone, the deep resonance of the Sequoia and Redwoods National Parks, the mysteries of the Everglades, and the profound history of the Ancestral Pueblo cliff dwellings are each a unique and vital part of the network of more than 400 parks covering 84 million acres.

The national parks are not only an opportunity for us to "be in nature," but they allow us to experience and be inspired by the vastness and beauty of nature. Monroy and Keltner (2023) note that "nature is one of the most common elicitors of awe," and they identify five pathways through which the experience of awe improves our well-being, including "shifts in neurophysiology, a diminished focus on the self, increased prosocial relationality, greater social integration, and a heightened sense of meaning." On the other hand, apathy threatens the natural world globally, and how we can get people to care actively about preserving nature is an ongoing concern. Part of the solution to apathy is education and engagement, but these factors are most impactful when they begin early. Programs like scouting, Youth Conservation Corps (NPS), Junior Rangers (NPS), Conservation Connect (virtual, US Fish and Wildlife), and Kids & Nature Programs (National Wildlife Federation) all provide programming to engage children and youth in environmental education, conservation, and outdoor activities. Local programs like City Kids Adventures in San Antonio, Texas, take inner city youth into the outdoors and engage them in recreation, education, skill-building, and mentoring, all focused on appreciation for the natural world (for more information, view the documentary "City Kids").

Our love for nature and our awe for its wonders have real impacts, not only on our wellness but on political and economic agendas. Climate change is a threat to our natural spaces as much as it is to our populated spaces. The NPS has identified climate change as a key driver of changes to the parks' ecosystems that threaten the welfare of plants and animals, as well as the natural landscapes (National Park Service, n.d.). Furthermore, national parks are extremely popular, and tourism can spoil the vistas, trails, landmarks, and cultural sites as well as disturbing the peace and activities of the wildlife. Tourists, Instagrammers, and adventure-seekers topple rock formations, dangerously approach buffalo and bears, immerse in protected springs, and litter. This is an opportunity not only for education and awareness, but for us all to come together with a renewed commitment to protecting the natural world…even from ourselves.

Environmental Activism. Social and political leaders only know how important environmental wellness is if we speak up/act up about it and vote accordingly. Not only can we vote, contact our political representatives, and participate in environmental demonstrations and campaigns, but we can also join or contribute to groups addressing issues like preserving and sustaining forests, rainforests, wildlife, ocean life, parks, and clean air and water.

Environmental Education. Awareness and action are intimately intertwined—the more we know about the threats to the natural environment and also the hazards it contains, the more effectively we can plan and act. By understanding what our risks are and what steps we can take (or not take) to deal with them, we can bring a sense of planful action and order to our wellness journey. For example, climate change is a known hazard to our health. Variations in temperature, weather patterns, and precipitation caused by climate change can increase the impact of toxins and allergens, exacerbate the effects of natural disasters, and expand the range and number of harmful pests and virulent diseases. Research suggests that education does work to change people's attitudes and behaviors. A 2020 study suggests that climate change education for young people can positively impact their sustainability practices over time, leading to lower carbon emissions over the lifespan (Cordero et al., 2020).

Natural Disasters and Discrimination

How can a storm or a flood be discriminatory? Of course, it is not the natural disaster itself that is discriminatory, but rather these disasters expose preexisting inequities in income, geography, access to resources, and social status. People of color are more likely to live in areas that are likely to be negatively affected by climate change-induced natural disasters, and Black people, in particular, have substantially higher mortality risk due to extreme tempera`Study after study finds inequity between people of color and white people in negative impacts experienced during and after natural disasters, such as increased chance of death for Black people due to hurricane impact (Sharkey, 2007), increased vulnerability of indigenous people and people of color to wildfires (Davies et al., 2018), and inequitable distribution of FEMA funds that assist with recovery and repair of damaged houses, with people of color receiving less financial assistance than white counterparts (Emrich et al., 2022). Further, there is evidence that as natural disasters increase in a given locale, there is a subsequent decrease in wealth accumulation for people of color and an increase in wealth for white people (Howell & Elliott, 2018).

Systemic racism affects employment, housing, financial institutions, education, and social supports for people of color in the best of times. In the worst of times, natural disasters reveal an array of structural vulnerabilities of people of color to death, disability, financial disaster, and inequitable social and financial governmental response, among others.

Sustainable Living. A sustainable way of living includes our lifestyle choices, social behaviors, and consumer habits, which impact not only our personal environment but the larger human environment. On a personal level, we can conserve water and energy at home, choose energy-efficient appliances, and purchasing reusable items are ways every person can engage in sustainable practices at home. Driving a more fuel-efficient car is also a good way to both help the environment and our pocketbook, reducing gas consumption and emissions. Another way we can live more sustainably while improving our wellness is to grow some of our own food, which gives us greater control over what does and does not go into the food we eat and also gives a sense of satisfaction that we are eating the fruits of our labor.

Urban Planning. There are many ways in which our wellness is impacted by the way we design the places we live. The car-centric design ideals of the twentieth century have led to a decline in public wellness, reducing both the need and desire to walk, be outdoors, and interact with our communities. Planning cities around cars, rather than people, makes it more difficult to interact with the community when we are in a car whizzing by from point to point. Furthermore, everyone shops at the same few big box stores with ample parking, while driving by smaller businesses with tighter parking lots. Walking and utilizing transit encourage us to stop in local shops and actually see people rather than taillights, fostering a greater sense of communal wellness. Wellness-based urban planning dedicates space for more "third places." A third place is a place other than work/school and the home, where people may gather in a setting such as a public square, cafe, or parks and green spaces. Car-centric design has turned the squares into intersections, cafes into drive-throughs, and green spaces into places we (confoundingly) must drive to. Walking and biking also have the obvious benefit of getting people outside and moving, a natural remedy to a sedentary lifestyle.

Ecotherapy

Ecotherapy or Nature Therapy is a mind-body technique emphasizing the powerful ability of the natural world to positively influence our physical, mental, and emotional well-being. Ecotherapy purposefully and mindfully explores our connection and interdependence with natural environments. This therapeutic practice is not only about "spending time outdoors," but rather it is a planful involvement with nature that has a healing, growth, or self-exploration goal in mind. Nurturing change through nature counterbalances the effects of urbanization and time spent indoors, thereby reducing anxiety, depression, and the physiological symptoms of stress (e.g., Bratman et al., 2015). An additional benefit of ecotherapy is that it encourages participants to recognize and act on the link between their well-being and the natural world through sustainable behaviors and environmental stewardship.

Lewis et al. (2022) reviewed the literature regarding ecotherapy and described different modalities of ecotherapy that appear to be related to positive mental health outcomes, which can include:

Horticulture Therapy: Includes farming, indoor and outdoor gardening, and flower arranging.
Adventure Therapy: Includes strenuous, technical, and/or higher-risk activities, like climbing, skydiving, rafting, diving, etc.
Wilderness Therapy: Encompasses a range of experiences from typical tent camping to skill-building camping to extreme camping.
Green Exercise: Can include exercising in nature, but also includes physical conservation work (i.e., planting trees or clearing trails).
Animal-Assisted Ecotherapy: Outdoor exploration, exercise, and adventure with animal companionship.

Environmental Justice. The most environmentally impactful aspects of industrialization, such as the production of toxic materials, emission of pollutants, and massive quantities of waste, have often disproportionately affected those of lower income and racial or ethnic minorities. For example, the "poor vs rich" parts of town are often determined by proximity to industrial areas and the prevailing direction of the wind—wealthier areas are upwind of industrial areas, and poorer areas are downwind, receiving the brunt of dirty, smelly, and toxic pollutants. A famous "dumping ground" for industrial toxins is "Cancer Alley" in Louisiana, a large tract of the state, largely populated by poor and working-class people, which is rife with oil, gas, and chemical plants. These plants are relatively poorly controlled, and the cancer rates of those in the region show it—residents experience a cancer rate of 45.8 per million, compared to 30.3 in the United States and 37.1 in Louisiana as a whole. This is well-known in the area, contributing to increased health anxiety. In areas like this, a fisherman may know it is not safe to eat their catch, a mother may be scared to let her children spend too much time outside, or a person may want to take a nice walk but be stopped by a horrible smell. Again, these health impacts are not equally shared across the population but rather are more likely to affect people living in poverty, racial minorities, and other marginalized groups. Equitable access to clean air, water, and soil should be the right of every person, not just a privileged few.

Wellness Tip—Taking a Screen Time Vacation

Do you always have one screen or another either on or at your fingertips? Is your phone your last interaction at night and the first thing you pick up in the morning? It's not unusual for students to identify screens as a barrier to getting things done and, particularly, as related to various sleep issues. Technostress is a type of stress related to our immersion in a society that requires us to interact consistently with technology, particularly new technology. In a digitized society, new technology comes to us quickly and is often required to efficiently complete our everyday tasks at home and at work. Technostress can also be experienced when we are constantly "tethered" to our devices via the need to be immediately available to work or family. Technostress can be felt intermittently or sporadically, when we have to interact with a new update for our screens, a different infotainment system in our new car, or a new type of tech (like a new user of a smart watch). However, it can also be more chronic, due to the pressures of incessant connectivity, the overload of both necessary and unnecessary information that is available (or pushed toward us) on smart devices. Sometimes it might seem like we are more in service to our technology than it is to us. This might leave us with feelings of frustration and anxiety, perhaps even interrupting our sleep resulting in fatigue and brain fog. Additional mental and physical outcomes of too much screen time can include:

- Eye/vision problems.
- Sleeping problems.
- Lack of attention to social relationships and loss of social skills.
- Sedentary weight gain.
- "Texting thumb" (tendonitis that causes pain and inflammation in the thumb)
- Procrastination.
- Reduced productivity.
- Digital motion sickness (typically caused by scrolling too much or too fast).
- Phantom phone vibration (feeling that your phone is vibrating in your pocket when it's not even in your pocket).

What can you do to keep the benefits of your screens for information, entertainment, and connectivity while minimizing the risks?

- Set screen time limits (use the phone's features for this, such as setting dark hours).
- When you must be around your screens, take frequent breaks—preferably, breaks where you move around.
- Screen-free zones, especially the bedroom.
- If you use your phone as an alarm, stop—get a separate alarm so you don't reach for your phone first thing.
- If you must use your phone or computer at night, reduce the brightness or use a blue light filter.
- No screens at meals.
- Family or friend "fun nights" with no phones allowed.
- Get rid of apps that suck you in and waste your time.
- Never use a device as a reward or punishment (for yourself or your kids, if any)—keep it neutral and focus on its practical aspects.

References

Bhattacharyya, A., Chattopadhyay, R., Mitra, S., & Crowe, S. E. (2014). Oxidative stress: An essential factor in the pathogenesis of gastrointestinal mucosal diseases. *Physiological Reviews, 94*(2), 329–354. https://doi.org/10.1152/physrev.00040.2012

Bratman, G. N., Hamilton, J. P., & Daily, G. C. (2012). The impacts of nature experience on human cognitive function and mental health. *Annals of the New York Academy of Sciences, 1249*(1), 118–136. https://doi.org/10.1111/j.1749-6632.2011.06400.x

Bratman, G. N., Hamilton, J. P., Hahn, K. S., Daily, G. C., & Gross, J. J. (2015). Nature experience reduces rumination and subgenual prefrontal cortex activation. *Proceedings of the National Academy of Sciences of the United States of America, 112*(28), 8567–8572. https://doi.org/10.1073/pnas.1510459112

Brown, V. J. (2014). Risk perception: It's personal. *Environmental Health Perspectives, 122*(10), A276–A279. https://doi.org/10.1289/ehp.122-A276

Brunekreef, B., & Holgate, S. T. (2002). Air pollution and health. *Lancet (London, England), 360*(9341), 1233–1242. https://doi.org/10.1016/S0140-6736(02)11274-8

Chen, C. C., & Petrick, J. F. (2013). Health and wellness benefits of travel experiences: A literature review. *Journal of Travel Research, 52*(6), 709–719. https://doi.org/10.1177/0047287513496477

Cordero, E. C., Centeno, D., & Todd, A. M. (2020). The role of climate change education on individual lifetime carbon emissions. *PLoS One, 15*(2), e0206266. https://doi.org/10.1371/journal.pone.0206266

Davies, I. P., Haugo, R. D., Robertson, J. C., & Levin, P. S. (2018). The unequal vulnerability of communities of color to wildfire. *PLoS One, 13*(11), e0205825. https://doi.org/10.1371/journal.pone.0205825

Drexler, M., & Institute of Medicine. (2010). *What you need to know about infectious disease.* National Academies Press. https://www.ncbi.nlm.nih.gov/books/NBK209704/

Emrich, C. T., Aksha, S. K., & Zhou, Y. (2022). Assessing distributive inequities in FEMA's disaster recovery assistance fund allocation. *International Journal of Disaster Risk Reduction, 74*, 102855.

Environmental Protection Agency (n.d.). *Indoor air quality.* https://www.epa.gov/report-environment/indoor-air-quality

Environmental Working Group (n.d.). *The 2024 Clean Fifteen™.* https://www.ewg.org/foodnews/clean-fifteen.php

EPA. (2021). *Climate change and social vulnerability in the United States: A focus on six impacts.* U.S. Environmental Protection Agency, EPA 430-R-21-003.https://www.epa.gov/cira/social-vulnerability-report

Gore, A. C., Chappell, V. A., Fenton, S. E., Flaws, J. A., Nadal, A., Prins, G. S., Toppari, J., & Zoeller, R. T. (2015). Executive summary to EDC-2: The Endocrine Society's second scientific statement on endocrine-disrupting chemicals. *Endocrine Reviews, 36*(6), 593–602. https://doi.org/10.1210/er.2015-1093

Howell, J., & Elliott, J. R. (2018). As disaster costs rise, so does inequality. *Socius, 4.*https://doi.org/10.1177/2378023118816795 (Original work published 2018).

Kaplan, S. (1995). The restorative benefits of nature: Toward an integrative framework. *Journal of Environmental Psychology, 15*(3), 169–182. https://doi.org/10.1016/0272-4944(95)90001-2

Lewis, O., Ohrt, J., Toomey, T., Linich, K., Wymer, B., & Newton, T. (2022). A systematic review of nature-based counseling interventions to promote mental health and wellness. *Journal of Mental Health Counseling, 44*(3), 191–208. https://doi.org/10.17744/mehc.44.3.01

Maslow, A. H. (1954). *Motivation and personality.* Harper and Row.

Monroy, M., & Keltner, D. (2023). Awe as a pathway to mental and physical health. *Perspectives on Psychological Science: A Journal of the Association for Psychological Science, 18*(2), 309–320. https://doi.org/10.1177/17456916221094856

National Park Service (n.d.). *Climate change.* https://www.nps.gov/im/ncpn/climate.htm

Pope, C. A., Ezzati, M., & Dockery, D. W. (2009). Fine-particulate air pollution and life expectancy in the United States. *The New England Journal of Medicine, 360*(4), 376–386. https://doi.org/10.1056/NEJMsa0805646

Rabbitt, M. P., Reed-Jones, M., Hales, L. J., & Burke, M. P. (2024). *Household food security in the United States in 2023* (Report No. ERR-337). U.S. Department of Agriculture, Economic Research Service. https://doi.org/10.32747/2024.8583175.ers.

Sexton, K., & Hattis, D. (2007). Assessing cumulative health risks from exposure to environmental mixtures—three fundamental questions. *Environmental Health Perspectives, 115*(5), 825–832. https://doi.org/10.1289/ehp.9333

Sharkey, P. (2007). Survival and death in New Orleans: An empirical look at the human impact of Katrina. *Journal of Black Studies, 37*(4), 482–501. https://www.jstor.org/stable/40034319

Taylor, C. L., Byrne, A., Coppinger, K., Fisher, D., Foreman, C., & Mahavier, K. (2022, May). *Synthesis of studies that relate amount of enforcement to magnitude of safety outcomes* (Report No. DOT HS 813 274-A). National Highway Traffic Safety Administration.

UNICEF (n.d.). *Childhood diseases*. https://www.unicef.org/health/childhood-diseases

World Health Organization (2018, September 13). *Preventing disease through healthy environments: A global assessment of the burden of disease from environmental risks.*. https://www.who.int/publications/i/item/9789241565196.

World Health Organization (n.d.-a). *Environmental health.* https://www.who.int/health-topics/environmental-health#tab=tab_1

World Health Organization (n.d.-b). WHO COVID-19 Dashboard. https://data.who.int/dashboards/covid19/cases

Zu, D., Zhai, K., Qiu, Y., Pei, P., Zhu, X., & Han, D. (2020). The impacts of air pollution on mental health: Evidence from the Chinese university students. *International Journal of Environmental Research and Public Health, 17*(18), 6734. https://doi.org/10.3390/ijerph17186734

Chapter 14
Wellness in Relationships and Social Situations

Many people are familiar with Aristotle's view on the social nature of human beings, which refers to us as "the social animal." It is not hard to see why. We spend a significant amount of time with other people, and social connections are a significant driver of our well-being. In fact, Rath and Harter (2010) describe five key factors that contribute to a great life: financial, physical, community, work, and social. It is hard to overstate just how important other people are for our sense of well-being. We strive for close connections with others, and these connections allow us to form friendships and, possibly, more intimate romantic relationships.

Social interactions are a central aspect of the human experience. When we attempt to think about someone who chooses to live a remote life with little to no contact with other people, we tend to think of someone like Ted Kaczynski—the Unabomber. We think of people like this as cautionary examples of the risks of social isolation. In Maslow's Hierarchy of Needs, once we have our physiological and safety concerns met, we seek out a sense of belonging and love. Our close connections can be family, friends, and romantic partners. We want to love and be loved, feel a sense of acceptance, and know we are part of a group or social network that cares and supports each other.

Early Attachment

Shortly after birth, we began the process of making strong connections to others. Attachment theory, born out of interest in the infant-caregiver bond, highlights the essential role the relationship with our primary caregiver has on us. This model looks at how the sense of safety and security we feel, or do not feel, from our caregivers impacts us over the course of our entire lives. From this work, we know that our expectations for adult relationships are influenced by our experiences as children. These early experiences with our primary caregivers provide us with beliefs

S. M. Henney, J. D. Hackett, *Mind-Body Wellness*,
https://doi.org/10.1007/978-3-031-91611-3_14

and expectations about how relationships work and what to expect out of them. In other words, they lay the foundation for what we think relationships should and will be like for us. As we get older, these expectations influence how we interact with the world and how we experience ourselves in relation to other people.

Early interactions create an "internal working model" of relationships for us. That is, from our caregivers' availability and responsiveness, we learn what to expect from others. These expectations are incorporated into the expectations we have for our significant partners later in life. This internal model consists of two key components: (1) How we view ourselves—do we see ourselves as worthy or unworthy of love and care? and (2) How we view the other person—are other people available, caring, and responsive? These internal models inform what we expect from other people, impact how we think about information, and produce approach or avoidance tendencies in us.

There are four attachment styles we can experience as adults. With a secure attachment, we feel comfortable displaying interested affection with our partners. People with this attachment style are comfortable being alone and see themselves as independent actors in their lives. Important relationships are prioritized, and they trust others. For securely attached toddlers, a caregiver serves as a "safe haven" they can return to for comfort. An anxious attachment type is reflected in constant nervousness or stress about relationships. These individuals need continuous reassurance and affection and do not feel comfortable being alone. Despite needing reassurances from their partner, they have issues trusting others and tend to be irrational and emotional. Many with this attachment type are in unhealthy relationships—they may monitor their partner to make sure no one else is receiving their attention or be so clingy and needy that they stifle their partner. Avoidant attachment is characterized by extreme independence and is often associated with unease with intimacy. They will feel like others are crowding them when trying to get close and will avoid intimate situations with others. Finally, the anxious-avoidant attachment style manifests in fear of intimacy and commitment, and a deep distrust of others. These individuals often spend a great deal of time alone, are low in self-confidence, and prefer to suppress their emotions. When they are in relationships, they tend to be dysfunctional and abusive. Unlike avoidant attachments, where they prefer to be alone, anxious-avoidant people avoid intimacy because they fear how it may hurt them to be so close to others. This theory provides a perspective on how our past relationship experiences influence our current relationships.

Attachment and Wellness

Attachment styles in adult relationships offer an interesting look at the connection between our relationships and our health and well-being. Our close connections—friends and romantic partnerships—serve as a key outlet for social interactions. They are the people in our lives we can self-disclose or discuss personal issues with and not fear rejection or ridicule. Furthermore, the quality of these relationships may impact how we feel. In other words, the positive benefits from close relationships may depend on attachment style.

Research has found attachment styles are an important health risk factor. Both anxious and avoidant attachment styles are related to depression, anxiety, loneliness, emotional regulation difficulties, and negative affect. Similarly, both of these attachment styles are related to less positive mental health indicators—less life satisfaction, positive affect, psychological well-being, and self-esteem. In contrast, secure attachments are associated with less depression, fewer symptoms of generalized anxiety disorder, and less trouble controlling emotions. When we feel threatened, upset, or in need of support, being in a securely attached relationship means our partner may help ease negative feelings and make us feel better. In contrast, those in less securely attached relationships (anxious and avoidant) do not have relationships that can help improve their sense of well-being. The positive health aspects of the relationship are minimized when we are less inclined to be emotionally connected and available for our partner.

Why Do We Affiliate with Others?

Models of affiliation propose a variety of reasons for why people are driven to connect with others. These include positive stimulation, emotional support, making social comparisons, and the good feelings engendered by attention from others. Interacting with others is typically a rewarding experience for us (Hill, 1987). Our evolutionary history "prepared" us to anticipate positive social interactions when we engage with others. Building connections served a critical evolutionary function by increasing the likelihood we would survive and pass on our genetic information to children. Living and working with others increased our chances of making it through tough winters, fighting off attacks from others, and hunting for food. We are the descendants of people who "played well with others." As a result, we are likely inclined to want to associate and be with other people. Brain imaging studies indicate social interactions can be physiologically rewarding for us. Areas of our brain that are active while we interact with others are the same areas activated when we receive food or money.

Interacting with others can provide us with much-needed emotional support. When a friend loses a loved one, we feel compelled to be there for them and to remind them we are there to help in any way they need. This can help provide the needed support to confront and work through terrible situations. In a much less significant manner, positive benefits can be seen through a quick connection with someone. A quick phone calls a few times a week has the ability to lower depression, loneliness, and anxiety (Kahlon et al., 2021). Simply keeping in touch with our loved ones can make meaningful impacts on them. You never know how much checking in with your friends and family can mean. For some, it may end up being the best part of their day!

Affiliating with others also gives us a glimpse into their attitudes, values, and behavioral tendencies, which can help us navigate confusing or ambiguous social situations. We also tend to compare ourselves to others. These comparisons can provide information on the accuracy of our own attitudes and skills and provide information on how we are expected to behave in uncertain situations. Finally, social interactions provide us with attention and can give us a sense of status. It feels good to associate with other people and to share our thoughts and ideas.

Social isolation, when we feel disconnected from others, increases depressive symptoms and all-cause mortality. In contrast, there is plenty of evidence that feeling supported and connected can help people improve and maintain their health, such as sustaining a healthy body mass index, increasing cancer survival, decreasing depression, and enhancing their mental health (e.g., Martino et al., 2015). These social relationships can also contribute to a longer life. In a large meta-analysis, researchers found strong social relationships to be associated with a 50% increase in our likelihood of survival (Holt-Lunstad et al., 2010). These findings indicate that our connections with other people have a comparable influence on mortality as other known factors (e.g., smoking and alcohol consumption) and have greater influence than a lack of physical exercise and obesity. Counselors may prescribe social interaction to encourage these benefits in clients. A lunch or a night out with friends provides more than a momentary good time. The unseen benefits of connecting with others are meaningful and can add to our lifespan and improve health and well-being over many years.

Building Positive Relationships

If we think about the happiest moments of our lives, many of these memories likely include other people. Watching a movie is more enjoyable when we are with our family, close friends, or romantic partner. Heading out to happy hour with our work colleagues after a hectic week gives us a sense of connection and "escape" from the demands of work. These moments, where we spend time with others, make the experiences more meaningful and impactful. This is not true for people in unhealthy or abusive relationships, which are not only physically and emotionally dangerous but also ruin normal enjoyable experiences and create a tremendous amount of stress.

To benefit from our close relationships, they need to be healthy and positive. So, what makes a healthy, positive relationship? Some characteristics of positive relationships include:

Communication. Many key aspects of our relationships require open and honest communication. As people, we are unable to read one another's minds, so it is essential that we are willing to communicate and express our thoughts and feelings with others. Without honest communication, misunderstandings are more likely, increasing the likelihood of conflict.

Respect. Respect is a critical component of positive relationships. Respect denotes a valuing of the worth and dignity of another person. When social interactions include mutual respect, we create environments based on positivity, empathy, compassion, and comfort.

Trust. In our relationships, trust indicates a willingness to be vulnerable to another person and expect that person to care enough for us that they'll work to help us, even when doing so may come at a cost (Righetti & Finkenauer, 2011). In romantic relationships with greater trust, we see our partners in a more positive light (Rempel et al., 2001), quickly associate them with positive traits (Murray et al., 2011), and show partner-specific memory bias by minimizing past negative issues (Luchies et al., 2013).

Mutual support. A critical aspect of every relationship is unwavering support. We want to know that our friends and our partners will always be there for us and are people we can always rely on for help and comfort. Likewise, we want to be that person for our close friends. While we seek equity in our relationships, where we get out of it what we put into it, there may be times we need to be more supportive. As our parents age, we are likely to be taking on a greater caregiving role to assist them. If our partner is ill, we know they need more from us than we need from them.

Intimacy/disclosure. When we self-disclose, we are revealing intimate and personal information to another person. Self-disclosure communicates our thoughts, beliefs, and experiences that we are not likely to share with many people. This vulnerable disclosure, according to Social Penetration Theory (Willems et al., 2020), is how we build intimacy and close connections with others. This is important for both friendships and our romantic relationships. In fact, when we stop self-disclosing, the close emotional bonds between people suffer and the relationship may become problematic.

Authenticity. When we are authentic, we are true to ourselves and our private or true-self matches our public-self. Said differently, we present ourselves in a manner that is true to who we are. Authenticity is related to better physical and mental well-being (Heppner et al., 2008; Wood et al., 2008) and more satisfying relationships (Brunell et al., 2010). Authenticity in our relationships refers to consistently engaging with our partners with our true and honest self. When we perceive our romantic partners as being authentic, we experience greater interpersonal trust, satisfaction, and commitment (Wickham, 2013).

Acceptance. In relationships, acceptance refers to valuing our differences. We are all unique in our own way and feeling valued and supported by our friends, family, and partners strengths connections. Acceptance is shown by treating someone with respect and love, and by embracing our flaws and differences.

Reciprocity. In close relationships, reciprocity refers to a mutual exchange of love, affection, and support. In every relationship, we will give and take, and it is important that we give as much as we take! An equal exchange of everything we put into our relationships makes us happier and more confident with our partner.

Affection, Intimacy, and Vulnerability

Our romantic relationships are an important aspect of health and well-being in adulthood. Struggling to maintain close intimate bonds with others can generate physical and emotional distress in us. So, what impacts intimacy? Part of the story is chemically based. Oxytocin, a hormone produced by the hypothalamus and released into our bloodstream by the pituitary gland, produces positive feelings, causing it to be referred to as the "love hormone" and the "cuddling chemical." Thus, it plays an important role in developing a bond between partners. Couples in the early stages of a relationship experience higher levels of oxytocin when compared to people not in relationships (Schneiderman et al., 2012). The impact of the drug expands beyond promoting a connection, as oxytocin is also involved in sexual arousal and orgasm for both women (Blaicher et al., 1999) and men (Thackare et al., 2006).

Our modern lives are incredibly busy and often require us to juggle not only our own schedule, but our partner's, and if you have children, their schedules as well. As a result, it is easy to overlook the simple things we can do with our partner that have surprising health benefits. Feeling a sense of intimacy—a strong connection to our partner—influences our sense of well-being (Pietromonaco & Collins, 2017). There are many things we can do to promote intimacy in our relationships, including physical touch. Some of the things we can do are rather simple but do convey the connection we feel to our partner: holding hands when you are walking together, a quick embrace when you are both home at the end of a busy day, or sitting close on the couch while streaming your favorite show.

Research has found a decrease in cortisol levels, an indication of lower stress, on days when people experience greater touch from their partners (e.g., holding hands and hugging; Ditzen et al., 2008). Elevated cortisol levels can increase both heart rate and blood pressure. Physical touch, more specifically hugging, can lower blood pressure. Women who frequently hugged their partners had lower blood pressure than those who reported less frequent hugging (Light et al., 2005). Intimacy impacts perceptions of pain as well. In a study by Stadler et al. (2012), an increase in intimacy over several days decreased reports of back pain, headaches, and insomnia.

Technology allows us to have a "virtual touch" as well. Gone are the days when people left in the morning for work and were unable to connect again until they arrived back home. Staying in touch via texts allows couples to experience intimate moments even while physically apart, whether that is a quick text checking in on your partner, hoping they are having a great day, or reminding them how excited you are for those dinner plans on Friday night!

The negative aspects of technology on relationships are important to understand as well. Social media provides a constant stream of social comparisons. We often see the "highlights" of others' lives, but what we do not see are the mundane moments of life or the negative moments in their lives. We see the amazing and fun times they experience, and we see a nearly always happy couple who seem to have a never-ending list of cool things to do, parties to attend, or places to visit. Wellness culture can create pressures to maintain a perfect, ideal relationship, but a perfect relationship—one that involves no conflict, compromise, or down moments—does not exist. Comparing our relationships to the unattainable and unrealistic ones, we see on social media can lead us to feel inadequate, guilty, and even less satisfied about our own.

Dating

Dating is an opportunity to find someone with whom we click and, perhaps, meet a life partner. While this prospect of dating can be daunting, meeting new people brings some positive mental health benefits. First and foremost, dating can be fun and exciting! When we meet new people, the anticipation of potentially meeting a romantic partner generates neurotransmitters (like Oxytocin!) making us feel good. This excitement often improves our sense of well-being and our overall mental health.

Meeting other people does give you the opportunity to understand yourself better. You learn what you want in a partner, develop a clearer understanding of the various expectations you have for someone else, and probably learn relatively quickly whether these are realistic. There is no perfect person out there. We all have our own unique traits, characteristics, and quirks that make us *us*. The trick is to find someone with whom we mesh and enjoy being with and spending time together. When we find that connection, we often experience greater emotional support, a stronger sense of belonging, and an increase in our overall life satisfaction.

Dating often pushes us outside of our comfort zones. We may try new activities, experience new foods, or watch a new movie genre that our date enjoys and wants to share with us. These may all be new adventures that we would not have tried had dates not pushed us in these directions. Trying new things can help us develop resiliency and allow us to be more adaptable to new situations. Personal growth comes through this self-expansion by developing a recognition in us that we can try new things and meet challenges. Both people in relationships may experience personal growth together through dates and other activities they do together.

An underappreciated impact of dating is its impact on the interpersonal skills that are important in all aspects of life. Successful dating or marriage requires strong communication skills. Healthy relationships require us to not only communicate our thoughts and concerns but to truly listen to our partner. Phubbing, a term combining "phone" and "snubbing," describes giving priority to a phone over interpersonal interaction. Many may relate to talking excitedly about something and looking over to see someone busy on their phone and ignoring what you were sharing. Checking your phone while your partner is talking to you makes them feel as if you don't care and are not listening to what they are saying. In fact, research has found it predicts less marital satisfaction and promotes feelings of distrust and ostracism (Kılıçarslan & Parmaksız, 2023; Knausenberger et al., 2022). Our smartphones are amazing, and the notifications we receive keep us up to date on not only our social media accounts but even current affairs happening around the world. The concern, however, is that people become reliant on their phones instead of on people for interaction and engagement. Teens experience a drug-like high when active on their phones, and this "addiction" is associated with greater physical and mental health issues (Ratan et al., 2022). Interestingly, phubbing creates a perspective that this behavior is normative, or something everyone does. When we are phubbed by our partner, and we phubb them, it creates a cycle where people are paying more attention to their phones than to their partners. Healthy relationships require communication, understanding, emotional regulation, as well as compromising and conflict resolution skills.

Boundary setting is important while dating. Being involved in a relationship can, at times, feel overwhelming. Our concern about being there for our partner may mean we lose our sense of self in the relationship. We become so focused on meeting someone else's needs and seeking their approval, that our needs and goals in the relationship are left unmet. Being well in a relationship may mean setting boundaries. We need to feel comfortable saying no at times and feel confident communicating how we are feeling in the relationship. Not setting boundaries can make burnout, resentment, and conflict within the relationship more likely,

Love, Marriage, and Long-Term Relationships

Love often seems like a mystical term that is hard to clearly define. I (JH) often ask my students, "How many of you have told someone that you love them?" Most students raise their hand to affirm they have said "I love you" to someone. What happens next is interesting. I asked them to indicate exactly what they meant when they said it. At this point, students struggle to clearly indicate what they meant. "That I care about them." "No, there is more to it than that. It means I'd do anything for you." "Well, kind of, but it is so much more than that!" It seems the only thing we can agree on is that it is hard to define and that, perhaps, defining it takes the magic out of it!

In 2021, the marriage rate in the United States hit a 50-year low, but it has been on the rise since then. There are many known benefits that come with marriage—tax benefits, access to insurance, medical rights, and inheritance. Important for this book, however, is a different question: Are there wellness benefits to being married? On average, married people tend to report more happiness than individuals who are single, divorced, or widowed (Dupre et al., 2009), better mental health (Horwitz et al., 1996), and reduced mortality (Liu, 2009). Marriage partners are often the strongest social support we have in our lives. This support gives us the ability to withstand many of the stressors we encounter in our lives and, as a result, leads to better health and well-being outcomes for us.

There is a bit of a caveat in the work highlighting the link between marriage and positive health outcomes. If we are in unhappy and unfulfilling marriages, rather than happy ones, it is not likely we'll reap many of the positive benefits of marriage. In other words, unhappy marriages will not improve our mental and physical health. When we are unhappy in our marriage, we likely pull away from our partners, and they will do the same. As a result, the social support we often see in marriage is minimized, and the marriage becomes a source of stress that impacts our cardiovascular, endocrine, and immune systems (Robles & Kiecolt-Glaser, 2003).

It is not uncommon for passion and sexual desire between partners to wax and wane over the course of a relationship. Many factors influence this fluctuation in passion, including focusing on our careers, financial concerns, and meeting the demands associated with raising children. Low sexual desire is associated with less relationship satisfaction. There are, however, things we can do to improve our sexual connection with our partner. Work by Muise et al. (2019) suggests self-expansion can play a role. According to theory, when we engage in activities that broaden our sense of self and our world perspective together (novel, exciting, and challenging activities), this can reignite passionate feelings that often characterize the love people feel earlier in their relationship. Their findings show when we do these things together, couples report an increase in sexual activity and greater sexual satisfaction. These fun and enriching activities positively impact the close emotional connection we feel—our intimacy! Fluctuations and changes in intimacy impact our passion and sexual desire. Want to change the passion between you and your partner, increase your emotional connection! If the intoxicating emotional high we experience in the early stages of a relationship will fade as these relationships change and develop over time, what is it that can help couples weather the storm when life is challenging and keep them together? As our relationships develop, they can take on a different type of love. Companionate love refers to a love characterized by a deep intimacy and sense of commitment between couples. Maintaining a strong emotional connection, and staying committed to our partner, helps relationships when times are tough. Relationships are more likely to end when we're feeling disconnected.

Emotional intelligence is often referred to as the secret for long-lasting intimate relationships. Emotional intelligence, a term popularized by psychologist Dr. Daniel Goleman, is our ability to perceive, use, understand, and manage emotions. Someone with high emotional intelligence can recognize emotional experiences in themselves and in others, and they can use this information to change how they are thinking and to change their behaviors to adapt to situations. When it comes to our relationships, emotional intelligence allows us to notice and understand the emotions our partner is experiencing and behave in ways that help support them. It improves our ability to communicate, understand, and support our significant others.

Love Languages

Dr. Gary Chapman's (2010) book on love languages describes ways that we can communicate love. Each "language" describes ways that we both give and receive love.

Gift Giving. Some people express their love through giving gifts to others. The act of giving the gift is more than just the "gift." It involves thinking about wanting to do something for someone else, deciding what it is you want to get, and then giving it to them in a way that conveys its meaning.

Quality Time. You've likely heard the phrase "Quality over quantity" before. The meaning is that we spend meaningful time together and not just lots of time together. In other words, put down your phone and engage with your partner. Making sure you are giving one another 100% of your focus and energy is incredibly powerful.

Physical Touch. Touch is one of the first forms of love we experience. The time right after a baby is born is referred to as "The Golden Hour." A time when skin-to-skin contact between mother and newborn promotes bonding between them. Many hospitals try to minimize any interruptions to focus on this special time. Later in life, touch between romantic partners is associated with relational, psychological, and physical well-being (Jakubiak & Feeney, 2017).

Words of Affirmation. Expressing our love through verbal or written communications emphasizing encouragement, love, support, and appreciation are another way we can show our love to someone. These expressions meet our desires to feel loved and supported.

Acts of Service. Engaging in helpful and thoughtful actions is another way we express our love. Being helpful expresses our love and, when it is done for us, makes us feel good!

Same-Sex Marriage

Same-sex marriage was legalized in the United States on June 26, 2015, through a Supreme Court ruling (Obergefell v. Hodges). While arguments were made that the decision would threaten the institution of marriage, no issues have emerged negatively impacting marriage. In fact, some research suggests the decision strengthened marriage. After the legalization, marriage rates went up by rates not explained through same-sex couples only. It seems the decision increased interest in marriage amongst the American population as a whole.

The positive health benefits seen in different-sex couples are found among same-sex couples as well. Research found lower psychological distress, improved stress, greater positive mood, and an overall improvement in life satisfaction amongst married same-sex couples when compared to those not married. Physical health improved as well. State-level rates of syphilis, HIV, AIDS, and reports of problematic substance use all significantly improved. Marriage provided many with greater access to health insurance, and mental health care visits and mental health care costs declined in sexual-minority men. Among sexual minority women, declines in perceived discrimination and depressive symptoms were reported, and hate crimes reported against LGBTQIA+ individuals declined.

Wellness in the LBGTQIA+ Community

Over the course of their lifespans, members of the lesbian, gay, bisexual, transgender, and queer communities (LBGTQIA+) face significant health and wellness disparities compared to heterosexual and cisgender individuals (Fredriksen Goldsen & de Vries, 2019). Stigmatization and a lack of representation in medical and wellness research have increased the difficulty for LGBTQIA+ individuals to access quality care (Flatt et al., 2022). Moreover, barriers exist regarding access to resources and social support, LBGTQIA+ affirming care (Donald et al., 2017), and open communication with knowledgeable professionals aware of the unique health and wellness challenges faced by members of the LBGTQIA+ Community.

The American Medical Association (AMA) supports access to quality evidence-based physical and mental healthcare for everyone and works at both the state and federal levels to expand healthcare access and address discriminatory barriers. The AMA opposes the use of any "conversion therapy." Conversion therapies are interventions involving an attempt to change a person's sexual orientation or gender identity. Use of these approaches is related to an increase in suicidal behaviors (Green et al., 2020), psychological distress (Turban et al., 2020), and internalized homophobia (Meanley et al., 2020). The AMA supports health insurance coverage for gender dysphoria and stands in opposition to denying coverage based on sexual orientation or gender identity. Gender-affirming care is linked to lower rates of suicide attempts and depression (Tordoff et al., 2022), anxiety (Chen et al., 2023), and decreased substance use. The AMA also opposes any attempt to limit access to basic human services and public facilities for transgender individuals.

If competent healthcare is difficult to find for LBGTQIA+ individuals, wellness-care that is relevant and appropriate is even more rare. Wellness care in the LGBTQIA+ community is essential for promoting overall health and well-being. It encompasses a variety of services and practices tailored to the unique needs and experiences of LGBTQIA+ individuals. Dr. Alex Keuroghlian, director of the education and training division at the Fenway Institute and an associate professor of psychiatry at Harvard Medical School, recognizes the inequities faced by LBGTQIA+ individuals: "The biggest obstacle to health equity for LGBTQIA+ people has been societal stigma and bias reflected in our health policies, systems, institutions and clinical practices. Clinicians do not receive adequate education in LGBTQIA+ health care during their formative professional training and therefore often have to play catch-up after they start practicing." Medical professionals and wellness practitioners alike must be provided with opportunities to increase their knowledge and improve the care provided to LBGTQIA+ individuals. Services and practices required for culturally sensitive care of LBGTQIA+ individuals include:

Competent and culturally relevant medical treatment and psychotherapy.
Peer support.
Inclusive providers.
Preventive care that is focused on unique needs of LBGTQIA+ individuals *and* needs shared with the CIS-gendered community.
Professionals skilled in working with intersectional identities.
Education on the healthcare rights and protections of LBGTQIA+ individuals.
Hotlines and helplines like the Trevor Project and LGBT National Help Center.

By prioritizing these aspects of wellness care, those within the LGBTQIA+ community can feel heard and acknowledged, which in turn will foster resilience, connection with needed health resources, and overall health and well-being.

Consensual Nonmonogamy

In consensual nonmonogamy relationships, all partners involved agree that relationships and sexual encounters outside of the relationship are okay (Conley et al., 2012). Three common consensual nonmonogamy relationships include swinging, open relationships, and polyamory. Swinging refers to couples who engage in sexual activities with other couples. In open relationships, partners are ok with one another having sexual encounters outside of the relationship. Polyamory relationships are characterized by people with multiple romantic and sexual partners with the consent of all involved. Interest in consensual nonmonogamy is growing (Scoats & Campbell, 2022).

In a 2023 Match Singles in America Report, 31% of singles have tried a consensual nonmonogamy relationship and, of them, 16% are interested in pursuing another consensual nonmonogamy relationship in the future. As the report suggests, these relationships are often stigmatized and viewed as dysfunctional. Empirical research, however, paints a different picture. Compared to those in monogamous relationships, people in consensual nonmonogamy relationships report equal levels of satisfaction with their relationships, trust, commitment, and psychological health (Conley et al., 2012). They also report low levels of jealousy and relationship insecurity (Ritchie & Barker, 2006). Consensual nonmonogamy does provide some benefits over monogamous relationships. Specifically, people in consensual nonmonogamy report getting more of their needs met, as well as personal growth and development (Moors et al., 2017).

Sex is one area where consensual nonmonogamy is strongly stereotyped. In the Match Singles Report, 37% of people perceived those in consensual nonmonogamy relationships as simply looking for casual sex. Compared to others, people engaged in consensual nonmonogamy report higher levels of safer sex strategies, including STI testing (Conley et al., 2012; Lehmiller, 2015). The research is quite clear—different relationship styles produce positive outcomes and are equally meaningful for those who are in them. Communication and understanding are critical for producing positive benefits from any relationship style.

Family Wellness

The concept of wellness extends to the whole family. Family wellness examines whether everyone in a family is healthy both physically and mentally, has productive activities to engage in, and whether the relationships between family members are positive. Strong family wellness makes everyone feel safe and healthy. Financial, housing, and food insecurity all negatively impact family wellness and can lead to physical and mental health issues. A key component of family wellness is the relationship between the parents. Healthy relationships between parents produce healthy parent-child relationships as well. The "Spillover Hypothesis" refers to the tendency for conflict between parents to spillover and negatively impact children, which, of course, is related to negative outcomes for everyone involved (Erel & Burman, 1995).

Interpersonal Conflict Management

It doesn't matter where you live, work, or go to school—as a person interacting with other people in the world, you will have encounters with frustrated, irate, and upset people. This includes conflict with our romantic partners. People are quirky, imperfect, messy, and irrational, and we must know how to deal with them. Even people who are normally calm may quickly reach the boiling point when illness or financial issues or issues related to family occur. Physical or emotional pain, fear, frustration, and distress can lead to increased stress, and anxiety, which can result in anger and even loss of control. Whatever the cause, interpersonal conflict is a stressor that most of us very much dislike to encounter.

The first step in conflict management is to practice conflict prevention; it is much more productive to prevent conflict than to manage it later. We must take care of our relationships in a way that "conflict-proofs" them to the extent possible. This includes taking steps to make sure that we are not part of the problem, such as being trustworthy, helpful, and kind. Conflict-proofing includes having reliable and useful communication patterns with others and being able to clearly state and enforce personal boundaries. It often, paradoxically, involves actively engaging with the topic, behavior, or emotions involved in the conflict, because avoiding the things that cause conflict doesn't solve anything.

It is also helpful to conceive of conflict as a puzzle, not a battle. If you think of it as a puzzle, then it has pieces and steps. First, you must be clear what the problem is before you can address it. Then, instead of limiting yourself to just one course of action, search for and evaluate a variety of possible alternative ways to address the conflict. You will ultimately implement the best alternative and tweak it as necessary for the outcome you want. Of course, mental illness and emotional crises are part of this puzzle. Mental illness can make people behave in erratic and irrational ways, ways that are often hard to anticipate and make it hard to plan or to converse with a client. You should always enlist help with dealing with someone with known or obvious mental health challenges.

Engaging people with empathy and compassion can go a long way toward preventing conflict and moderating it when it occurs. Empathy is typically defined as having three foundational elements—emotion, thought, and action. The emotional or affective part of empathy occurs when we resonate and emotionally connect with others' emotions. This allows us to authentically feel what the other is feeling and to interact with genuine affinity. The thinking or cognitive part of empathy occurs when we use our imagination and reasoning to fully understand what the other is feeling. This allows us to "walk in their shoes" and thereby to comprehend their emotions and behaviors. Finally, the action or empathetic concern component of empathy occurs when we are motivated to assist, help, and support another, based on our understanding of their situation and our resonance with their feelings. It's important to note that empathy does not require your agreement, approval, or that you have experienced the same thing as the person you are supporting. Empathy is an approach that can be used to engage people compassionately, thereby reducing or even preventing conflict, and Table 14.1 shows some examples of how this can happen.

Being calm and in control of our emotions is always our role when dealing with conflict. Although it is challenging, we must try not to let people's anger or outbursts make us reactive; calmly finding out why the other person is frustrated, anxious, and agitated goes a long way toward diffusing high emotions. It's ok to ask questions to try to find out what is really bothering them, as it is sometimes not the thing they are yelling about. Also remember that defensiveness when challenged by someone is not productive, especially when coupled with return aggression (defensive engagement) or withdrawing/leaving (defensive disengagement). This highlights the importance of effective communication strategies within high-emotion situations. For example, call the person by their name, and speak to them in a mild voice to diffuse tension. Employ active listening by summarizing or paraphrasing what they are saying back to them, so that they are very clear that you have heard them. Identifying the emotions behind the words is a great strategy, such as, "It sounds like you are going through some feelings of sadness and depression about being a burden on your family. Is that right?"

Table 14.1 Engaging people with empathy

Parts of empathy	Empathetic response	Non-empathetic response
Acknowledge how they feel	"It's really hard to hear that you have this problem."	"You are lucky—At least there is a solution to your problem."
Share how you feel	"I am sad to have to deliver this bad news."	"When my mother/daughter/sister found out they had cancer, it was totally devastating to me. I cried about it for days."
Honor that they have opened up to you	"This is hard to talk about. I'm glad we are discussing it."	"Don't worry so much…just be happy and focus on the good things."
Show interest in the person (not just the problem)	"What has college been like for you?"	"Your college is so easy…you shouldn't have to do much to keep up."
Focus on uplifting them	"I'm in your corner, and I am so proud of you!"	"Most people don't have such a hard time with this. Just change your attitude!"
Be a source of encouragement	"It's hard, but you can do this. I will help."	"I'm sorry that this is so difficult, but you really have no one to blame but yourself for your problems."
Behave in a supportive manner	"What can I do to help you right now?" (then follow through)	"Feel free to reach out."

Finally, always be safe and protect yourself in conflictual situations—ask for help, don't be alone, don't allow gaslighting, and have a path to the door. When conflict occurs at work, it is appropriate also to protect our reputation and our job by being assertive in protecting our rights, challenging incorrect statements, refusing to tolerate abuse, documenting conflictual interactions (including microaggressions), and filing a grievance if necessary.

Wellness Tip—Sexual Wellness

Sexual wellness refers to physical, emotional, mental, and social well-being when it comes to our sexuality. Many factors impact our sexual wellness, and it is important for us to think about how to improve our wellness in this area. In an article in *The Lancet*, a leading medical journal, Dr. Kirstin Mitchell et al. (2021) describe four key areas of sexual wellness.

Sexual Health. Sexual health refers to our ability to make decisions on fertility and pregnancy, preventing sexually transmitted infections, sexual violence prevention, and addressing issues related to sexual functions. These areas of sexual health impact our physical, mental, emotional, and social well-being when we think about our sexuality.

Sexual Pleasure. This addresses the physical and psychological satisfactions associated with sexual experiences. This satisfaction is related to our ability to give consent, maintain privacy, feel safe, and engage in open and honest communication.

Sexual Justice. This aspect of sexual wellness includes our ability to access public health services and to combat any restriction placed on people due to sexual orientation or gender identity.

Sexual Well-Being. This well-being relates to developing a sense of comfort with our sexuality, respecting others' sexuality, understanding past sexual events and experiences, and feeling free in making our own sexual decisions.

These four domains represent a holistic view of sexual wellness and are important for our overall sense of well-being. Like other aspects of health and wellness, we can take steps to address our sexual wellness. The first step toward sexual wellness is to self-assess your status in the domains above. For instance, when was the last time you went to a doctor for a check-up that included reproductive health? Do you have access to birth control options? Are there health care locations in your community that are accessible and affordable (e.g., a Planned Parenthood facility)? Are you able to make decisions regarding sexual experiences without someone else's influence? Have you explored your sexual history and experiences through therapy, journaling, reflection, or other clarity-enhancing practices? Great educational materials, medical advice, therapeutic help, and a wide variety of programs, products, and methods are available to enhance sexual wellness—make sure to take advantage of the resources available to you!

References

Blaicher, W., Gruber, D., Bieglmayer, C., Blaicher, A. M., Knogler, W., & Huber, J. C. (1999). The role of oxytocin in relation to female sexual arousal. *Gynecologic and Obstetric Investigation, 47*(2), 125–126. https://doi.org/10.1159/000010075

Brunell, A. B., Kernis, M. H., Goldman, B. M., Heppner, W., Davis, P., Cascio, E. V., & Webster, G. D. (2010). Dispositional authenticity and romantic relationship functioning. *Personality and Individual Differences, 48*(8), 900–905. https://doi.org/10.1016/j.paid.2010.02.018

Chapman, G. D. (2010). The 5 love languages: The secret to love that lasts. Northfield.

Chen, D., Berona, J., Chan, Y.-M., Ehrensaft, D., Garofalo, R., Hidalgo, M. A., Rosenthal, S. M., Tishelman, A. C., & Olson-Kennedy, J. (2023). Psychosocial functioning in transgender youth after 2 years of hormones. *The New England Journal of Medicine, 388*(3), 240–250. https://doi.org/10.1056/NEJMoa2206297

Conley, T. D., Moors, A. C., Ziegler, A., & Karathanasis, C. (2012). Unfaithful individuals are less likely to practice safer sex than openly nonmonogamous individuals. *Journal of Sexual Medicine, 9*(6), 1559–1565.

Ditzen, B., Hoppmann, C., & Klumb, P. (2008). Positive couple interactions and daily cortisol: On the stress-protecting role of intimacy. *Psychosomatic Medicine, 70*(8), 883–889. https://doi.org/10.1097/PSY.0b013e318185c4fc

Donald, C. A., DasGupta, S., Metzl, J. M., & Eckstrand, K. L. (2017). Queer frontiers in medicine: A structural competency approach. *Academic Medicine: Journal of the Association of American Medical Colleges, 92*(3), 345–350. https://doi.org/10.1097/ACM.0000000000001533

Dupre, M. E., Beck, A. N., & Meadows, S. O. (2009). Marital trajectories and mortality among US adults. *American Journal of Epidemiology, 170*(5), 546–555.

Erel, O., & Burman, B. (1995). Interrelatedness of marital relations and parent-child relations: A meta-analytic review. *Psychological Bulletin, 118*(1), 108–132. https://doi.org/10.1037/0033-2909.118.1.108
Flatt, J. D., Cicero, E. C., Kittle, K. R., & Brennan-Ing, M. (2022). Recommendations for advancing research with sexual and gender minority older adults. *The Journals of Gerontology: Series B, 77*(1), 1–9. https://doi.org/10.1093/geronb/gbab127
Fredriksen Goldsen, K., & de Vries, B. (2019). Global aging with pride: International perspectives on LGBT aging. *International Journal of Aging & Human Development, 88*(4), 315–324. https://doi.org/10.1177/0091415019837648
Green, A. E., Price-Feeney, M., Dorison, S. H., & Pick, C. J. (2020). Self-reported conversion efforts and suicidality among US LGBTQ youths and young adults, 2018. *American Journal of Public Health, 110*(8), 1221–1227. https://doi.org/10.2105/AJPH.2020.305701
Heppner, W. L., Kernis, M. H., Nezlek, J. B., Foster, J., Lakey, C. E., & Goldman, B. M. (2008). Within-person relationships among daily self-esteem, need satisfaction, and authenticity. *Psychological Science, 19*(11), 1140–1145. https://doi.org/10.1111/j.1467-9280.2008.02215.x
Hill, C. A. (1987). Affiliation motivation: People who need people… but in different ways. *Journal of Personality and Social Psychology, 52*(5), 1008–1018. https://doi.org/10.1037/0022-3514.52.5.1008
Holt-Lunstad, J., Smith, T. B., & Layton, J. B. (2010). Social relationships and mortality risk: A meta-analytic review. *PLoS Medicine, 7*(7), e1000316–e1000316. https://doi.org/10.1371/journal.pmed.1000316
Horwitz, A. V., White, H. R., & Howell-White, S. (1996). Becoming married and mental health: A longitudinal study of a cohort of young adults. *Journal of Marriage and the Family, 58*(4), 895–907.
Jakubiak, B. K., & Feeney, B. C. (2017). Affectionate touch to promote relational, psychological, and physical well-being in adulthood: A theoretical model and review of the research. *Personality and Social Psychology Review, 21*(3), 228–252. https://doi.org/10.1177/1088868316650307
Kahlon, M. K., Aksan, N., Aubrey, R., Clark, N., Cowley-Morillo, M., Jacobs, E. A., Mundhenk, R., Sebastian, K. R., & Tomlinson, S. (2021). Effect of Layperson-delivered, empathy-focused program of telephone calls on loneliness, depression, and anxiety among adults during the COVID-19 pandemic: A randomized clinical trial. *JAMA Psychiatry, 78*(6), 616–622. https://doi.org/10.1001/jamapsychiatry.2021.0113
Kılıçarslan, S., & Parmaksız, İ. (2023). The mediator role of effective communication skills on the relationship between phubbing tendencies and marriage satisfaction in married individuals. *Computers in Human Behavior, 147*, 107863. https://doi.org/10.1016/j.chb.2023.107863
Knausenberger, J., Giesen-Leuchter, A., & Echterhoff, G. (2022). Feeling ostracized by others' smartphone use: The effect of phubbing on fundamental needs, mood, and trust. *Frontiers in Psychology, 13*, 883901–883901. https://doi.org/10.3389/fpsyg.2022.883901
Lehmiller, J. J. (2015). A comparison of sexual health history and practices among monogamous and consensually nonmonogamous sexual partners. *Journal of Sexual Medicine, 12*(10), 2022–2028.
Light, K. C., Grewen, K. M., & Amico, J. A. (2005). More frequent partner hugs and higher oxytocin levels are linked to lower blood pressure and heart rate in premenopausal women. *Biological Psychology, 69*(1), 5–21. https://doi.org/10.1016/j.biopsycho.2004.11.002
Liu, H. (2009). Till death do US part: Marital status and US mortality trends, 1986–2000. *Journal of Marriage and Family, 71*(5), 1158–1173.
Luchies, L. B., Wieselquist, J., Rusbult, C. E., Kumashiro, M., Eastwick, P. W., Coolsen, M. K., & Finkel, E. J. (2013). Trust and biased memory of transgressions in romantic relationships. *Journal of Personality and Social Psychology, 104*(4), 673–694. https://doi.org/10.1037/a0031054
Martino, J., Pegg, J., & Frates, E. P. (2015). The connection prescription: Using the power of social interactions and the deep desire for connectedness to empower health and wellness. *American Journal of Lifestyle Medicine, 11*(6), 466–475. https://doi.org/10.1177/1559827615608788

Match (2023). *Singles in America*. https://www.singlesinamerica.com/home

Meanley, S., Haberlen, S. A., Okafor, C. N., Brown, A., Brennan-Ing, M., Ware, D., Egan, J. E., Teplin, L. A., Bolan, R. K., Friedman, M. R., & Plankey, M. W. (2020). Lifetime exposure to conversion therapy and psychosocial health among midlife and older adult men who have sex with men. *The Gerontologist, 60*(7), 1291–1302. https://doi.org/10.1093/geront/gnaa069

Mitchell, K. R., Lewis, R., O'Sullivan, L. F., & Fortenberry, J. D. (2021). What is sexual wellbeing and why does it matter for public health? *The Lancet. Public Health, 6*(8), e608–e613. https://doi.org/10.1016/S2468-2667(21)00099-2

Moors, A. C., Matsick, J. L., & Schechinger, H. A. (2017). Unique and shared relationship benefits of consensually non-monogamous and monogamous relationships: A review and insights for moving forward. *European Psychologist, 22*(1), 55–71. https://doi.org/10.1027/1016-9040/a000278

Muise, A., Harasymchuk, C., Day, L. C., Bacev-Giles, C., Gere, J., & Impett, E. A. (2019). Broadening your horizons: Self-expanding activities promote desire and satisfaction in established romantic relationships. *Journal of Personality and Social Psychology, 116*(2), 237–258. https://doi.org/10.1037/pspi0000148

Murray, S. L., Pinkus, R. T., Holmes, J. G., Harris, B., Gomillion, S., Aloni, M., Derrick, J. L., & Leder, S. (2011). Signaling when (and when not) to be cautious and self-protective: Impulsive and reflective trust in close relationships. *Journal of Personality and Social Psychology, 101*(3), 485–502. https://doi.org/10.1037/a0023233

Pietromonaco, P. R., & Collins, N. L. (2017). Interpersonal mechanisms linking close relationships to health. *The American Psychologist, 72*(6), 531–542. https://doi.org/10.1037/amp0000129

Ratan, Z. A., Parrish, A. M., Alotaibi, M. S., & Hosseinzadeh, H. (2022). Prevalence of smartphone addiction and its association with sociodemographic, physical and mental well-being: A cross-sectional study among the young adults of Bangladesh. *International Journal of Environmental Research and Public Health, 19*(24), 16583. https://doi.org/10.3390/ijerph192416583

Rath, T., & Harter, J. (2010). *The five essential elements of well-being*. Gallup. https://www.gallup.com/workplace/237020/five-essential-elements.aspx

Rempel, J. K., Ross, M., & Holmes, J. G. (2001). Trust and communicated attributions in close relationships. *Journal of Personality and Social Psychology, 81*(1), 57–64. https://doi.org/10.1037/0022-3514.81.1.57

Righetti, F., & Finkenauer, C. (2011). If you are able to control yourself, I will trust you: The role of perceived self-control in interpersonal trust. *Journal of Personality and Social Psychology, 100*(5), 874–886. https://doi.org/10.1037/a0021827

Ritchie, A., & Barker, M. (2006). 'There aren't words for what we do or how we feel so we have to make them up': Constructing polyamorous languages in a culture of compulsory monogamy. *Sexualities, 9*(5), 584–601.

Robles, T. F., & Kiecolt-Glaser, J. K. (2003). The physiology of marriage: Pathways to health. *Physiology & Behavior, 79*(3), 409–416. https://doi.org/10.1016/s0031-9384(03)00160-4

Schneiderman, I., Zagoory-Sharon, O., Leckman, J. F., & Feldman, R. (2012). Oxytocin during the initial stages of romantic attachment: Relations to couples' interactive reciprocity. *Psychoneuroendocrinology, 37*(8), 1277–1285. https://doi.org/10.1016/j.psyneuen.2011.12.021

Scoats, R., & Campbell, C. (2022). What do we know about consensual non-monogamy? *Current Opinion in Psychology, 48*, 101468. https://doi.org/10.1016/j.copsyc.2022.101468

Stadler, G., Snyder, K. A., Horn, A. B., Shrout, P. E., & Bolger, N. P. (2012). Close relationships and health in daily life: A review and empirical data on intimacy and somatic symptoms. *Psychosomatic Medicine, 74*(4), 398–409. https://doi.org/10.1097/PSY.0b013e31825473b8

Thackare, H., Nicholson, H. D., & Whittington, K. (2006). Oxytocin—Its role in male reproduction and new potential therapeutic uses. *Human Reproduction Update, 12*(4), 437–448. https://doi.org/10.1093/humupd/dmk002

Tordoff, D. M., Wanta, J. W., Collin, A., Stepney, C., Inwards-Breland, D. J., & Ahrens, K. (2022). Mental health outcomes in transgender and nonbinary youths receiving gender-affirming care. *JAMA Network Open, 5*(2), e220978. https://doi.org/10.1001/jamanetworkopen.2022.0978

Turban, J. L., Beckwith, N., Reisner, S. L., & Keuroghlian, A. S. (2020). Association between recalled exposure to gender identity conversion efforts and psychological distress and suicide attempts among transgender adults. *JAMA Psychiatry, 77*(1), 68–76. https://doi.org/10.1001/jamapsychiatry.2019.2285

Wickham, R. E. (2013). Perceived authenticity in romantic partners. *Journal of Experimental Social Psychology, 49*(5), 878–887. https://doi.org/10.1016/j.jesp.2013.04.001

Willems, Y. E., Finkenauer, C., & Kerkhof, P. (2020). The role of disclosure in relationships. *Current Opinion in Psychology, 31*, 33–37. https://doi.org/10.1016/j.copsyc.2019.07.032

Wood, A., Linley, P., Maltby, J., Baliousis, M., & Joseph, S. (2008). The authentic personality: A theoretical and empirical conceptualization and the development of the authenticity scale. *Journal of Counseling Psychology, 55*(3), 385–399.

Chapter 15
The Potential of Mind-Body Wellness

The promise of mind-body wellness offers us a path forward to prioritize physical, mental, and emotional well-being not only personally, but also in our society, community, and environment. Vitality, mindful living, and balance are not only things we achieve within ourselves, but they are motivators of action and models of how human beings can center well-being in the modern world. The promise of mind-body wellness is also empowerment to make informed choices and to be involved in the systems that affect our well-being so that we all have an equitable and health-enhancing range of choices available to us. As we realize that mind-body wellness not only has individual purposes and outcomes but also has community and societal implications, we can forge a path that includes work toward resilient communities, social cohesion, environmental justice, and public investment in human well-being.

One option for investing in wellness is creating programs that reach people where they are and how they are at this moment in time. Workplace wellness programs are an example of a positive approach for meeting people where they are. Due to inactivity, poor health decisions, and our use of alcohol and tobacco products, health issues (e.g., heart disease, diabetes, chronic pulmonary disease) are impacting people at younger ages. As a result, working-aged Americans are both missing work and are less productive while they are working. Concerns about employee health and well-being, coupled with the rising costs of health care coverage, have encouraged many employers to focus on health promotion and prevention strategies through offering wellness programs at work.

It is common for employers with wellness programs to screen their employees for health risks and, based on these results, create interventions addressing the identified health risks and work on developing and promoting a healthier lifestyle. These programs should meet people where they are in life in the present moment. Someone who has led a fairly sedentary life with little exercise built into their weekly schedule is not likely to run a marathon anytime soon. Meeting people where they are involves a consideration of their current fitness level and lifestyle and developing a plan that begins to work for them. Perhaps starting with walking or light stretching

S. M. Henney, J. D. Hackett, *Mind-Body Wellness*,
https://doi.org/10.1007/978-3-031-91611-3_15

and working up to jogging or a more strenuous yoga class. Working within someone's current state makes lifestyle changes more manageable and less daunting. A surefire way to discourage active lifestyle changes is to encourage behaviors that are too challenging and make the whole process feel unattainable for people. When this happens, any motivation to continue these health promotion behaviors is lost.

The prevention and preventative strategies that are a core aspect of wellness programs encourage healthy lifestyle changes. A healthier society allows communities to thrive economically, socially, and environmentally. Economically, healthier societies are more productive, tend to have a larger workforce, save on healthcare costs, and produce a sustainable and strong economy. Wellness programs have meaningful economic impact themselves. Research by Baicker et al. (2010) suggests that every $1 spent on wellness programs produces $3.27 in medical cost savings and an additional $2.73 in savings from a reduction in employee absenteeism. The return on investment for these programs makes them economically appealing for companies. The American Heart Association (AHA, 2015) recognizes companies that focus on employee health by including them on their list of "Fit-Friendly Worksites." The goal of this list is for the AHA to reward companies for their progressive leadership and concern for the health of their staff.

Technology

It is worth noting the business and marketing aspects involved in wellness as well. Wearable devices, apps for our phones, and artificial intelligence will all continue to impact health and wellness. Wearable devices allow us to monitor our fitness by providing us with health metrics. Some examples of these include smartwatches, fitness trackers, blood pressure monitors, and glucose monitors. Fitness apps on our phones make it easier for us to track our fitness level and activity throughout the day. The number of fitness app users doubled from 2019 to about 749.9 million today (Statista, n.d.). There is clearly a lot of interest in how this technology can improve our activity level throughout the day. Many people like to make sure they achieve their step goal every day, and there are multiple free or low-cost apps available for activity tracking. The market for these apps is expected to grow to $33 billion by 2027.

The role of artificial intelligence will continue to expand and has the potential to improve how we manage our personal health. In fact, AI technology can analyze our heartbeat, breathing patterns, activity level, and make personalized health recommendations. The Alter Mirror, a smart fitness mirror introduced in 2021, analyzes users' DNA and biometrics to provide daily workout recommendations. The AI technology used in the mirror even provides form correction advice to ensure users are working out safely. It is exciting to think about how AI will continue to improve how we approach our health and wellness.

Overall, the advances in technology—from apps and wearable devices to AI—contribute to a trend called personalized or individualized health. These advances allow for personally tailored and individually relevant health and wellness plans that address the unique needs of the person; in other words, they allow for "customized" wellness approaches. This is very attractive to people who are drawn to the potential of wellness to address problems that conventional medicine has been (so far) unable to resolve. People want to feel like they are being heard and treated as an individual with distinct needs, different from the "average," and many wellness practitioners and approaches offer (or appear to offer) such customized care.

There is, however, a caveat when it comes to health and wellness technology. We may be losing control over some of our health information and, as a result, it may be used in ways we did not intend. The genetic testing service 23andMe has over 14 million customers and it is sitting on the verge of financial collapse (Turner, 2024). The concern is what will happen to all of the genetic information the company has in its research database? That information, private as it is, could be sold to another company that may use it in a manner different than originally intended. Learning that our DNA information could be used in ways beyond our control is understandably concerning. Our information related to blood pressure, glucose levels, sleeping patterns, and heart health might seem less important than our DNA, but they are not. Letting other people have our health information has unknown consequences for future insurability.

Social Capital

Healthier communities are characterized by a more socially engaged citizenry, and the involvement of community members in health-promoting community activities helps them to develop greater social capital. Social capital refers to the positive connections that develop amongst people living in a community together. With social capital, communities have stronger ties, trust, and increased social support, all of which lead to stronger health outcomes for residents. Feeling well, physically and mentally, allows us to build stronger connections with others and engage more in our local communities. Research shows social capital is linked to lower mortality rates, improved mental health, and is linked to healthier decision-making (Eriksson, 2011).

Social capital has a direct link to community resilience and the ability to weather traumatic experiences. Community resilience refers to "the ability to prepare for anticipated hazards, adapt to changing conditions, and withstand and recover rapidly from disruptions. Activities, such as disaster preparedness—which includes prevention, protection, mitigation, response and recovery—are key steps to resilience" (National Institute of Standards and Technology, n.d.). Work on community resilience has considered the unique role that social capital plays in establishing networks to help provide access to resources in disaster situations. These resources include accessing and transmitting essential information, providing needed aid, accessing financial resources, providing childcare, and helping to ensure emotional and psychological support for those impacted by the disaster.

Many of the issues confronting people around the world (e.g., the disruptive impact of war, climate change, refugee crises, and the spread of COVID-19) have significant health and wellness implications and require a united global response to address them. There is growing interest amongst researchers and the general public in feelings of connection to the global community and identification with large, superordinate groups. The concept called Identification with All Humanity (IWAH) measures the extent to which one identifies with all humanity, feels connected to other people all over the world, perceives them as members of the same group, and cares deeply about their welfare. During the COVID-19 crisis, IWAH predicted the prosocial motivation to wear masks and maintain physical distance in public (Barragan & Meltzoff, 2023). IWAH represents a psychological variable that can be targeted to encourage more cooperative health behaviors. These behaviors have implications for the health and wellness of all people.

With many conflicts raging across the globe, public health researchers view war as a significant public health problem. War impacts humans through direct violence—guns and bombings—and in more indirect, albeit still significant, ways—poverty, famine, and loss of educational opportunities. It also disrupts social and economic systems used to maintain health and address health problems. During conflict, health systems collapse, medical supply chains are interrupted, and health care workers flee. It is easy to see how health and peace are interrelated concepts. In fact, for the World Health Organization (WHO), 80% of its humanitarian cases and 70% of disease outbreaks where the WHO intervenes occur in conflict zones. The WHO's Global Health and Peace Initiative was established in 2019 to assist with protecting the health of populations in conflict zones and other fragile situations (World Health Organization, n.d.). This initiative's slogan, "there can be no health without peace and no peace without health" reflects its commitment to integrating health into peacebuilding processes.

Focusing on individual health and wellness has the potential to improve society at large. Societal health promotion refers to a systemic approach addressing social determinants of health to encourage positive social change. These social determinants refer to our ability to access quality health care, live in healthy neighborhoods and environments, experience economic stability, and access educational opportunities. Social health promotion has generated a greater awareness of mental health issues. These changes have decreased the stigma associated with receiving mental health care and increased the accessibility of services available. Societal change generates communities supportive of healthy choices and provides individuals with the opportunity to take action for their own health and well-being. For many, these changes are transformative and produce significant improvements in their lives.

Transformative Social Change

Both our mental and physical well-being are impacted in the short and long term by cultural, social, economic, political policies, systems, and institutions. Transformative social change occurs when efforts to improve our health and well-being result in significant positive shifts in our social norms, shared values, and institutions. These changes are often the result of movements that demand social justice and equitable distribution of the costs and benefits of social and political policy. For example, the

United States has a long history of movements to secure environmental justice and sustainability. The environmental justice movement arose out of the observation that environmental policies and the effects of industrial activities disproportionately affect minoritized people and marginalized communities (Bullard, 2005).

In recent years, we've seen a rising interest in clean water and air, organic food, and a growing concern about safe consumer products. In 2014, the city of Flint, Michigan switched its water supply from Detroit's system to the Flint River. The switch did not go as planned and families in Flint suffered poor water quality for 4 years and 9 months. The Michigan Civil Rights Commission found the weak government response to be based on systemic racism. Another example is the media coverage on the negative health effects of pesticides that have encouraged greater interest in organic foods. For food to earn the organic label, the United States Department of Agriculture requires these products to be grown without the use of synthetic pesticides, genetic engineering, antibiotics, growth hormones, artificial colors, flavors, preservatives, or irradiation. Activists and citizens have influenced food policies in the United States for over 100 years.

Transformative social change typically has three foundational aspects:

Institutional change. This type of change addresses the social systems that provide structure and even legitimacy to social and political policies that create and maintain social and economic disparities. An example is that people who live in communities comprised predominantly of racial minorities can have less access to obstetric care and trauma centers.

Social change. This involves shifts in social and cultural beliefs, attitudes, normative behaviors, and even daily habits. Sometimes social change is so gradual that one hardly notices it happening, and other times there is a seismic transformation in our social norms. In recent years, we've seen a significant movement to destigmatize mental health care. Historically, people seeking mental health care were viewed as weak, vulnerable, and unstable. Data from the World Health Organization suggests at some point in their life, 1 in 4 people will experience a mental health issue. Destigmatizing mental health care encourages people to seek care when they need it.

Collective action. When people work together in an organized fashion toward a common cause, impressive change can occur. In 1987, the AIDS epidemic had killed 60,000 people and another 40,000 were HIV-positive in the United States. ACT UP (the AIDS Coalition to Unleash Power), an organization founded in 1987 to help push for a cure for AIDS and bring awareness about the disease through education and nonviolent protest, was one of the first movements to advocate for designing healthcare solutions based on the population being treated. Through their efforts, ACT UP helped generate new regulations for drug approval and access to drugs still in clinical trials.

Transformative social change with a focus on health and well-being can cause us to be more susceptible to misinformation. In our desire for better living and searching for healthy options and products to help us in our pursuit, we may put down our defense as we strive for optimal wellness. As a result, we need to understand how wellness culture is marketed.

The Marketing of Wellness Culture

Being a part of wellness culture doesn't only mean feeling healthy and well, it's also about gobbling down experiences—often expensive, high-end experiences, if you can afford them (and sometimes even if you can't). People pursue the most unique mud or clay for facials or body masks, the most exclusive spas and retreats, the rarest essential oils, custom diets, and detoxes, machines for cryotherapy, hypobaric treatments, and laser treatments, plunge baths, saunas, red light treatment, and so on. The endless array of specialty supplements from IV drips to deer antler velvet to ox bile to horny goat weed offer youth, vitality, sexual stamina, and the perfect body (with no effort). Wellness culture is a lot about consumerism, but it is even more about seeking and searching for a special version of the self and a perfected ideal of the body.

The matching of these things—high cost along with exclusivity, prestige, and increased social status—makes us vulnerable to unsubstantiated claims, the placebo effect, and our own desire to remake ourselves. Someone is marketing and selling these products, supplements, and programs to consumers who are willing and eager to purchase wellness. Are there some evidence-based wellness products and programs that are in fact beneficial? Of course. However, there is also true-believer misinformation and marketing disinformation that take advantage of our propensity to avoid sunk costs (reluctance to abandon something you have invested heavily in), to believe in people with dubious expertise, and investment in the naturalistic fallacy. Let's also not forget the power of cognitive dissonance, because when we invest heavily in a product, we search for every reason to like it and ignore every reason not to so that we don't feel disappointed or (worse) that we have wasted our hard-earned money.

It's important to keep the business and marketing aspect of wellness culture at front-of-mind so that people can be informed and discerning consumers of the products and services they choose. Don't be a wellness impulse-buyer; take time to research and explore options. Most of all, remember that there is no product that will make or keep us healthy, thin, beautiful/handsome, and young—these cannot be found inside a red-light sauna pod or via a supplement or health drink, but rather they result from a lifetime of making healthy choices every day that prioritize well-being.

What Wellness Can't Do

Wellness in general, and the mind-body approach in particular, has obvious limitations. Mind-body wellness is and should be more nuanced than true believers would have us think, both in understanding the field of mind-body wellness and in implementing it. One key limitation of mind-body wellness is the emphasis on individual change and personal responsibility. We focus on actively engaging in decisions and behaviors that improve our overall health. While it is true that we can take a more active involvement in our health, and there are many meaningful reasons for doing so discussed throughout this book, it does not guarantee we will have all the success we desire. Placing the focus on individual decision-making does have implications for how we may judge our own success. If we are implementing changes but not seeing the desired results, we may be quick to "blame" ourselves and think we are simply not trying hard enough. Self-blame, and the behaviors that could result from judging ourselves so negatively, could have the opposite effect of what we intend (e.g., unhealthy exercising, limiting our diet in a way that has a negative impact on our health). Many factors we are unable to control have meaningful impacts on us. We cannot outrun our genetic blueprint, and family histories for diseases and cancer may indicate our own predisposition to these illnesses. Knowing this, we can choose to engage in preventive health behaviors. Environmental factors, like living in food deserts or areas where access to nature is limited, may make consistent healthy decisions challenging.

Mind-body wellness is complex, challenging, and without guarantees. Living in wellness does not guarantee we will remain healthy for an extended period of time. Cancer cannot be cured with a supplement, or with a specific diet, or with a strenuous workout routine. Our individual choices are not able to solve all complex health problems. That doesn't mean we should choose to simply lead an unhealthy life. While we can certainly make decisions that promote wellness (e.g., stop smoking, monitor our drinking), it is important to recognize the complex nature of health.

The pursuit of wellness can create an expectation for perfection that, entwined with our ever-increasing access to health-related products and information (or misinformation), creates unrealistic expectations for us. These unrealistic expectations cause us to pursue goals where the goalposts are always moving away from us. We may see some positive changes, but a moving goalpost puts us in a cycle of never-ending investments. These pursuits encourage us to "double down" and continue our monetary and emotional investments in products and wellness plans. Our socio-economic status may mean we have to be very mindful in how we budget our money. Pursuing quick guarantees or the next big fad in health and wellness can cause us to spend money in areas that are not going to bring about the return we are led to believe will follow. Falling short of our health and wellness goals, unrealistic as they may be, can generate feelings of anxiety, depression, self-blame, and low self-worth.

There are aspects to our wellness that are often overlooked. Wellness culture markets itself to us in ways that focus on physical health, beauty, and attractiveness. We often overlook the importance of our mental health and the positive benefits of a strong and supportive social network. The destigmatization of mental health care (discussed earlier) is important. Recognizing that many people will deal with a mental health issue, or someone close to them will, it is important to seek the help from a professional and support those who do. Having a close social network of friends and colleagues provides us with ongoing support and people we can turn to when we need help, advice, or a fun night out.

One last aspect of wellness to think about is the villainization of doctors and other medical personnel, medication, medical tests, and medical treatment. Wellness cannot replace evidence-based approaches and treatments. Wellness should not be defined as a "stand-alone" approach. It is best conceptualized as an approach that can be integrated with or occur in conjunction with evidence-based approaches.

Improved Quality of Life

The potential of mind-body wellness to improve an individual's quality of life is profound, offering tools to optimize well-being and maximizing the ability to thrive and flourish across all aspects of life. We are moving away from equating mind-body wellness with simply "feeling good" or "being happy." Rather, we acknowledge that mind-body wellness is a multidimensional concept that is complex to understand and study, let alone to enact diligently in our own lives. However, the benefits of prioritizing our wellness cannot be overlooked, because they meaningfully impact our quality of life. The World Health Organization defines quality of life as an "...individuals' perception of their position in life in the context of the culture and value systems in which they live and in relation to their goals, expectations, standards and concerns. It is a broad ranging concept affected in a complex way by the person's physical health, psychological state, level of independence, social relationships, personal beliefs and their relationship to salient features of their environment" (World Health Organization, 1997, p. 1). This definition for quality of life highlights the broad array of factors that play into mind-body wellness and how we subjectively view our lives. Mind-body wellness addresses many of these factors!

Wellness is a journey and does not have an end result that means we've achieved all the wellness we'll ever need. It does not work like that! If it did, this would be a much shorter book. As a result, many people benefit from having a Wellness Coach to help navigate the wellness terrain. In the wellness coaching process, we examine our behaviors and work to make healthy decisions a regular part of how we approach life. A Wellness Coach is someone who can help us make informed and meaningful choices. They are not our therapist—they typically are not trained to provide mental health services. Instead, they work with clients on improving their wellness through guiding internal processes associated with goal setting, building self-awareness, focusing on self-care, and helping to develop sustainable healthy decisions and behaviors. The focus is not on being prescriptive, telling clients exactly what they need to do, but rather working with them to develop healthy habits and the confidence to make decisions that meaningfully impact wellness. Work by Clark et al. (2014) found wellness coaching significantly improved clients' quality of life, mood, and stress levels. While it may not be necessary for everyone, a Wellness Coach can help guide the wellness space and develop the confidence needed to focus on our well-being.

Our minds and our bodies are intricately connected with one another. Supporting one often has positive implications for the other. Acknowledging the limitations of mind-body wellness does not mean we should ignore the positive impact wellness decisions can have for us. This book has provided a science-based perspective when considering wellness issues. Taking positive actions for ourselves can improve our own wellness, but there are a lot of "wellness traps" that will consume our time, energy, and money if we let them. Being a critical consumer of information helps us navigate these pitfalls in the wellness space, but the good news is that achieving wellness in mind and body is possible. If we assess our current state of wellness, identify sound, evidence-based wellness practices, and practice them consistently, we can be the authors of our own story of health and well-being.

References

American Heart Association (2015, October 2). *Fit-friendly worksites program encourages healthy workforce.* https://www.yourethecure.org/fit-friendly-worksites-program-encourages-healthy-workforce

Baicker, K., Cutler, D., & Song, Z. (2010). Workplace wellness programs can generate savings. *Health Affairs, 29*, 304–311. https://doi.org/10.1377/hlthaff.2009.0626

Barragan, R. C., & Meltzoff, A. N. (2023). Prosociality and health: Identification with all humanity is a replicable predictor of prosocial motivation for health behaviors. *Frontiers in Psychology, 13*, 1–11. https://doi.org/10.3389/fpsyg.2022.1052713

Bullard, R. D. (2005). *The quest for environmental justice: Human rights and the politics of pollution.* Sierra Club Books.

Clark, M. M., Bradley, K. L., Jenkins, S. M., Mettler, E. A., Larson, B. G., Preston, H. R., Liesinger, J. T., Werneburg, B. L., Hagen, P. T., Harris, A. M., Riley, B. A., Olsen, K. D., & Vickers Douglas, K. S. (2014). The effectiveness of wellness coaching for improving quality of life. *Mayo Clinic Proceedings, 89*(11), 1537–1544. https://doi.org/10.1016/j.mayocp.2014.04.028

Eriksson, M. (2011). Social capital and health—Implications for health promotion. *Global Health Action, 4*, 5611. https://doi.org/10.3402/gha.v4i0.5611

National Institute of Standards and Technology (n.d.). *Community resilience.* https://www.nist.gov/community-resilience

Statista. (n.d.). *Fitness Apps—United States: Statista Market Forecast.* https://www.statista.com/outlook/dmo/digital-health/digital-fitness-well-being/health-wellness-coaching/fitness-apps/united-states#users

Turner, E. (2024, November 20). *DNA dilemma: How to protect your data if 23andMe Shuts Down.* https://www.actionnewsjax.com/news/local/dna-dilemma-how-protect-your-data-if-23andme-shuts-down/ZBDBG5UTENDEHHZPNFFPVNTEV4/

World Health Organization. (1997). Measuring quality of life: The World Health Organization quality of life instruments. *Quality of Life for People with Disabilities: Models, Research and Practice*, 116–150.

World Health Organization (n.d.). *WHO Global Health and Peace Initiative.* https://www.who.int/initiatives/who-health-and-peace-initiative

Index

S. M. Henney, J. D. Hackett, *Mind-Body Wellness*,
https://doi.org/10.1007/978-3-031-91611-3